Electromagnetic and Acoustic Waves in Bioengineering Applications

Authored by Ivo Čáp, Klára Čápová, Milan Smetana and Štefan Borik

Published in London, United Kingdom

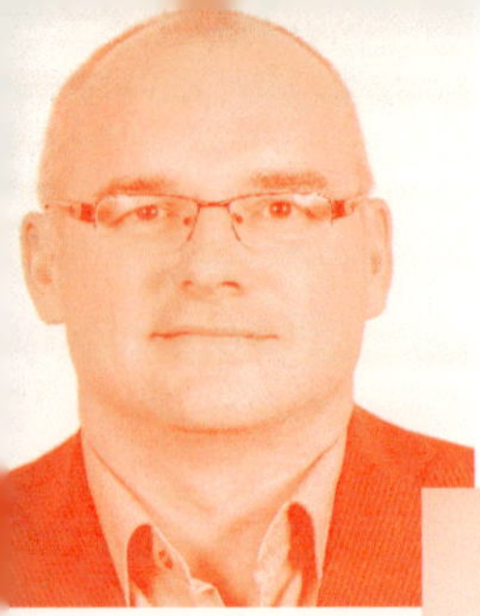
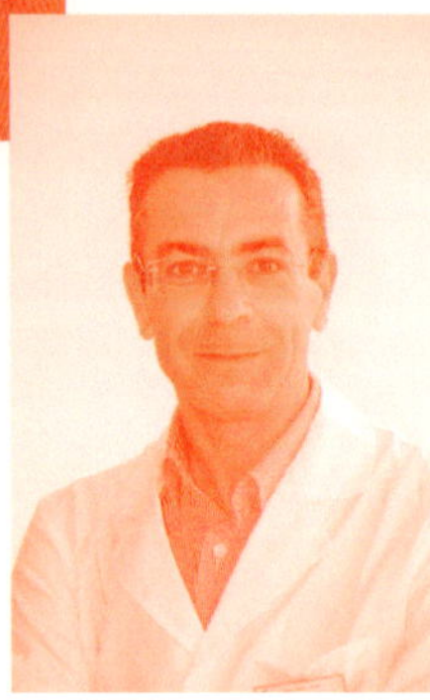
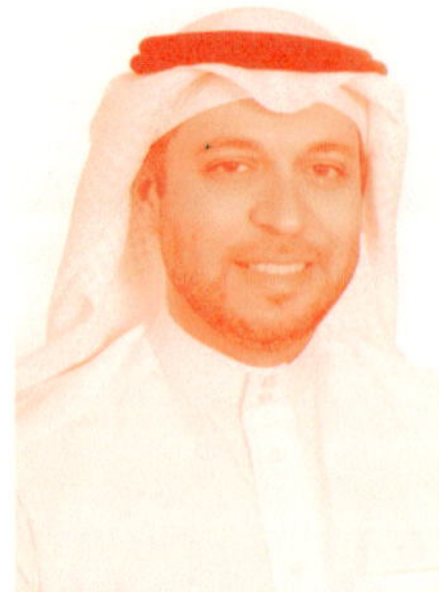
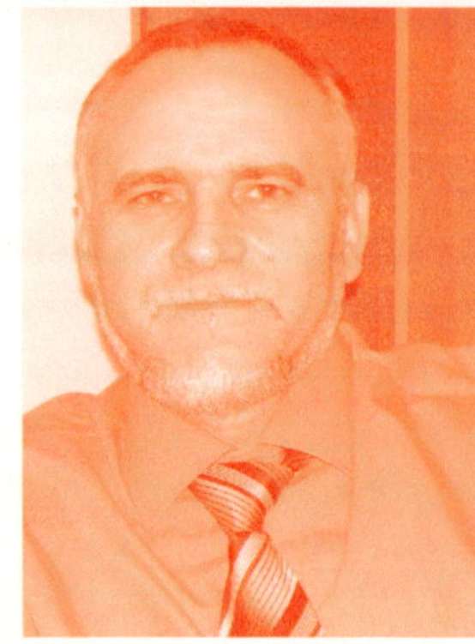
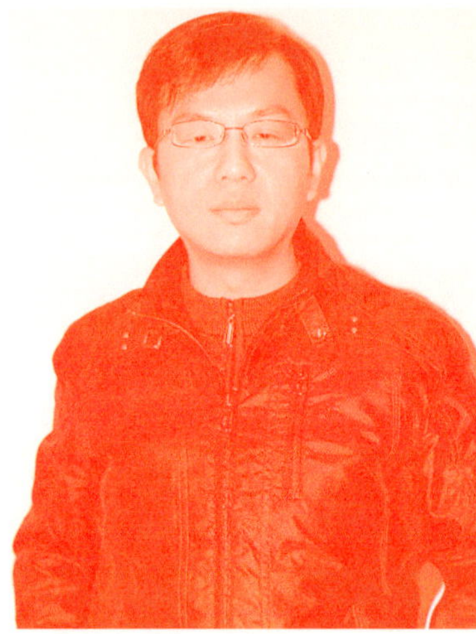
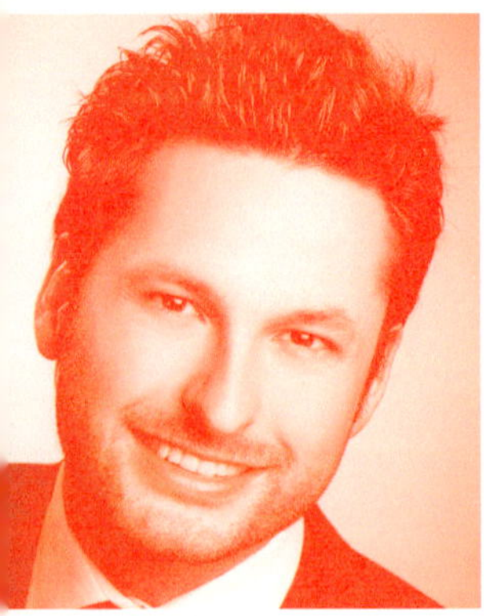
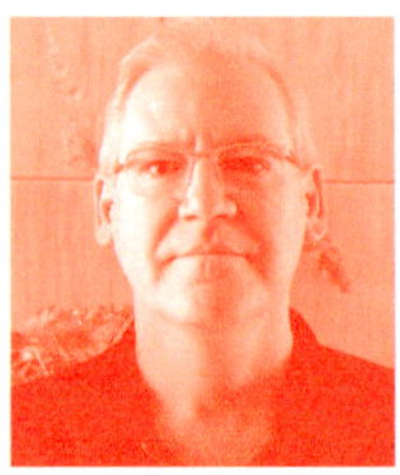

IntechOpen

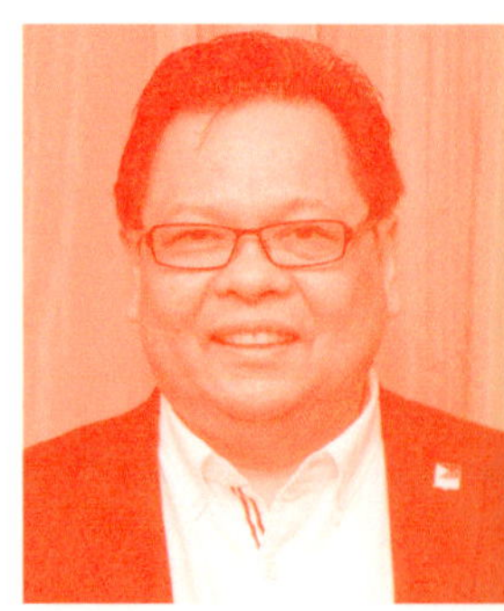
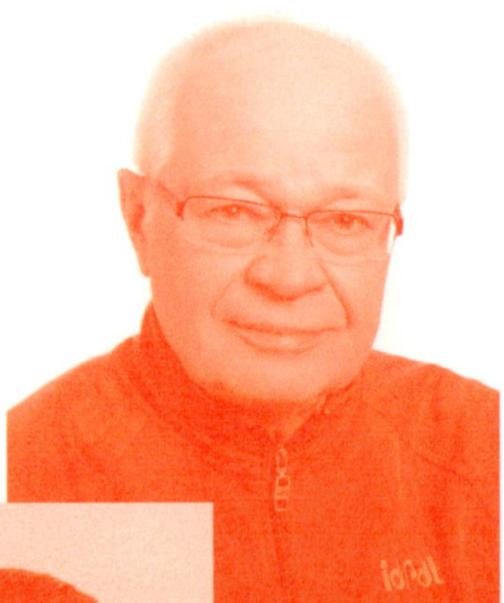
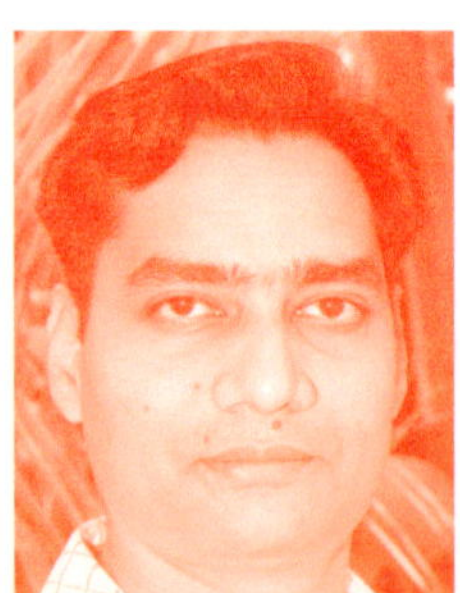
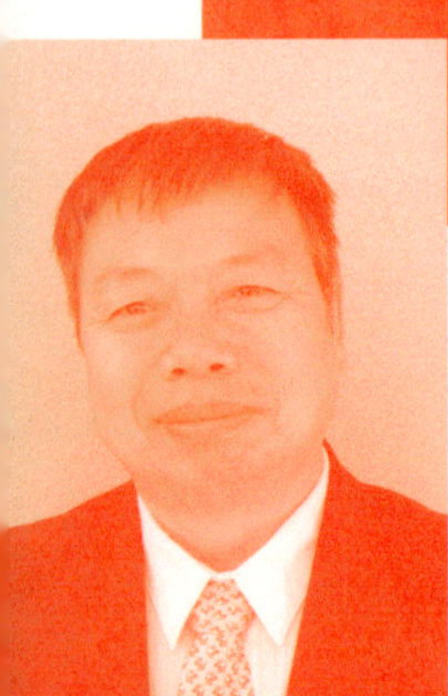
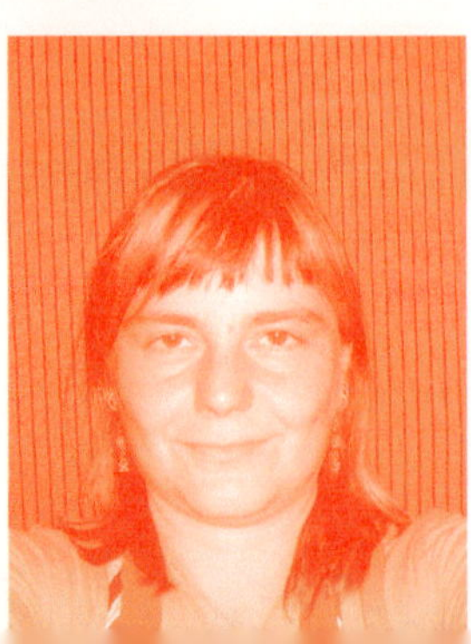
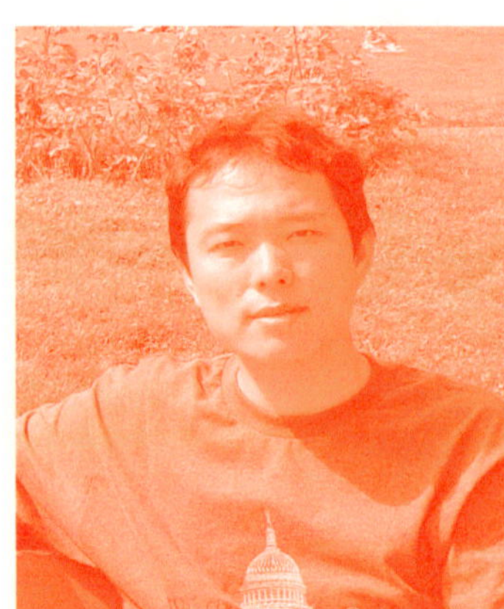

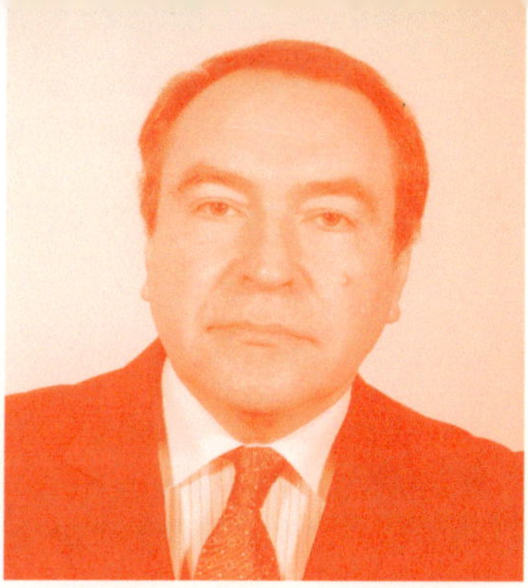
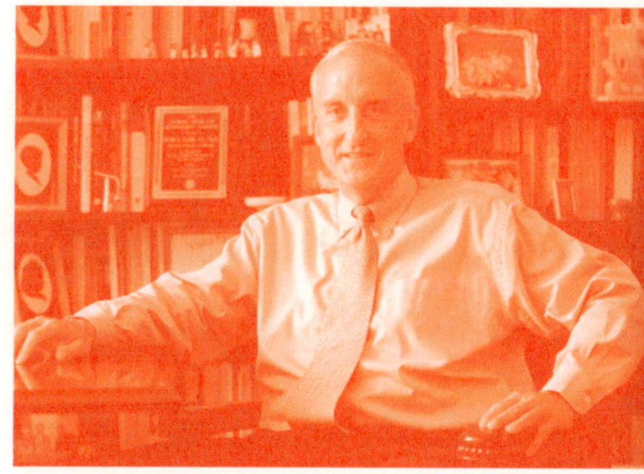
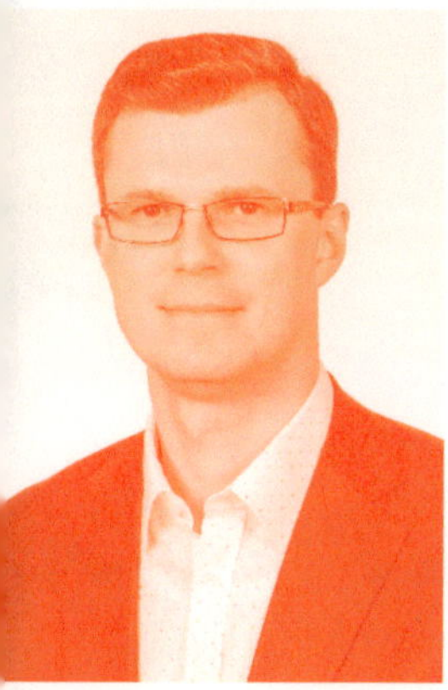
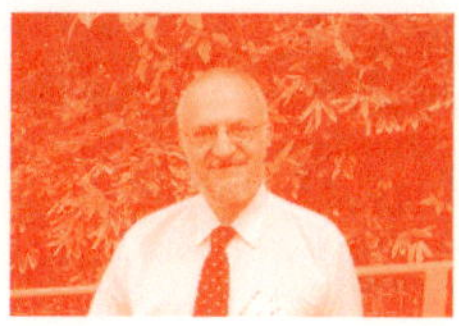
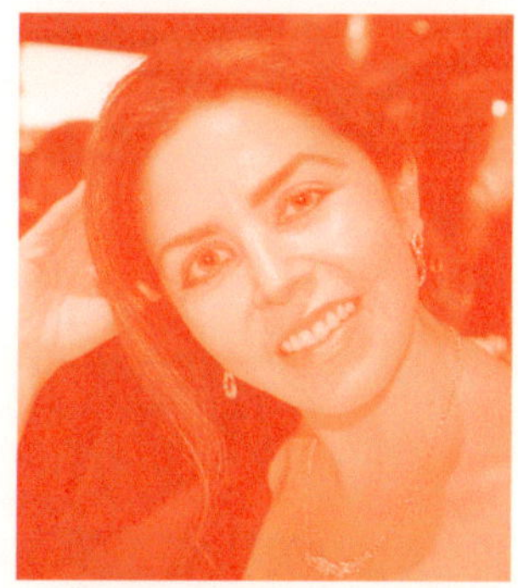

Supporting open minds since 2005

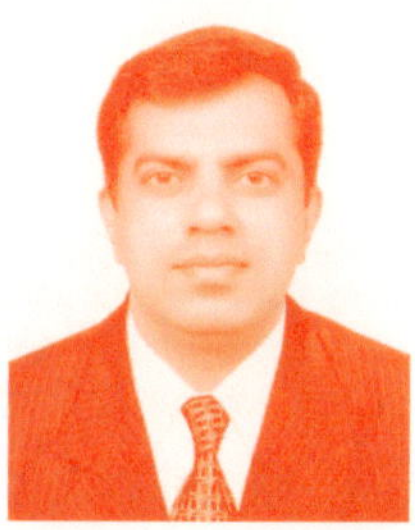
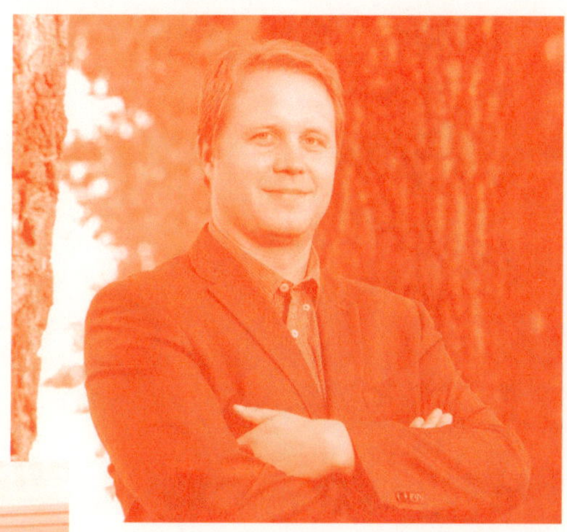
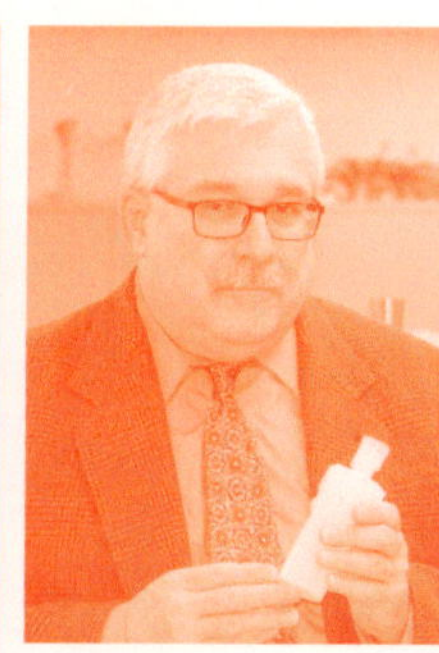
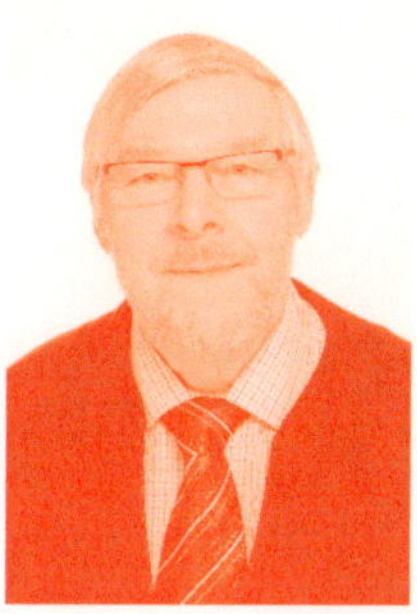
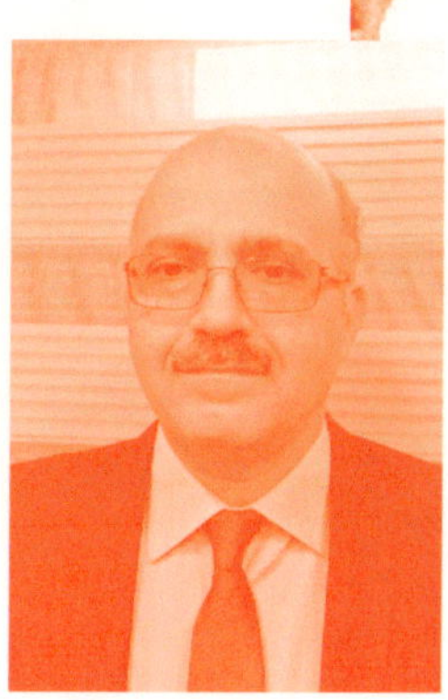
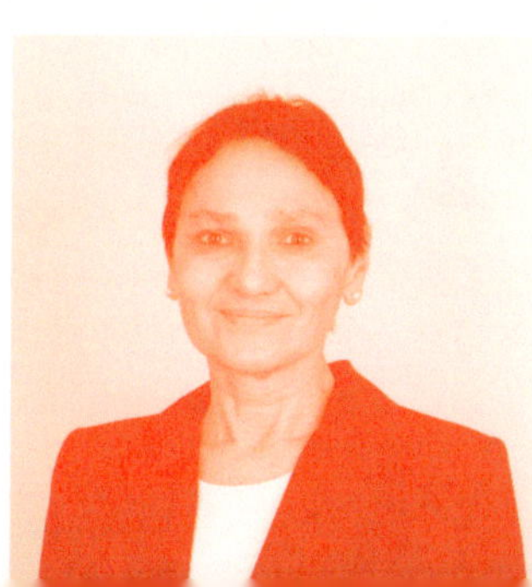
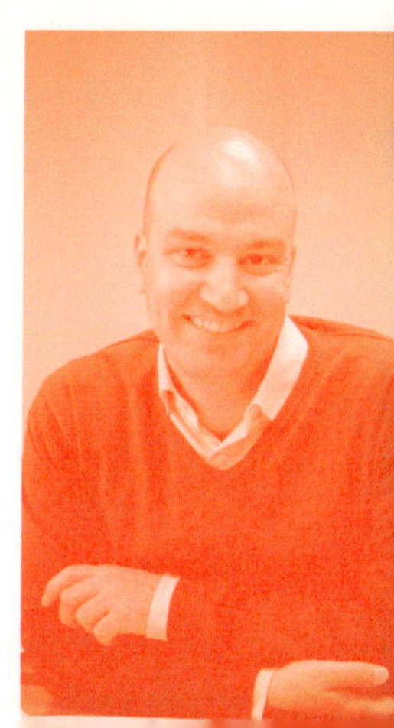

Electromagnetic and Acoustic Waves in Bioengineering Applications
http://dx.doi.org/10.5772/intechopen.90379
Authored by Ivo Čáp, Klára Čápová, Milan Smetana and Štefan Borik

Contributors
Ivo Čáp, Klára Čápová, Milan Smetana, Štefan Borik

First published in London, United Kingdom, 2021 by IntechOpen
IntechOpen is the global imprint of INTECHOPEN LIMITED, registered in England and Wales, registration number: 11086078, 5 Princes Gate Court, London, SW7 2QJ, United Kingdom
Printed in Croatia

British Library Cataloguing-in-Publication Data
A catalogue record for this book is available from the British Library

Additional hard and PDF copies can be obtained from orders@intechopen.com

Electromagnetic and Acoustic Waves in Bioengineering Applications
Authored by Ivo Čáp, Klára Čápová, Milan Smetana and Štefan Borik
p. cm.
Print ISBN 978-1-78985-347-6
Online ISBN 978-1-78985-348-3
eBook (PDF) ISBN 978-1-78985-723-8

An electronic version of this book is freely available, thanks to the support of libraries working with Knowledge Unlatched. KU is a collaborative initiative designed to make high quality books Open Access for the public good. More information about the initiative and links to the Open Access version can be found at www.knowledgeunlatched.org

For EU product safety concerns:
IN TECH d.o.o., Prolaz Marije Krucifikse Kozulić 3, 51000 Rijeka, Croatia, info@intechopen.com or visit our website at intechopen.com.

Meet the authors

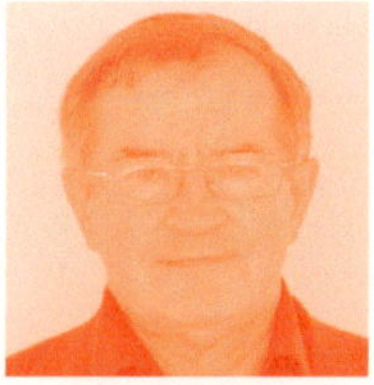

Prof. Ivo Čáp, MSc, Ph.D., graduated in Electrical Engineering from the Czech Technical University Prague. He was engaged in the physics of solids for thirty years. Currently, he is a Professor of Biomedical Engineering at the University of Žilina, Slovakia. His research focus is on modeling the cardiovascular system using an electromagnetic analogy, optical plethysmography, and interaction of the electromagnetic field with living organisms. He is the author of more than 100 scientific publications and six textbooks on the physics of solids, ultrasonic methods, and electromagnetic and biomedical phenomena. He is the national head of the Physics Olympiad in Slovakia.

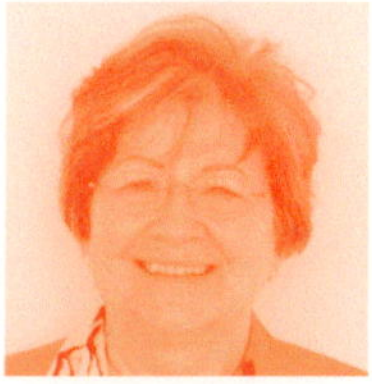

Prof. Klára Čápová, MSc, Ph.D., graduated in Communications from the Czech Technical University Prague. She obtained her Ph.D. in Theory of Electrical Engineering from the Slovak Academy of Science in 1982. She is currently a Professor of Electromagnetic Engineering at the University of Žilina, Slovakia, where she founded the biomedical engineering study field in the Faculty of Electrical Engineering and Information Technology. Her education focuses on the theory of electromagnetism and biomedical sensors. Her research interests include the non-destructive investigation of conductive materials and the interaction of the electromagnetic field with living organisms.

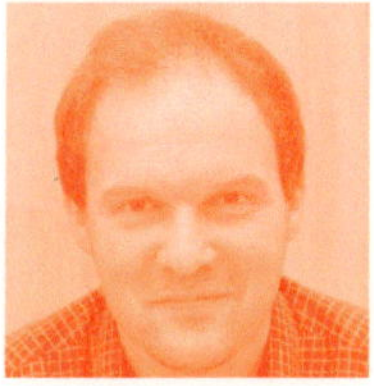

Prof. Milan Smetana, MSc, Ph.D., graduated in Biomedical Engineering from the University of Žilina, Slovakia. He holds a Ph.D. in Theory of Electrical Engineering. He is currently employed at the Department of Electromagnetic and Biomedical Engineering, University of Žilina, Slovakia. His education focuses on electrical circuits, electromagnetic fields, and sensors in biomedicine. In his research, Dr. Smetana deals with the non-destructive evaluation of conductive biomaterials by electromagnetic methods, particularly the eddy current testing. His area of scientific interest is the application of new approaches to the study of biocompatible prosthetic replacements by both direct and inverse methods.

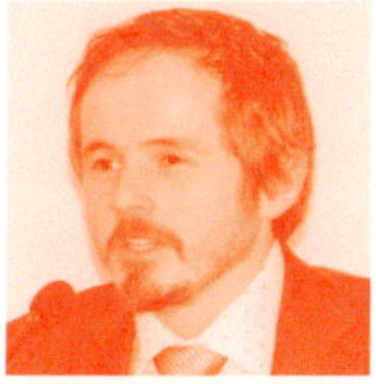

Prof. Štefan Borik, MSc, Ph.D., graduated in Biomedical Engineering from the University of Žilina, Slovakia. He received his MSc in Biomedical Engineering in 2011 and a Ph.D. in Theory of Electrical Engineering in 2014. He underwent habilitation in 2021 and was appointed an associate professor in the Department of Electromagnetic and Biomedical Engineering, Faculty of Electrical Engineering and Information Technology, University of Žilina. His education focuses on biomedical engineering and research of biomedical sensors, biosignal measurement techniques and processing, and cardiovascular diagnostics.

Contents

Preface

In nature, various events take place all the time. From a human point of view, these events can be divided into internal (intracorporeal) and external (extracorporeal) events. The human organism as well as its components are in interaction with its surroundings. This interaction, on the one hand, affects the state of the organism and, on the other hand, reveals everything about the state of the organism. This is the basis of different methods of treatment (therapy), such as targeted action on the body to eliminate disease and methods of examination (diagnosis) in which the doctor seeks to detect the disease and its causes.

In addition to the mechanical, thermal, electrical, and magnetic forms of interaction used in diagnostics and therapy, the richest interaction channels are waves, such as mechanical (sound, infrasound, ultrasound) and electromagnetic (radio waves, microwaves, visible light, infrared, ultraviolet, X-ray, radioactive gamma radiation). Radiation of various kinds is used in medical diagnostics and therapy. Today, highly sophisticated devices such as ultrasonography (USG), computed tomography (CT), magnetic resonance imaging (MRI), positron emission tomography (PET), single-photon emission tomography (SPECT), and many others are used. For a correct and thorough understanding of the principles of such devices, it is necessary to know the properties of the abovementioned types of waves as well as the methods of their generation and detection.

To understand the laws of generation, propagation, and detection of waves, we must first get acquainted with oscillations, which are the source of waves. The oscillations take place in one place, while the waves represent the propagation of oscillations into the surrounding space in a given transmission medium. The first part of this book, therefore, focuses on an analysis of oscillations, which is followed by an analysis of the waves themselves. We describe mechanical waves in material substances, and electromagnetic waves, which can also propagate in a vacuum. The description of the behaviour of waves is followed by a simple explanation of waves' quantum character, which is important for understanding phenomena such as ionization, spectroscopy, generation of laser radiation, and the like.

The authors of this book explain the theoretical fundamentals of phenomena that apply in medical diagnostics and therapy, and that are important for explaining the function of sophisticated devices of medical radiology and nuclear medicine. This book is not an introduction to the topic, thus knowledge of mathematics, physics, electrical circuits, and electromagnetic phenomena is recommended.

This book is a useful resource for university students in the field of biomedical engineering, as well as readers interested in taking a closer look at the technical means used by modern medicine.

Ivo Čáp, Klára Čápová, Milan Smetana and Štefan Borik
Faculty of Electrical Engineering and Information Technology,
University of Žilina,
Žilina, Slovakia

Chapter 1

Electromagnetic and Acoustic Waves in Bioengineering Applications

Ivo Čáp, Klára Čápová, Milan Smetana and Štefan Borik

Abstract

The textbook deals with the analysis of oscillations, mechanical and electromagnetic waves and their use in medicine. The individual chapters are based on the theoretical foundations of the issue and describe the use of relevant disciplines in medical practice. The chapter on oscillations is a starting point for explaining the basic principles of waves and focuses on explaining the nature of magnetic resonance. The chapter on mechanical waves explains the nature and properties of sound, infrasound, ultrasound, and medical applications, such as lithotripsy or ultrasonography. The chapter on electromagnetic waves discusses their basic principles, origin and properties, and applications of individual frequency bands from long wavelengths to gamma radiation in therapy and diagnostics. The chapter on wave manifestations explains phenomena such as interference and diffraction and their use in applications such as optical imaging systems, holography, virtual reality, etc. The description complements the explanation of the quantum properties of radiation, which are essential for understanding applications such as laser scalpel, fluorescence microscopy, spectroscopy, generation and detection of X-rays and gamma rays. Special attention is paid to the perception of EM waves by the human eye and the perception of sound by the human ear.

Keywords: oscillations, resonance, attenuation, waves, acoustic waves, sound, ultrasound, ultrasonography, lithotripsy, MRI, magnetic resonance, hearing apparatus, audiometry, auscultation, piezoelectric transducers, electromagnetic waves, radiofrequency, microwaves, infrared radiation, visible light, ultraviolet radiation, X-radiation, gamma radiation, quantum properties, radiodiagnostics, ionizing radiation, therapy by radiation, optical methods, photoplethysmography, photometry, colorimetry, human eye, microscopy, endoscopy, fibroskopy, laparoscopy, interference, diffraction, refraction, standing waves, wave resonance, waves transmission, energy of waves, photo-acoustic imaging, waves generators, waves sensors, wave detectors

1. Foreword

In nature, various events take place all the time. From a human point of view, these events can be divided into internal (intracorporeal) and external (extracorporeal). The human organism, as well as its components, is in interaction with its surroundings. This interaction, on the one hand, affects the state of the organism, on the other hand, reveals everything about the state of the organism. This is the basis of different methods of treatment (therapy), such as targeted action on the body to eliminate the disease, and methods of examination (diagnosis), in which the doctor seeks to detect the disease and its causes.

In addition to the mechanical, thermal, electrical, and magnetic forms of interaction used in diagnostics and therapy, the richest interaction channel are waves - mechanical (sound, infrasound, ultrasound) and electromagnetic (radio waves, microwaves, visible light, infrared, ultraviolet, X-ray, radioactive gamma radiation). Radiation of various kinds is used in medical diagnostics and therapy. Today, highly sophisticated devices such as USG (Ultrasonography), CT (Computed Tomography), MRI (Magnetic Resonance Imaging), PET (Positron Emission Tomography), SPECT (Single Photon Emission Tomography), and many others are used. For a correct and thorough understanding of the principles of such devices, it is necessary to know the properties of mentioned types of waves as well as the methods of their generation and detection.

To understand the laws of generation, propagation, and detection of waves, we first get acquainted with oscillations that are the source of waves. The oscillations take place in one place, while the waves represent the propagation of oscillations into the surrounding space in a given transmission medium. The first part of this textbook, therefore, focuses on an analysis of oscillations. It is followed by an analysis of the waves themselves. We will describe especially mechanical waves in the material substances, and electromagnetic waves, which can also propagate in a vacuum. The wave behavior of waves is followed by a simple explanation of their quantum character, which is important for understanding phenomena such as ionization, spectroscopy, generation of laser radiation, and the like.

The authors of this textbook aim to explain the theoretical fundamentals of phenomena that apply in medical diagnostics and therapy, and which are important for explaining the function of sophisticated devices of medical radiology and nuclear medicine. To master the problems of this textbook, knowledge acquired in the subjects of mathematics, physics, electrical circuits, and electromagnetic phenomena is supposed. The introductory chapters only briefly summarize this basic knowledge without a deeper detailed explanation. For more information on some special topics we recommend, e.g., Bronzino [1], Bronzino [2], Čápová [3], Hall [4], Rubin [5], Street [6], Webb [7], Wise [8].

The textbook is intended mainly for university students in the field of biomedical engineering, but it will also serve others interested in a closer look at the technical means used by modern medicine.

Author details

Ivo Čáp*, Klára Čápová, Milan Smetana and Štefan Borik
Faculty of Electrical Engineering and Information Technology, University of Žilina, Slovakia

*Address all correspondence to: ivo.cap@fel.uniza.sk

References

[1] Bronzino JD. The Biomedical Engineering Handbook – Medical Devices and Systems. Boca Raton: CRC Press; 2006

[2] Bronzino JD. The Biomedical Engineering Handbook – Biomedical Engineering Fundamentals. Boca Raton: CRC Press; 2006

[3] Čápová K, Čáp I. Sensors in Biomedical Engineering. Žilina: EDIS Press, University of Žilina; 2008

[4] Hall J. Textbook of Medical Physiology. Amsterdam: Elsevier Inc.; 2011

[5] Rubin A. Fundamentals of Biophysics. New Jersey: Wiley-Blackwell; 2014

[6] Street LJ. Introduction to Biomedical Engineering Technology. Boca Raton: CRC Press; 2016

[7] Webb AG. Introduction to Biomedical Imaging. New Jersey: John Wiley & Sons; 2017

[8] Wise DL. Bioinstrumentation and Biosensors. Boca Raton: CRC Press; 1991

Chapter 2

Simple Oscillating Systems

Ivo Čáp, Klára Čápová, Milan Smetana and Štefan Borik

1. Introduction

A wave is a disturbance (deviation from equilibrium) that propagates through space. This disturbance can be caused by an impulse excitation (shock wave) or by a time-varying excitation (e.g., the sound generated by vocal cords). The most frequent cause of wave excitation is a source with periodical time dependence—*oscillations*. The simplest one is *harmonic oscillation*. For example, we can express any periodic function of time as a sum of the harmonic functions (*Fourier series*). Thus, the excitation by the harmonic oscillations is a matter of specific interest. In this chapter, attention is, therefore, paid to the description of the physical nature of oscillations and their properties, see also Halliday [1].

Oscillations represent a very wide group of processes, which are generally characterised by their regular state repeating caused by the internal dynamics of a system. Such systems, whose internal couplings allow oscillations, are called *oscillating systems*. From the energy point of view, the oscillations are conditioned by the existence of two conservative forms of energy, which can *reversibly* exchange due to the internal dynamics of the system. There is, for example, potential energy—kinetic energy (oscillations of mass on a spring) or electric field energy of capacitor—magnetic field energy of inductor (an oscillating LC circuit). A special case represents the 'oscillations' in a rotating system, such as the movement of a conical pendulum where energy exchanges between two perpendicular kinetic components of $\frac{1}{2}mv_x^2$ and $\frac{1}{2}mv_y^2$, or the precession of a rotating body where energy exchanges between two perpendicular rotational components of kinetic energy $\frac{1}{2}J_x\omega_x^2$ and $\frac{1}{2}J_y\omega_y^2$. Some of these cases will be described below as examples.

If the oscillating system is isolated from external influences, it oscillates spontaneously after the initial energy supply (*excitation*). Thus, we are talking about *self-sustained oscillations*. The oscillation amplitude remains almost constant if the energy losses of the oscillations in the system are negligibly small. The oscillations of the ideal lossless system are called *undamped self-oscillations* and represent only theoretical idealisation. There exist loss mechanisms in each real system. They cause the *irreversible* transformation of the conservative form of the system energy into another *non-conservative* one, for example, friction, heat losses due to internal friction, energy losses of the electrical system by radiation, etc. As the total energy of the conservative components decreases, the amplitude of oscillations gradually decreases over time too. We call them *damped self-oscillations*. Due to the damping, these self-oscillations disappear after some time. Thus, they are a transient phenomenon in the system, for example, the vibrations of the string of the musical instrument fade; a swinging of pendulum stops after a certain time; oscillations of an LC circuit gradually disappear, etc.

The system may oscillate permanently without damping if there is a mechanism capable to cover the energy losses from an energy storage device. Such systems are different types of *oscillators*. Examples are pendulum clocks with weights or watches with a spring. In modern watches, a precisely sharpened crystal represents the oscillating system. In this case, a small lithium cell covers the energy losses caused by damping.

Specific phenomena arise when the system is exposed to periodic force. When such a force acts, the system, after attenuating the transient event, enters a steady state, characterised by oscillations with a constant amplitude and a period equal to the excitation period. These oscillations are called *forced oscillations* of the system. The magnitude of the response to periodic excitation depends on the period or frequency of excitation. Significant is the *resonance* phenomenon that occurs when the excitation frequency is equal to the frequency of the system's undamped oscillations.

The following sections focus on the different types of oscillations in simple systems, that is, in systems in which two conservative forms of energy occur in oscillations. This textbook presents a summary of the knowledge with an emphasis on application. A more detailed analysis of the mentioned phenomena can be found in physics textbooks.

1.1 Undamped self-oscillations

As the basic model of the oscillating system, we use a particle bound to the equilibrium position by the reversing conservative force of the springs (**Figure 1**).

At the top of the figure, the particle is in equilibrium, and the resulting force acting on it is zero. If the particle shifts from the equilibrium position by the displacement of x, there arises a force of $F(x)$ which depends on the x displacement, is reversible, and has the opposite direction as the displacement.

If the particle is displaced from the equilibrium position and released, it starts to move back to the equilibrium position. Its velocity is a derivative of the displacement

$$v = \frac{dx}{dt} = \dot{x} \text{ (a dot over } x \text{ describes the time derivative).} \tag{1}$$

Displacing particle from equilibrium by x, we perform a work of W, which represents the potential energy of the particle

$$E_p(x) = W = \int_0^x F(\xi) d\xi. \tag{2}$$

A moving particle has a kinetic energy

$$E_k(v) = \frac{1}{2} m v^2. \tag{3}$$

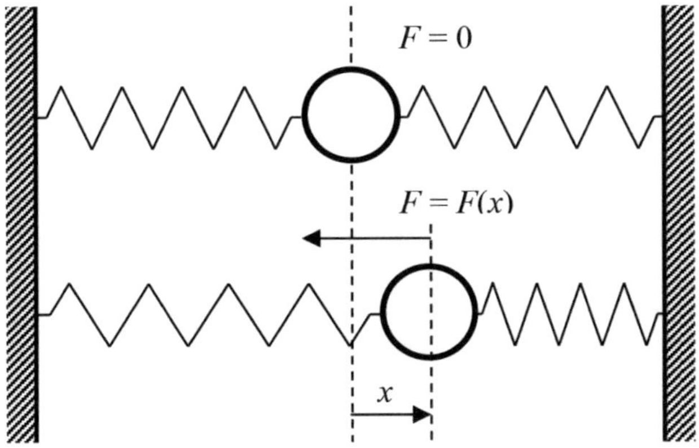

Figure 1.
Particle bound to the equilibrium by the restoring force.

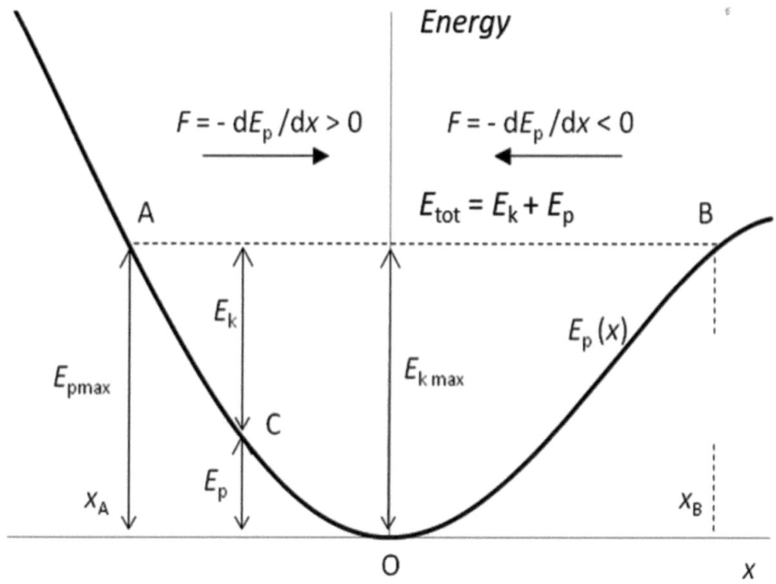

Figure 2.
Total potential and kinetic energy of a particle moving along the x*-axis under conservative forces (law of conservation of mechanical energy).*

Reversible energy exchange occurs between the energy components of E_p and E_k. It is a system with two degrees of freedom. If we consider no loss mechanisms, the sum of the $E_p + E_k$ energy components remains constant. The situation is in **Figure 2**. It indicates the potential energy as a function of the displacement x (solid line). We can see that in the equilibrium position ($x = 0$) the potential energy is minimal, and thus, at a constant sum, $E_{tot} = E_p + E_k$, the kinetic energy is maximal. It means that the particle moves due to inertia until its kinetic energy drops to zero. The particle thus moves periodically between the extreme positions of A and B, which are given by the total energy E_{tot}.

We can express a function of the potential energy $E_p(x)$ near the minimum, that is, equilibrium position, by the Taylor power series

$$E_p(x) = \frac{1}{2!}kx^2 + \frac{1}{3!}lx^3 + \frac{1}{4!}nx^4 + \cdots, \tag{4}$$

where $k = \left.\frac{d^2E_p}{dx^2}\right|_{x=0}$ represents the *stiffness* of the system, $l = \left.\frac{d^3E_p}{dx^3}\right|_{x=0}$ expresses *asymmetry* of the potential energy function regarding the equilibrium position. Other coefficients such as $n = \left.\frac{d^4E_p}{dx^4}\right|_{x=0}$ and higher (odd and even derivatives) have similar characteristics but they change function course in the larger distance of x from the equilibrium position. The first power term of x is zero because it is the local minimum of the $E_p(x)$.

A negative potential energy gradient defines the force acting on a particle as follows

$$F(x) = -\frac{dE_p(x)}{dx} = -kx - \frac{1}{2!}lx^2 - \frac{1}{3!}nx^3 - \cdots. \tag{5}$$

We distinguish the *linear* and *non-linear* oscillating systems depending on the number of force or energy terms that are considered in the motion. If the displacement x approaches zero, the higher powers of x^n decrease faster than the first one.

Then, the higher terms of the function $F(x)$ are negligibly small, and the system appears to be linear. However, the terms with higher powers apply, and the system behaves as non-linear if displacement x *significantly increases*.

1.1.1 Undamped self-oscillations of linear system

A system is *linear* if the restoring force is a linear function of the displacement of x from the equilibrium position. According to Eqs. (4) or (5), it follows

$$F(x) \approx -kx, \text{ or } E_p(x) \approx \frac{1}{2}kx^2. \tag{6}$$

Potential energy is a quadratic function of the displacement x and is called a *quadratic potential well*. Its graph is a quadratic parabola. **Figure 3** shows a replacement of the real function $E_p(x)$ by a quadratic function. This replacement fits well only in the near vicinity of the minimum, that is, only for small variations of x around the equilibrium. Oscillations within the range of the fitted region are sometimes called *small oscillations*.

Equation of motion of the particle $ma = F$, where $a = \ddot{x}$ is an acceleration, has form for the linear system as follows

$$\ddot{x} + \omega_0^2 x = 0, \text{ where } \omega_0 = \sqrt{\frac{k}{m}}. \tag{7}$$

The solution of this equation is the function

$$x(t) = x_m \sin(\omega_0 t + \alpha), \tag{8}$$

where x_m and α are integration constants and their values are determined from initial conditions $x(0) = x_0$ and $v(0) = \dot{x}(0) = v_0$ at $t = 0$.

It is a harmonic motion where the x_m is an amplitude of oscillations and α is a phase constant (initial phase).

Oscillations with harmonic time dependence are called *harmonic oscillations*. It follows from the previous description that harmonic oscillations occur when a particle (body) moves in a quadratic potential well.

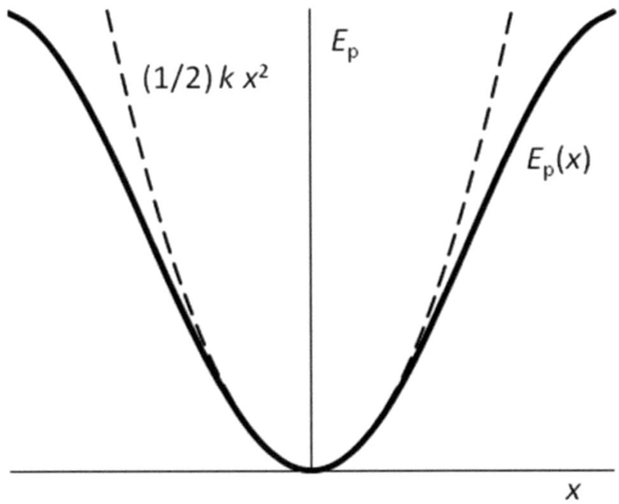

Figure 3.
Quadratic fitting (dashed) of the potential energy function.

The quantity

$$\omega_0 = 2\pi f_0 = \frac{2\pi}{T_0} \tag{9}$$

represents the angular frequency, where f_0 is frequency and T_0 is the period of the *undamped self-oscillations* of the system. According to Eq. (7), these quantities depend on the stiffness k of the system, and the inertia given by the mass m of the particle. As the stiffness increases, the frequency f_0 increases as well, and the period T_0 decreases. With the mass increase, the frequency f_0 decreases, and the period T_0 increases. For example, as a body hung on the spring oscillates with the period of order seconds, an atom in the crystal lattice with the period of the order of 10^{-14} s.

Example 1. Oscillations in an electrical LC circuit.

Let us assume one loop electrical circuit consisting of an inductor L and a capacitor C. Electrical current $i(t)$ flows through this circuit, and we can express the energy of an electrical field of the capacitor and a magnetic field of the inductor as follows:

$$E = \frac{1}{2}\frac{1}{C}\ Q^2 + \frac{1}{2}L\ i^2,$$

where the electrical charge Q of the capacitor relates to the current i of the inductor $i = \dot{Q}$. We can see the analogy between electrical and mechanical systems, in case $x \to Q$, $k \to 1/C$ and $m \to L$. If we do not consider the power losses, the energy E is constant, and by differentiating it, we get the equation

$$\frac{1}{C}\ Q\ \frac{\mathrm{d}Q}{\mathrm{d}t} + L\ i\ \frac{\mathrm{d}i}{\mathrm{d}t} = 0.$$

Dividing the equation by i = dQ/dt, we get

$$\frac{d^2Q}{dt^2} + \frac{1}{LC}Q = 0,$$

which has the same form as (7). Then, the solution is

$$Q(t) = Q_m \sin(\omega_0 t + \alpha), \text{where } \omega_0 = \sqrt{\frac{1}{LC}}.$$

The capacitor voltage is

$$u_C(t) = \frac{Q(t)}{C} = \frac{Q_m}{C}\sin(\omega_0 t + \alpha) = U_m \sin(\omega_0 t + \alpha)$$

and the inductor current equals to

$$i(t) = \frac{dQ(t)}{dt} = \omega_0 Q_m \cos(\omega_0 t + \alpha) = I_m \sin\left(\omega_0 t + \alpha + \frac{\pi}{2}\right).$$

Thus, there are the harmonic undamped oscillations of the circuit quantities with the angular frequency of ω_0.

Example 2. Pendulum.

Consider a small body suspended on a long fibre (**Figure 4**). After the initial excitation, the body oscillates around the equilibrium position, and thus performs a

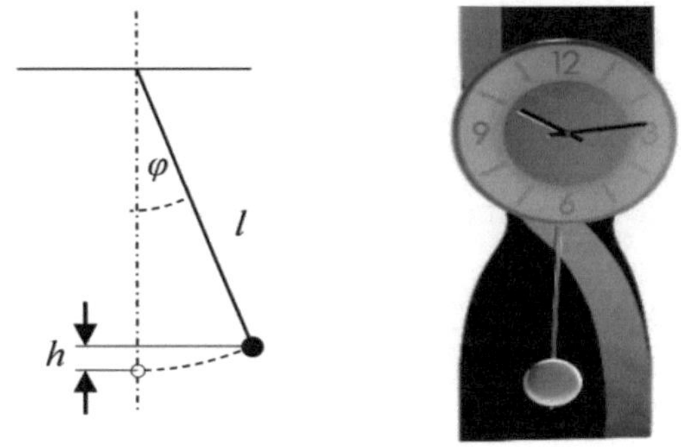

Figure 4.
Pendulum.

circular motion with a radius equal to the fibre length of the l. If we displace the fibre by an angle φ from the equilibrium position, then the potential energy of the body changes as

$$E_{\mathrm{p}}(\varphi) = mgh = mgl\ (1 - \cos\varphi).$$

The $E_p(\varphi)$ function is not quadratic, and therefore, we can use a decomposition using the power series

$$E_{\mathrm{p}}(\varphi) = mgl\ \left(\frac{\varphi^2}{2!} - \frac{\varphi^4}{4!} + \cdots\right).$$

We can neglect the series terms of the higher order for $\varphi < < 1$, and then the potential energy is

$$E_{\mathrm{p}}(\varphi) = \frac{1}{2} mgl\ \varphi^2.$$

Additionally, the kinetic energy is

$$E_{\mathrm{k}}(v) = \frac{1}{2} m\ v^2 = \frac{1}{2} m\ l^2\ \dot{\varphi}^2.$$

We can see the analogy to (7) again, if $x \to \varphi$, $k \to mgl$ and $m \to ml^2$.
Pendulum displacement is described by the function

$$\phi(t) = \phi_m \sin(\omega_0 t + \alpha), \text{where } \omega_0 = \sqrt{\frac{g}{l}}.$$

Hence, the body oscillates with the period

$$T_0 = 2\pi\sqrt{\frac{l}{g}}.$$

By measuring the oscillation period, it is possible to determine the length of the pendulum if we do not have a measuring tool. Alternatively, with a pendulum of a certain length, we can realise a periodic movement with the required period, such as in the case of the pendulum clock.

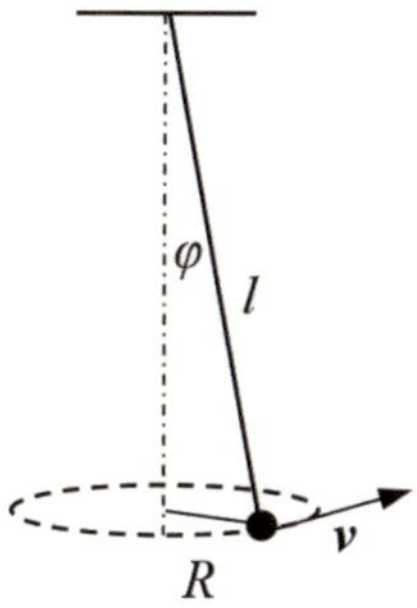

Figure 5.
Cone pendulum.

Example 3. Cone pendulum.

Consider the same case as in the previous example, but let the body move along a circle in the horizontal plane (x, y). The pendulum copies a conical surface as it moves. Thus, the deviation angle from the vertical axis is φ, as shown in **Figure 5**. The radius of motion of the body is $R = l \sin \varphi$. The kinetic energy of the body is

$$E_k = \frac{1}{2}mv^2 = \frac{1}{2}m\left(v_x^2 + v_y^2\right),$$

where v is the velocity of the circular motion.

The force acts on the body and equals to $F_d = -m\omega^2 r$, where the angular velocity is $\omega = v/r$. The centrifugal force composes of gravitational force $F_g = mg$, while the resultant force has the direction of the pendulum fibre that means $tg\varphi = F_d/F_g$. For small displacement, when $\varphi < < 1$ rad, it follows that $tg\varphi \approx \sin\varphi = r/l$. From the $F_d/F_g = r/l$, we obtain $\omega = \sqrt{g/l}$, which is similar to the previous example.

Potential energy connected with the centrifugal force is given as

$$E_p = \frac{1}{2}m\omega^2 r^2 = \frac{1}{2}m\omega^2\left(x^2 + y^2\right).$$

And finally, the total energy can be expressed

$$E_k + E_p = \left(\frac{1}{2}mv_x^2 + \frac{1}{2}m\omega^2 x^2\right) + \left(\frac{1}{2}mv_y^2 + \frac{1}{2}m\omega^2 y^2\right).$$

In this case, the motion can be considered as a superposition of two mutually perpendicular oscillations in the x- and y-direction, which are phase-shifted by $\pi/2$ rad. The total energy $(E_k + E_p)$ is constant and is the sum of the total energy of oscillations in the x- and y-direction.

Example 4. Precession of magnetic dipole in the magnetic field.

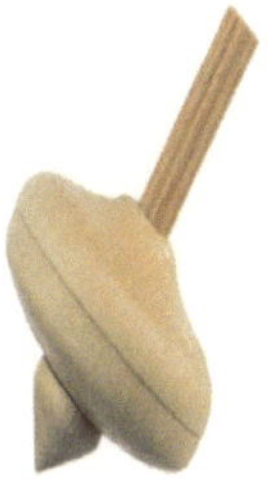

Another specific case of periodic movement is the precession (rotating axis of a rotating body). We can observe it looking at a children's toy, such as a spinning top.

By spinning and laying it on the pad, the toy axis rotates, see the illustration. The precession occurs due to the gravitational force.

Similarly, the magnetic dipole, here the proton, is affected by an external magnetic field. One of the proton parameters is the angular momentum $\boldsymbol{L}$, which describes its mechanical rotation. The rotation of the charged particle is associated with the accompanying magnetic field. Thus, the proton behaves like an elemental magnet (the magnetic dipole) with a magnetic moment $\boldsymbol{m}$. The ratio of magnetic moment to mechanical angular momentum is called the gyromagnetic ratio $\gamma = \boldsymbol{m}/\boldsymbol{L}$ (see **Table 1**). If the dipole is in an external magnetic field, then the moment of the force acting on it is.

$\boldsymbol{M} = \boldsymbol{m} \times \boldsymbol{B}$, where $\boldsymbol{B}$ is the magnetic induction.

The moment of force determines the dynamics of the dipole movement. The basic equation of rotational motion (impulse theorem II) has the form

$$\frac{\boldsymbol{dL}}{\boldsymbol{dt}} = \boldsymbol{M}.$$

Combining both equations, we get $\boldsymbol{dL} = \boldsymbol{m} \times \boldsymbol{B}\ \boldsymbol{dt} = \gamma\ \boldsymbol{L} \times \mathbf{B}\ \mathrm{d}t$.

The d$\boldsymbol{L}$ vector is perpendicular to the vector $\boldsymbol{L}$, and therefore its magnitude does not change but the direction only.

As shown in **Figure 6**, the end of the $\boldsymbol{L}$ vector moves along a circle with a radius equal to $L \sin\alpha$. The angle $\mathrm{d}\varphi$ over the time $\mathrm{d}t$ determines the magnitude of change of $\mathrm{d}L = L \sin\alpha\, \mathrm{d}\varphi$. The magnitude of the $\mathrm{d}L$ change according to the equation of motion is $\mathrm{d}L = mB \sin\alpha\, \mathrm{d}t$. By comparing these two expressions, we get the angular velocity of the endpoint of the $\boldsymbol{L}$ vector

$$\omega_L = \frac{d\phi}{dt} = \gamma B.$$

Core	s (spin)	γ [$\times 10^8$ s^{-1}·T^{-1}]
^{1}H (proton)	1/2	2.68
^{13}C	1/2	0.67
^{19}F	1/2	2.52
^{31}P	1/2	1.08
Free electron	1/2	−1758

Table 1.
Properties of selected nuclei of atoms and electron.

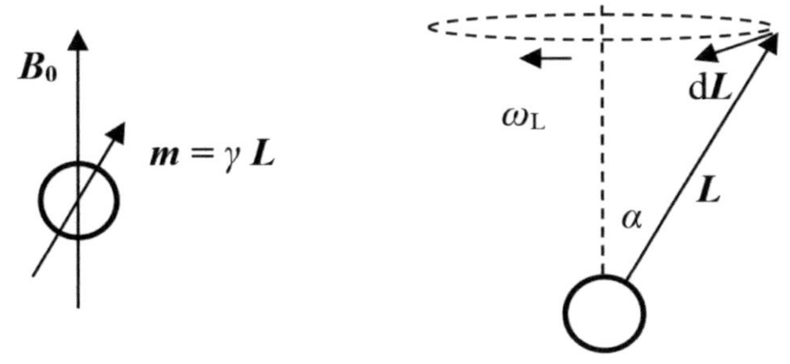

Figure 6.
Precession movement of a magnetic dipole in a magnetic field.

Thus, the dipole axis performs a circular (funnel) motion in the magnetic field, called the Larmor's precession. The frequency of $f_L = \omega_L/2\pi$ of this motion depends on the type of particle represented by its gyromagnetic ratio γ and the induction B of the magnetic field but does not depend on the angle α. As we show later, this phenomenon is used in magnetic resonance imaging and magnetic resonance spectroscopy. The nature of the phenomenon is like that of a conical pendulum.

Example 5. Ion oscillations in the crystal.

Crystals represent a simple or more complex regular arrangement of atoms of solids. For example, aluminium consists of an arranged lattice of positive ions. There are Al^+ ions and electron gas. The ions are subjected to electric forces by the surrounding particles. The equilibrium ion position is given by the zero resultant force or by the minimum value of the potential energy. If the ion deviates from the equilibrium position, it begins to oscillate around it.

As a simple model, consider three monovalent ions, of which two are fixed, and the third can move between the other two. In equilibrium, the distance of the central ion from the extreme ones is a (see **Figure 7**).

Let us move the central ion displacing it from the equilibrium. Then, the force acting on the ion is

$$F = F_1 - F_2 = k\ \frac{e^2}{a+x} - \ k\ \frac{e^2}{a-x} = -k\ \frac{2ae^2}{a^2-x^2}\ x,$$

where $k \approx 9.0 \times 10^9$ m·F^{-1} is Coulomb's law constant and $e \approx 1.6 \times 10^{-19}$ C is the elementary charge.

If the displacement is $x < < a$, then we can express the resultant force by the linear approximation as

$$F \approx -\frac{2ke^2}{a}\ x = -\ K\ x.$$

As shown, if a particle with a mass m exerted by a reversing force proportional to the displacement x, the particle oscillates around an equilibrium position with a frequency

$$f = \frac{1}{2\pi}\ \sqrt{\frac{K}{m}} = \frac{1}{2\pi}\ \sqrt{\frac{2ke^2}{ma}}.$$

The oscillating of a charged particle is the source of the electromagnetic wave at this frequency and the wavelength of this wave is

$$\lambda = \frac{c}{f} = 2\pi\ c\ \sqrt{\frac{ma}{2k\ e^2}}.$$

For example, if we use the typical values for aluminium: $m \approx 4.5 \times 10^{-26}$ kg, $a \approx 2.8 \times 10^{-10}$ m, while $c \approx 3.0 \times 10^8$ m·s^{-1}, we get $\lambda \approx 31$ μm.

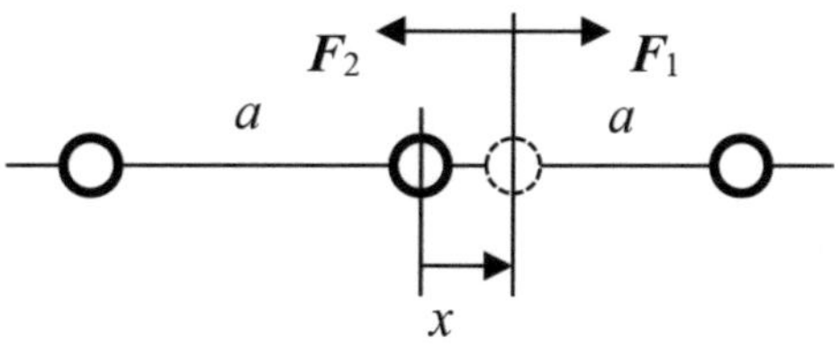

Figure 7.
Three monovalent ions.

The result corresponds to the wavelength of infrared (thermal) radiation. Oscillations of crystal lattice ions are the cause of the thermal radiation of the bodies.

There are many similar examples of oscillating systems, all of which have a similar physical nature. It is always a periodic exchange of energy between the various conservative forms of energy caused by the internal dynamics of the system.

1.1.2 Undamped self-oscillations of non-linear system

We find the system as non-linear if we cannot neglect its non-linearity. This means that we consider other higher terms in the expression of force by the power series [Eq. (5)]. Since the terms of the series generally gradually decrease with an increasing exponent of power, we can now consider the first higher non-zero member only. If the $E_p(x)$ function is odd (it means asymmetric potential well), we consider the term with the l coefficient, that is., quadratic term in the force expression. If the potential well is symmetrical, it is $l = 0$, the first non-linear term of the series is a cubic one. Accordingly, we are solving single cases by using this simplification.

In the following section, we analyse the case of oscillations in an *asymmetric potential well*, for which we express the force acting on a particle in the form

$$F(x) \approx -k\ x - \frac{1}{2!}\ l\ x^2. \tag{10}$$

Then the equation of motion is

$$ma = -kx - \frac{1}{2}\ l\ x^2. \tag{11}$$

We can rewrite the equation to the form

$$\ddot{x} + \omega_0^2\,(1 + \lambda x)x = 0, \tag{12}$$

where $\omega_0^2 = \frac{k}{m}$.

The coefficient $\lambda = \frac{l}{2k}$ is the degree of asymmetry of the potential well.

Figure 8 shows an example of the asymmetric potential well and it illustrates the fitting of the well by a quadratic function (dashed line). This function fits the well only in the near vicinity of the equilibrium position. Cubic function correction is

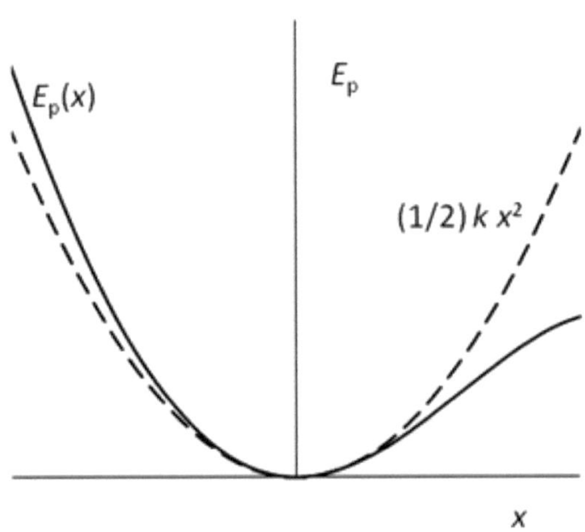

Figure 8.
Asymmetric potential well with asymmetry of the type l < o *or* λ < o.

positive on the left side and negative on the right side, which means that the asymmetry coefficient is $l < 0$.

Equation (12) represents a non-linear differential equation. When solving it, we use the physical nature of the phenomenon, which means the particle motion is periodic with an unknown angular frequency ω. We know, the periodic function can be expressed in the form of a Fourier series. If we choose for the start time $t = 0$ the moment when the particle displacement crosses the extreme value, then we can describe the course of the time dependence as an even function (symmetrical around the beginning $t = 0$).

For an even function, the Fourier series contains only even (cosine) terms.

$$x(t) = a_0 + \sum_{n=1}^{\infty} a_n \cos n\,\omega t. \tag{13}$$

The a_0 value represents the mean value of the particle displacement, the a_n are amplitudes of the individual harmonics with frequencies of $n\,\omega$.

The solution procedure is such that we substitute the function (13) into the differential equation and arrange the terms according to the angular frequency. If the expression on the left side is to be equal to the right side of the equation (i.e., zero), all terms must be zero at corresponding frequencies—harmonics with angular frequencies ω, 2ω, etc. So, we get a set of equations for unknown parameters ω, a_0, and a_n for $n = 1, 2, \ldots$

Assuming the weak non-linearity of the system, which is given by $\lambda\, x_m \ll 1$, where x_m is the maximal displacement from the equilibrium position, we get

$$\omega = \omega_0 \sqrt{1 - \frac{5}{6}(\lambda a_1)^2}, a_0 \approx -\frac{1}{2}(\lambda a_1) a_1, a_2 \approx \frac{1}{6}(\lambda a_1) a_1 \text{ etc.,} \tag{14}$$

where a_1 is the amplitude of the first harmonic with the frequency of ω. Thus, non-linearity influences the frequency of the self-oscillations. It causes the shift of the mean value of the position a_0, and it causes the higher harmonics involved in oscillations.

Example of the derivation:

After substituting into the differential equation, we get the equation

$$-\sum_{n=1}^{\infty} a_n n^2 \omega^2 \cos n\omega t + \omega_0^2 a_0 + \omega_0^2 \sum_{n=1}^{\infty} a_n \cos n\omega t$$
$$+\omega_0^2 \lambda \left(a_0 + \sum_{n=1}^{\infty} a_n \cos n\omega t \right) \left(a_0 + \sum_{k=1}^{\infty} a_k \cos k\omega t \right) = 0$$

and then

$$\omega_0^2 a_0 + \omega_0^2 \lambda a_0^2 + \sum_{n=1}^{\infty} (\omega_0^2 - n^2 \omega^2) a_n \cos n\omega t + 2\omega_0^2 \lambda a_0 \sum_{n=1}^{\infty} a_n \cos n\omega t +$$
$$+\omega_0^2 \lambda \sum_{n=1}^{\infty} \sum_{k=1}^{\infty} a_k a_n \cos k\omega t \cos n\omega t = 0$$

and then

$$\omega_0^2 a_0 (1 + \lambda a_0) + \sum_{n=1}^{\infty} (\omega_0^2 - n^2 \omega^2 + 2\omega_0^2 \lambda a_0) a_n \cos n\omega t +$$
$$+\omega_0^2 \lambda \sum_{n=1}^{\infty} \sum_{k=1}^{\infty} \frac{1}{2} a_k a_n [\cos (k+n)\omega t + \cos (k-n)\omega t] = 0$$

Equality must be met separately for each harmonic component and for the constant component.

For constant terms of the equation, we have

$$\omega_0^2 a_0(1+\lambda\ a_0)+\frac{1}{2}\omega_0^2\lambda\ \sum_{n=1}^{\infty}a_n^2\quad=0.$$

For terms with a fundamental angular frequency ω, we get the equation

$$\left(\omega_0^2-\omega^2+2\omega_0^2\lambda a_0\right)\ a_1+\omega_0^2\lambda\ \sum_{n=1}^{\infty}a_n a_{n+1}=0.$$

Then, the terms with the frequency of 2ω (second harmonic)

$$\left(\omega_0^2-4\omega^2+2\omega_0^2\lambda a_0\right)a_2+\frac{1}{2}\omega_0^2\lambda a_1^2+\omega_0^2\lambda\sum_{n=1}^{\infty}a_n a_{n+2}=0,\text{ etc.}$$

From the second equation, we get after neglecting higher terms

$$\left(\omega_0^2-\omega^2+2\omega_0^2\lambda a_0+\omega_0^2\lambda\ a_2\right)\ a_1=0,$$

from where

$$\omega^2=\omega_0^2\ \left[1+\lambda(2a_0+a_2)\right]\approx\omega_0^2.$$

It yields from the first equation

$$a_0(1+\lambda a_0)+\frac{1}{2}\lambda a_1^2=0,\text{ and approximately } a_0\approx-\frac{1}{2}\lambda a_1^2.$$

From the third equation, we obtain

$$\left(\omega_0^2-4\omega^2\right)a_2+\frac{1}{2}\omega_0^2\lambda a_1^2=0\text{ and } a_2\approx\frac{1}{6}\lambda a_1^2.$$

By substituting a_0 and a_2 to relation for ω^2, we get a more precise result in the form

$$\omega^2=\omega_0^2[1+\lambda(2a_0+a_2)]=\omega_0^2\left[1-\frac{5}{6}(\lambda a_1)^2\right].$$

Example 6. Thermal expansion of substances.

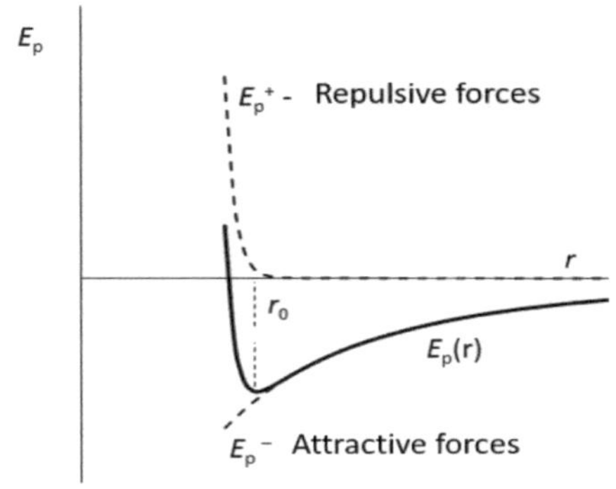

Atoms or molecules of solids or liquids are arranged in ordered structures. Attractive electric forces ensure the consistency of the substance. Approaching or moving the molecules or atoms together causes repulsive forces, which, along with attractive forces, provide equilibrium distances. The potential energy of the particle relative to the adjacent particle is shown in the figure. We can see that the potential well is asymmetrical. The minimum potential energy corresponds to the equilibrium distance of the particles of the substance. If we supply the particles with energy (e.g., in the form of heat), the amplitude of the oscillations of the particles increases.

Moreover, due to the non-linearity of the binding potential, the mean interatomic distance also increases. It means the macroscopic elongation of the material. According to the Eq. (14), the displacement of the mean distance of a_0 is proportional to the square a_1^2 of the amplitude of the fundamental harmonic. This amplitude square is proportional to the energy of the oscillations and the temperature. Hence, the thermal expansion of the substances is

$$\frac{\Delta l}{l_0} = \alpha(T - T_0), \text{resp.} l = l_0[1 + \alpha(T - T_0)],$$

where α is the coefficient of the length thermal expansion.

1.2 Oscillations in the linear system with viscous damping

In real systems, oscillation damping occurs because of irreversible energy loss of the system during the oscillation process. The loss mechanism describes the force that depends on the movement state of the system. In mechanical systems, it is mainly friction or resistance of the environment. In electrical circuits, there are Joule losses when current is passing through a resistor or emitting EM waves to the surrounding space. **Figure 9** shows an example of a damped oscillation model.

Let us consider the loss mechanism that often occurs in oscillating systems, which is a viscous resistance. A resistive force proportional to the velocity of movement characterises it, or in other words, the viscous resistance depends on power

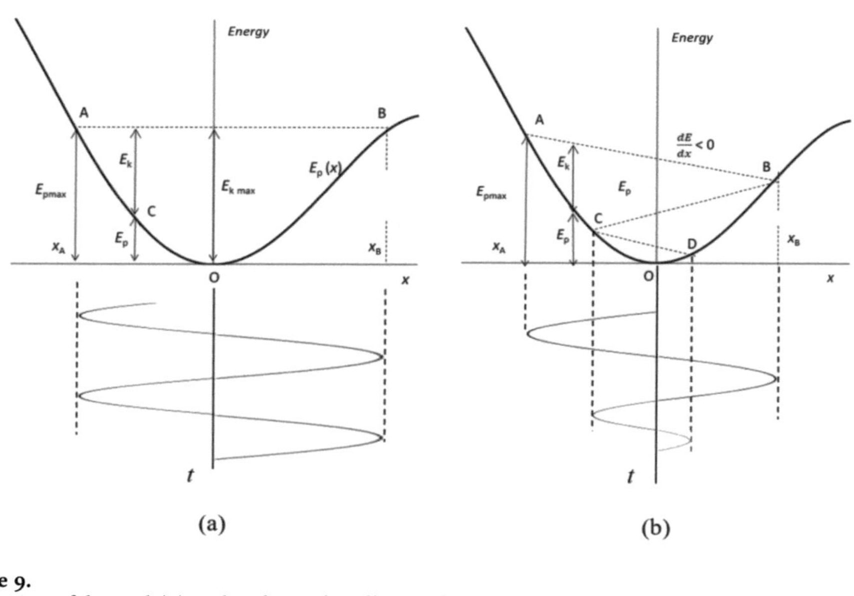

Figure 9.
Comparison of damped (a) and undamped oscillations (b).

dissipation proportional to the square of the velocity (in electric circuits, it is the square of the current). Thus,

$$F_o = -rv \tag{15}$$

where r is the coefficient of resistance. In the case of mechanical resistance, the viscous resistance depends on the dimension and shape of the body. It depends on the surrounding medium viscosity in which the body moves.

Power of the resistive force (power dissipation)

$$P_s = F_o v = -rv^2 \tag{16}$$

is a quadratic function of the velocity. In the case of the electrical circuit, the power dissipation is expressed as $P = Ri^2$. If the electrical current is analogous to the speed of motion, see Example 1, then this equation is analogous to Eq. (16) for viscous losses.

Motion equation $ma = F$ for the linear system with viscous damping has a form

$$ma = -kx - rv, \tag{17}$$

which can be rearranged to

$$\ddot{x} + 2b\dot{x} + \omega_0^2 x = 0, \tag{18}$$

where $v = \dot{x}$ and $b = r/(2\,m)$ is damping coefficient.

This equation is a linear differential equation with constant coefficients, and we find the solution in a form of the exponential function $e^{\lambda t}$. We obtain the values of the λ from the characteristic equation

$$\lambda^2 + 2b\lambda + \omega_0^2 = 0, \tag{19}$$

which solution is

$$\lambda_{1,2} = -b \pm \sqrt{b^2 - \omega_0^2}. \tag{20}$$

The type of motion of this oscillatory system depends on the ratio of the b, and ω_0 values, which defines the quality factor

$$Q = \frac{\omega_0}{2b}. \tag{21}$$

1.2.1 Underdamped oscillation system

Underdamping occurs in systems with a quality factor of $Q > 1/2$. Characteristic equation solution corresponds to a complex number $\lambda = -b \pm j\omega$, where $\omega = \sqrt{\omega_0^2 - b^2}$. Then, the solution can be expressed as

$$x(t) = Ae^{-bt} \cos(\omega t + \alpha), \tag{22}$$

where A and α are integration constants and they depend on the initial conditions of the movement, which are the initial particle displacement of x_0 and initial velocity of v_0 in time $t = 0$

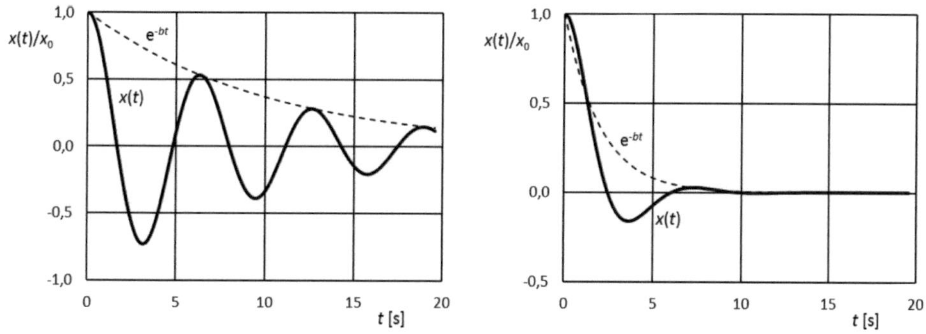

Figure 10.
Time course of subcritical damped oscillations for two values of the attenuation on the left is $\omega_o = 1.0\ rad\ s^{-1}$, $b = 0.1\ s^{-1}$, $v_o = 0\ m\ s^{-1}$, *on the right* $\omega_o = 1.0\ rad\ s^{-1}$, $b = 0.5\ s^{-1}$, $v_o = 0\ m\ s^{-1}$.

$$x_0 = A\cos\alpha \text{ and } v_0 = -bA\cos\alpha - \omega A\sin\alpha, \tag{23}$$

from where $\tan\alpha = -\frac{1}{\omega}\left(\frac{v_0}{x_0} + b\right)$ and $A = \sqrt{x_0^2 + \left(\frac{v_0}{\omega}\right)^2\left(1 + \frac{bx_0}{v_0}\right)^2}$.

See **Figure 10** as example, where are underdamped oscillations for different values of the attenuation coefficients $b = 0.1\ \text{s}^{-1}$ and $b = 0.5\ \text{s}^{-1}$, or for quality factors $Q = 5$ and $Q = 1$, respectively, at $\omega_0 = 1$ rad•s^{-1}, and initial conditions $x_0 > 0$ and $v_0 = 0$ m•s^{-1}.

In the case of the underdamped system, the particle displacement overshoots the zero value (see the negative values in the graphs).

The value of

$$\tau = \frac{1}{b} = \frac{2Q}{\omega_0} \tag{24}$$

is *damping time constant* and it indicates the time when the e^{-bt} function decreases to the value of $1/e \approx 0.37(=37\%)$. This constant provides information about the time when the oscillations disappear. Usually, we consider the disappearance time of 3τ, when the maximal particle displacement reaches $e^{-3} \approx 5\%$ of its initial value, or the time of 5τ, at which the displacement drops to $e^{-5} < 1\%$.

The ratio

$$\frac{\tau}{T} = \frac{\omega}{2\pi b} = \frac{1}{\pi}\ Q\ \sqrt{1 - \frac{1}{4Q^2}} \tag{25}$$

represents the oscillation count during the time of τ. We can see that there are no oscillations in the system if $Q \le 1/2$.

1.2.2 Critical damping

Critical damping occurs if $b = \omega_0$, and Eq. (19) has only one double solution. In this case, the solution of the equation is

$$x(t) = (A_1 + A_2 t)\ e^{-bt}, \tag{26}$$

where initial conditions are $x = x_0$ and $v = v_0$ at $t = 0$ s to determine A_1 and A_2. **Figure 11** shows typical time courses for different initial conditions.

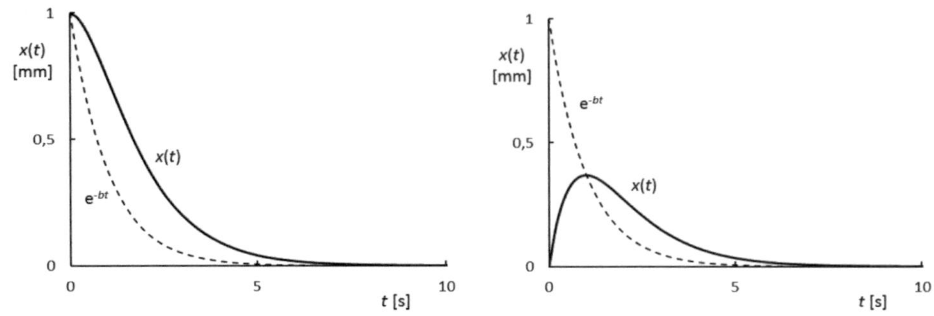

Figure 11.
Time course of critical damped oscillations for $\omega_o = b = 1\ s^{-1}$ (on the left $x_o = 1$ mm, $v_o = 0$, on the right $x_o = 0$, $v_o = 1\ mm\ s^{-1}$).

The importance of critical damping is that the system returns from the non-equilibrium state to the equilibrium fast and without overshooting. Various systems utilise critical damping, for example, shock absorbers for vehicles such as cars, motorcycles, etc. Critical damping is also used in the impulse electrical circuits to minimise distortion of the rising and falling edges of the impulse signal.

1.2.3 Overdamped oscillation system

Overdamping is given by $b > \omega_0$. If we denote $a = \sqrt{b^2 - \omega_0^2}$, then the solution of the Eq. (18) has a form as

$$x(t) = e^{-bt}(A_1 e^{at} + A_2 e^{-at}), \tag{27}$$

where A_1 and A_2 result from the initial conditions. The particle displacement over the time consists of two exponential functions while one function has a short relaxation time $\tau_1 = 1/(b + a)$ and the second function has a time of $\tau_2 = 1/(b - a)$. **Figure 12** shows examples of critical damped systems for different initial conditions.

Dashed lines in the graphs indicate both exponential components with different time constants. We can see that this is an aperiodic event with no overshoot through the equilibrium position.

Viscous damping occurs especially in the case of small oscillations of a mass in the liquid, when there is laminar flow, or in the case of capillary damping devices. Linear damping is also typical for oscillations of atoms due to heat exchange, or for damping of oscillations in electrical circuits. In the case of the mass movement in a

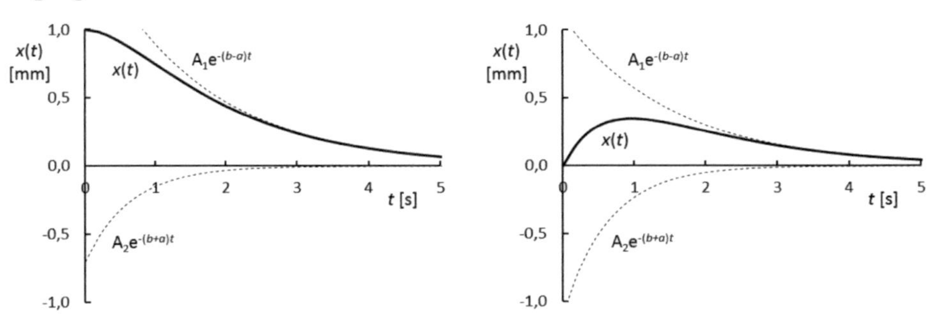

Figure 12.
Overdamped oscillation system for $\omega_o = 1.00\ rad\ s^{-1}$, $b = 1.10\ s^{-1}$ (on the left $x_o = 1$ mm, $v_o = 0\ mm\ s^{-1}$, on the right $x_o = 0$ mm, $v_o = 1\ mm\ s^{-1}$).

gaseous medium, for example, the pendulum in the air, the aerodynamic drag force $F \sim v^2$ usually applies, which is characterised by a quadratic dependence on speed. This means that it is no longer a linear system, and the solution leads to a non-linear differential equation even at small oscillations.

Example 7. Pendulum in a liquid.

Consider a pendulum (Example 2), whereby the suspended ball moves in water in a dish. For low velocities, the viscous resistance force for the ball-shaped body is given by the Stokes relation

$$F = -6\pi\eta r v,$$

where η is the dynamic viscosity of the liquid, r is the ball radius and v is the velocity of the motion.

The attenuation coefficient follows from (18):

$$b = \frac{3\pi\eta r}{m} = \frac{9\eta}{4\rho r^2},$$

where ρ is the ball density.

For example, the water has η = 1.0 × 10^{-3} Pa·s (at 20°C), the density of steel is 7.8 × 10^3 kg·m^{-3} and the ball radius r = 5.0 mm. Then, we get $b \approx 1.2 \times 10^{-2}$ s^{-1}.

If the ball hangs on the thread of the length l = 1.0 m, then $\omega_0 \approx 3.1$ s^{-1}.

The Q-factor is $Q \approx 130$. It is, therefore, subcritical damping and according to (25)

$$\frac{\tau}{T} = \frac{\omega}{2\pi b} = \frac{1}{\pi} Q \sqrt{1 - \frac{1}{4Q^2}} \approx 41.$$

It means that the oscillations are damped to the ratio of $1/e \approx 37\%$ after 41 periods.

Example 8. Oscillation damping in electrical RLC circuit.

Consider a single loop of series-connected elements of an inductor L, a capacitor C, and a resistor R. Assume that initially, the capacitor was charged to a U_0 voltage, and the current in the circuit was zero (RL connection to the charged C capacitor).

The energy of the conservative energy components is then

$$E = \frac{1}{2}\frac{Q^2}{C} + \frac{1}{2}Li^2.$$

The time change of this energy is equal to the power of Joule's losses

$$\frac{dE}{dt} = \frac{Q}{C}\dot{Q} + Li\dot{i} = -Ri^2,$$

where $\dot{Q} = i$. If we divide the equation by the current i, and knowing the $\dot{i} = \ddot{Q}$, we get

$$\frac{Q}{C} + L\ddot{Q} = -R\dot{Q}, \text{resp.} \ddot{Q} + 2\frac{R}{2L}\dot{Q} + \frac{1}{LC}Q = 0,$$

where $\omega_0 = \frac{1}{\sqrt{LC}}$ and $b = \frac{R}{2L}$.

For example, L = 50 mH, C = 20 μF, and R = 10 Ω, we obtain $\omega_0 \approx 1.0 \times 10^3$ s^{-1} and $b \approx 1.0 \times 10^2$ s^{-1}.

Thus, there are subcritically damped oscillations.

The charge time response is then

$$Q(t) = Q_0 \mathrm{e}^{-bt} \cos \omega t,$$

where $\omega = \sqrt{\omega_0^2 - b^2} \approx 0.99 \times 10^3\ \mathrm{s}^{-1}$.

$$\frac{\tau}{T} = \frac{\omega}{2\pi b} = \frac{1}{\pi} Q \sqrt{1 - \frac{1}{4Q^2}} \approx 1.6.$$

We can see that the angular frequency ω differs only slightly from the angular frequency ω_0 of the non-attenuated oscillations. However, the motion is significantly attenuated. The relative decrease to $1/e \approx 37\%$ of the initial value occurs after 1.6 periods of oscillations.

1.3 Oscillation of damped system with harmonic excitation

If an external periodic excitation force acts on the oscillation system, the system responds, after the transient process has disappeared, with a periodic answer. If the excitation is harmonic and the system is linear, then the steady answer is also harmonic with the same frequency. Any periodic stimulus of the linear system represents a superposition of harmonic components in terms of the Fourier series. Therefore, we will pay special attention to the response of the linear oscillation system to the external harmonic excitation.

1.3.1 Spectral characteristics of linear system with harmonic excitation

The harmonic force acting on linear oscillation system with viscous damping is given by the equation of motion

$$F_\mathrm{v} = F_\mathrm{m} \sin \Omega t, \tag{28}$$

where F_m is force amplitude and Ω is its angular frequency.
Then the equation of motion has a form

$$ma = -kx - rv + F_\mathrm{v}, \tag{29}$$

which we can rewrite to

$$\ddot{x} + 2b\dot{x} + \omega_0^2 x = f_\mathrm{m} \sin \Omega t, \tag{30}$$

where $f_m = F_m/m$ is external force amplitude related to the mass of the system.
The solution of the homogeneous equation corresponds to some of the results of the section 1.2 depending on the type of the system damping. A particular solution respects the right side. The homogeneous solution is a transient that fades out over time. The particular solution represents a process that lasts as long as the exciting force acts. There are steady harmonic oscillations in the system. In the case of harmonic excitation, the particular solution has a form

$$x_\mathrm{p}(t) = x_\mathrm{m} \sin(\Omega t + \beta), \tag{31}$$

where

$$x_m = \frac{f_m}{\sqrt{\left(\omega_0^2 - \Omega^2\right)^2 + (2b\Omega)^2}}, \text{and } \beta = -\text{arctg}\left(\frac{2b\Omega}{\omega_0^2 - \Omega^2}\right). \tag{32}$$

The x_m is the amplitude of oscillations and β is the phase shift of the response compared to the phase of the excitation force (28). These results can be convinced by directly substituting the solution (31) into the Eq. (30). The linear oscillation system must respond to a harmonic response with the same angular frequency. As can be seen from the previous relationships, the amplitude and phase shift of the response depends on the Ω angular frequency of the excitation.

A special case is the excitation response with an angular frequency which is equal to the angular frequency $\Omega_r = \omega_0$ of the undamped system. This case is called *resonance*. For the resonance state, we get values from relations (32)

$$x_{\text{mr}} = \frac{f_{\text{m}}}{2b\omega_0} = x_0 Q, \text{ and } \beta_r = -\frac{\pi}{2}\text{rad}, \tag{33}$$

where $x_0 = F_m/k$ is the displacement from the equilibrium while the constant force F_m acts on the system (zero angular frequency $\Omega = 0$). In the case of a system with a high Q-factor of $Q \gg 1$, the amplitude of the response in the resonance state is significantly greater than the displacement of x_0 caused by the constant force. The response is phase-delayed by $\pi/2$ rad compared to excitation. **Figure 13** shows the frequency response characteristics for different Q-factor values.

We can see from these characteristics that if the resonant amplification of the system oscillations is undesirable, it is necessary to choose critical or overcritical damping. In this case, however, considerable energy losses occur in the system because of the resistance force. On the other hand, there are systems with low internal losses and characterised by a very high Q-factor (in hundreds to thousands). In the case of high values of the quality factor ($Q \gg 1$), the frequency bandwidth of the resonant maximum can be determined at a level of 3db decrease relative to the maximum value (i.e., decrease to approximately 0.707 x_{mr})

$$\Delta\Omega = \frac{\omega_0}{Q}. \tag{34}$$

The resonant maximum increases proportionally with the Q-factor and narrows inversely with it. Therefore, the systems with a very high Q-factor have high selectivity, and we can use them, for example, for the spectral analysis of an unknown signal or for controlling pendulum clocks, resonant crystal clocks, atomic

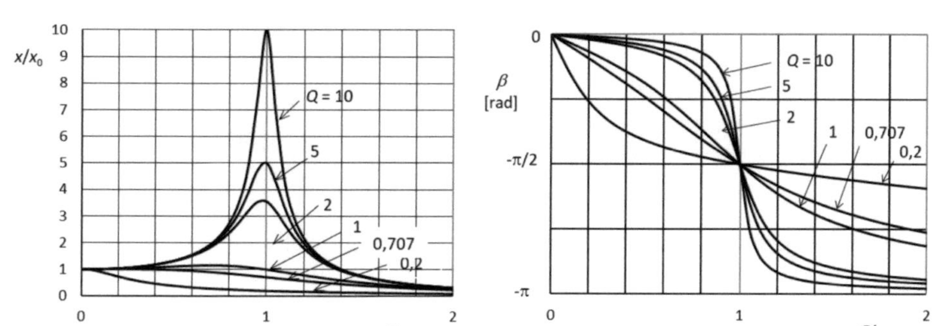

Figure 13.
Amplitude and phase shift response of the oscillating system versus a relative angular frequency for different values of the quality factor.

clocks, etc. An undesirable consequence of resonance in mechanical devices can be the occurrence of vibrations, for example, when the engine rpm corresponds to the resonant frequency of the mechanical system. These phenomena are not limited to mechanical systems only. Similarly, resonance phenomena occur in electrical circuits or electromagnetic systems. An example, to be mentioned later, is magnetic resonance used in medical diagnostics. In a very simplified view, the human auditory organ is a complicated resonant system too that allows different sound frequencies (pitch of tones) to be distinguished.

1.3.2 Non-linear oscillating system with harmonic excitation

The situation is more complex in the case of a non-linear oscillating system exposed to external harmonic excitation. As an example, consider the non-linear system with the asymmetric potential well described in Section 1.1.2, with harmonic excitation and viscous damping. The equation of motion expressed in a standard form, see Eqs. (12) and (30), has a form

$$\ddot{x} + 2b\dot{x} + \omega_0^2(1 + \lambda x)x = f_{\mathrm{m}} \sin \Omega\, t. \tag{35}$$

We are interested again in the steady-state response of the system described by the particular solution of the differential equation. The response of a non-linear system to harmonic excitation is no longer harmonic but remains periodic with the same angular frequency. The periodic response function is expressed as a superposition of harmonic components using the Fourier series

$$x(t) = x_0 + \sum_{n=1}^{\infty} x_{\mathrm{m}n} \sin(n\Omega t + \beta_n). \tag{36}$$

After substituting this assumed solution into the differential equation, we obtain the values of the individual quantities. In the case of weak non-linearity ($\lambda x_{\mathrm{m}1} << 1$), the results have the form of

$$x_{\mathrm{m}1} = \frac{f_{\mathrm{m}}}{\sqrt{\left(\omega_0^2 - \Omega^2 + 2\lambda\omega_0^2 B_0\right)^2 + (2b\,\Omega)^2}} \approx \frac{f_{\mathrm{m}}}{\sqrt{\left(\omega_0^2 - \Omega^2\right)^2 + (2b\,\Omega)^2}}, \tag{37}$$

$$x_0 = -\frac{1}{2}\lambda x_{\mathrm{m}1}^2 \tag{38}$$

$$x_{\mathrm{m}2} \approx -\frac{\lambda\omega_0^2}{2}\frac{x_{\mathrm{m}1}^2}{\sqrt{\left(\omega_0^2 - 4\Omega^2\right)^2 + (4b\,\Omega)^2}} \tag{39}$$

$$x_{\mathrm{m}3} \approx \frac{\lambda\omega_0^2}{2}\frac{B_{\mathrm{m}1}}{\sqrt{\left(\omega_0^2 - 9\Omega^2\right)^2 + (6b\Omega)^2}} x_{\mathrm{m}2}, \text{ etc.} \tag{40}$$

The fundamental harmonic having amplitude $x_{\mathrm{m}1}$ dominates. Its properties are similar to those of the linear system. Also, the mid-position x_0 is shifted due to the system's non-linearity. Furthermore, the resonance occurs at subharmonic frequencies, an integer fraction of the fundamental harmonic frequency ($\Omega_n = \omega_0/n$). They are expressed by response amplitudes $x_{\mathrm{m}n}$. The subharmonics components have an origin caused by excitation having a specific subharmonic frequency Ω_n. But the response has the fundamental resonance frequency ω_0 since there is the response of

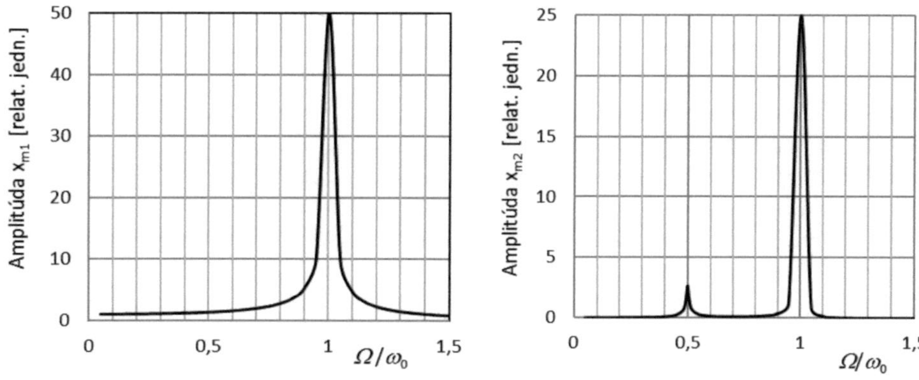

Figure 14.
Frequency amplitude characteristics of the first and second harmonic components for values of $\lambda = 0.06\ m^{-1}$*,* $Q = 50$*.*

specific harmonic defined as $n\Omega_n = \omega_0$. **Figure 14** shows the frequency amplitude characteristics of the first and second harmonics.

The subharmonic resonance is important to explain the perception of musical chords by the non-linear system of the auditory organ. For example, if we hear two tones with frequencies in the ratio 2:1 (octave), the tone with the angular frequency ω_{01} produces a signal with the second harmonic of $2\omega_{01}$. If this frequency is not equal to the frequency of ω_{02}, the auditory organ sensitively detects the difference between ω_{02} and $2\omega_{01}$ and evokes a feeling of non-tuned music interval.

1.3.3 Harmonic interaction in a non-linear oscillating system

In practice, we encounter cases, in which the oscillating system is simultaneously excited by several harmonic signals with different frequencies.

As a simple example, we will excite the system with two harmonic signals and determine its response to this excitation.

The equation of the response has the form

$$m\ddot{x} + r\dot{x} + k\ x + (l/2)\,x^2 = F_{\mathrm{m1}}\sin\Omega_1 t + F_{\mathrm{m}2}\sin\Omega_2 t, \tag{41}$$

where the Ω_1 and Ω_2 are angular frequencies of the harmonic components of the excitation.

We can rewrite the equation to

$$\ddot{x} + 2\,b\,\dot{x} + \omega_0\,(\omega_0 + \lambda x)x = f_{\mathrm{m}1}\sin\Omega_1 t + f_{\mathrm{m}2}\sin\Omega_2 t, \tag{42}$$

where $f_{m1} = F_{m1}/m$ and $f_{m2} = F_{m2}/m$.

Since the excitation signal is periodic, the response must also be periodic.

Considering the weak non-linearity when $\lambda \ll \omega_0 x_{\mathrm{m}}$, harmonic components with excitation angular frequencies dominate in response. Therefore, the steady response has the dominant components

$$x_1 = x_{\mathrm{m}1}\sin\ (\Omega_1 t + \beta_1) + x_{\mathrm{m}2}\sin\ (\Omega_2 t + \beta_2). \tag{43}$$

If we substitute this function into a quadratic term in the Eq. (42), there are elements with combinational frequencies $\Omega_1 \pm \Omega_2$ on the left side of the equation

$$x_1^2 = \frac{1}{2}\,x_{\mathrm{m}1}^2\,[1 - \ \cos\ (2\,\Omega_1 t + 2\beta_1)] + \frac{1}{2}\,x_{\mathrm{m}2}^2\,[1 - \ \cos\ (2\,\Omega_2 t + 2\beta_2)] +$$
$$+ x_{\mathrm{m}1}x_{\mathrm{m}2}\,[\cos\ ((\Omega_1 - \Omega_2)\,t + \beta_1 - \beta_2) - \ \cos\ ((\Omega_1 + \Omega_2)\,t + \beta_1 + \beta_2)]\ .$$

Due to non-linearity, components with frequencies 2 Ω_1, 2 Ω_2, $\Omega_1 + \Omega_2$, and $\Omega_1 - \Omega_2$ appear in the equation. Including these components together with the original components in the overall system response, the non-linearity (quadratic term) results in the second generation of components with twice the frequencies and with all combinations, for example, $3\Omega_1$, $3\Omega_2$, $2\,\Omega_1 \pm \Omega_2$, $\Omega_1 \pm 2\,\Omega_2$. The solution is very complex, and therefore, we will focus on the approximate determination of combination components of the first generation.

In the time response of the system, we consider only the most significant components

$$x(t) = x_0 + x_{m1,0}\sin\left(\Omega_1 t + \beta_{1,0}\right) + x_{m0,1}\sin\left(\Omega_2 t + \beta_{0,1}\right) +$$
$$+ x_{m2,0}\sin\left(2\Omega_1 t + \beta_{2,0}\right) + x_{m0,2}\sin\left(2\Omega_2 t + \beta_{0,2}\right) +$$
$$+ x_{m1,1}\sin\left((\Omega_1 + \Omega_2)t + \beta_{1,1}\right) + x_{m1,-1}\sin\left((\Omega_1 - \Omega_2)t + \beta_{1,-1}\right),$$

where numbered indices correspond to frequency combinations, for example, $Q_{mk,l}$ relates to the frequency of $\Omega_{k,l} = k\Omega_1 + l\Omega_2$.

If we substitute these components into the equation of motion and separate the corresponding harmonic elements on the left and right sides, we get a response for the amplitudes of the harmonic components

$$x_{m1,0} = f^*_{m1}\frac{1}{\sqrt{\left(\omega_0^2 - \Omega_1^2 + 2\lambda\omega_0 Q_0\right)^2 + (2b\,\Omega_1)^2}}$$

$$x_{m\ 0,1} = f^*_{m2}\frac{1}{\sqrt{\left(\omega_0^2 - \Omega_2^2 + 2\lambda\omega_0 Q_0\right)^2 + (2b\,\Omega_2)^2}},$$

which corresponds to the frequency response of the linear system (resonant characteristics with a maximum at the resonant frequency of ω_0).

Considering the dominant components with angular frequencies Ω_1 and Ω_2, the constant component is

$$x_0 \approx -\frac{1}{2}\lambda\frac{x^2_{m\ 1,0} + x^2_{m0,1}}{\omega_0 + \lambda Q_0} \approx -\left(\frac{\lambda}{2\omega_0}\right)\left(x^2_{m\ 1,0} + x^2_{m\ 0,1}\right).$$

Components with double frequencies of 2 Ω_1 and 2 Ω_2 shall be determined as in the case of simple harmonic excitation and with the same results.

For the lowest combination frequencies, we get a relationship

$$x_{m1,\pm 1} \approx \lambda\omega_0\frac{x_{m\ 1,0}\ x_{m\ 0,1}}{\sqrt{\left[\omega_0^2 - (\Omega_1 \pm \Omega_2)^2 + 2\lambda\omega_0 Q_0\right]^2 + \left[2b\,(\Omega_1 \pm \Omega_2)\right]^2}}.$$

From this relationship, we can see that the cause of combination frequencies is non-linearity, which occurs in the result as $\lambda\omega_0$. Similarly, we can determine the amplitudes of the response components with higher combinational frequencies. As with resonance at *subharmonic* frequencies, resonance occurs when combinational frequencies are

$$|\Omega_1 \pm \Omega_2| = \sqrt{\omega_0^2 + 2\lambda\omega_0\,Q_0} \approx \omega_0.$$

In this case, the response amplitude with an angular frequency of ω_0 is given by equation

$$x_{\mathrm{m}1,\pm 1} \approx \left(\frac{\omega_0}{2b}\right)\left(\frac{\lambda}{\omega_0}\right) x_{\mathrm{m}1,0} x_{\mathrm{m}0,1}.$$

System resonances also occur at higher combinational frequencies. Non-linearity and the resulting response components with combinational frequencies increase at higher excitation. There are systems where the combinational frequencies are undesirable. For example, the acoustic loudspeakers are load overrated, which means that the effects of system non-linearity under operating loads are negligible.

As indicated in Section 1.3.2, resonances with combinational frequencies or resonances at subharmonic frequencies are important, for example, in explaining the perception of musical chords by the non-linear system of the human auditory organ. For example, if we hear two tones with frequencies in the ratio of 2 (octave 2:1), the tone with the angular frequency of ω_{01} produces a signal with the second harmonic of $2\omega_{01}$. If this frequency is not equal to the frequency of ω_{02}, the auditory organ sensitively detects the difference of $\omega_{02} - 2\omega_{01}$ and creates a sense of non-tuned music interval. It is like other music intervals such as small third 6:5, big third 5:4, fourth 4:3, fifth 3:2, small sixth 8:5, big sixth 5:3, small seventh 16:9, and big seventh 15:8. These music intervals have the ratio of frequencies equal to the integer ratio. Due to the non-linearity of the auditory organ, the music listener can distinguish a pure (harmonic) or impure (disharmonic) chord and thus perceive the beauty of musical compositions.

1.3.4 Power losses and the nature of spectroscopy

The oscillations relate to the exchange of energy between conservative elements of the system. The total energy of the system is equal to the sum of kinetic and potential energy or their equivalents. In the case of forced harmonic oscillations of a linear system with the fundamental frequency of ω_0 and excitation frequency of Ω, the total energy of the system at a steady state is

$$E = \frac{1}{2} m v^2 + \frac{1}{2} k x^2 = \frac{1}{2} m v_{\mathrm{m}}^2 \cos^2(\Omega t + \beta) + \frac{1}{2} k x_{\mathrm{m}}^2 \sin^2(\Omega t + \beta) =$$
$$= \frac{1}{4} m \left(\Omega^2 + \omega_0^2\right) x_{\mathrm{m}}^2 + \frac{1}{4} m \left(\Omega^2 - \omega_0^2\right) \cos(2\Omega t + 2\beta).$$

The mean value of this energy is

$$\langle E \rangle = \frac{1}{4} m \left(\Omega^2 + \omega_0^2\right) x_{\mathrm{m}}^2 = \frac{1}{4}\left(1 + \frac{\Omega^2}{\omega_0^2}\right) k x_{\mathrm{m}}^2. \tag{44}$$

The second (alternating) component is directly proportional to the difference $\Omega^2 - {\omega_0}^2$ and corresponds to the periodic energy exchange between the source and the system with an angular frequency of $2\,\Omega$.

If we consider the viscous losses in the system, the energy losses in one period of T are as follows

$$W_T = \int_0^T P\,\mathrm{d}t = \int_0^T F v\,\mathrm{d}t = \int_0^T F_{\mathrm{m}} v_{\mathrm{m}} \sin \Omega t \ \cos(\Omega t + \beta)\,\mathrm{d}t =$$
$$= \frac{T}{2} F_{\mathrm{m}} v_{\mathrm{m}} \ \sin \beta = \pi \ F_{\mathrm{m}} x_{\mathrm{m}} \ \sin \beta.$$

In the state of resonance at frequency $\Omega = \omega_0$, $\beta = -\pi/2$ rad and the alternating component of energy E is zero.

Then, active power supplied to the system in the case of the steady state of forced oscillations is

$$\langle P \rangle = \frac{W_T}{T} = \frac{1}{2} F_m x_m \ \Omega \ \sin\beta = \frac{F_m^2}{2m} \frac{2b\Omega^2}{\left(\omega_0^2 - \Omega^2\right)^2 + (2b\Omega)^2} \tag{45}$$

Figure 15 shows the graph of the active power spectral function [see Eq. (45)] for two Q-values. These figures show that an oscillating system with a high Q-factor absorbs the energy of the source only in a narrow interval around the resonant frequency and changes it most often into heat.

There are various bonds of atoms and molecules in biological tissues. These bonds represent microscopic oscillating systems with characteristic resonant frequencies. If these tissues are irradiated with monochromatic electromagnetic waves with a frequency corresponding to a resonant frequency of coupling, then energy is supplied to these coupled systems. This energy can stimulate tissues at low-power applications, for example, phototherapy. At higher power, the absorbed energy increases the temperature of the tissue structures, and thus, it can lead to their destruction used, for example, in the treatment of cancer.

Example 9. Spectroscopy.

The above phenomenon explains the physical nature of *spectroscopy*. In systems with a higher Q-factor, the resonance state relates either to dynamically increased oscillations or to power absorption of the source.

The conservative forces bond the atoms of the matter and determine their equilibrium position. The oscillations around the equilibrium position are at the natural frequency and depend on the properties of the particle (mass) and the features of the bond (stiffness). Thus, differently bound particles have different oscillation frequencies. Each material has characteristic frequencies according to its composition.

When an electromagnetic wave interacts with a material, it acts on its atoms. If the EM wave frequency equals one of the resonant frequencies of the substance, then it significantly absorbs and attenuates this wave. For example, if we observe the white light of the Sun on the surface of the Earth using a spectrometer, we find in the continuous visible light spectrum black lines that correspond to the absorption of light with the appropriate frequencies of gas molecules in the atmosphere. In this way, we can measure the concentration of greenhouse gases in the atmosphere.

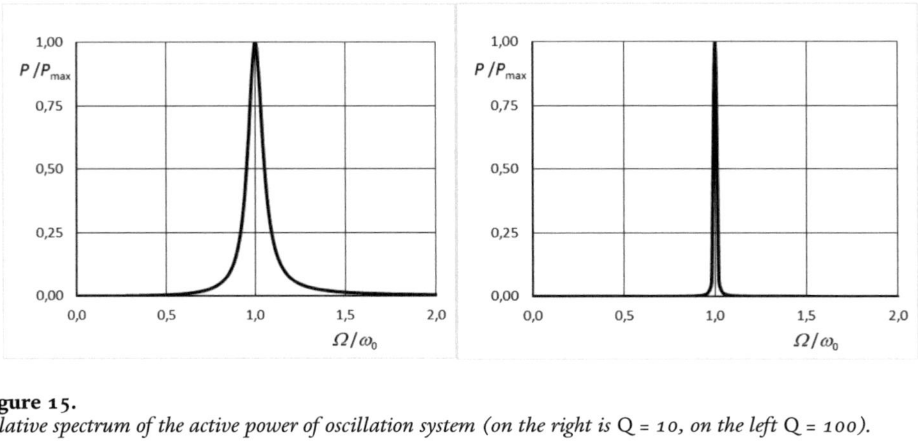

Figure 15.
Relative spectrum of the active power of oscillation system (on the right is Q = 10, on the left Q = 100).

Another example is optical spectroscopy used in biochemistry, pathology, or the investigation of blood plasma. As an example, let us pass the adjustable wavelength light through the liquid cuvette to search for wavelengths at which the liquid has a resonant absorption. Then, the found wavelengths or frequencies determine the presence of the individual substances of the material and their concentration in the solution.

Another example is magnetic resonance imaging, as discussed in the following paragraph.

1.3.5 Magnetic resonance

1.3.5.1 Nature of magnetic resonance

We talk about resonance if the frequency of external excitation on the oscillating system is the same as the frequency of its self-oscillations, and the mechanism of action can supply the oscillating system with energy. In the linear system, it is the frequency of its undamped oscillations. In the case of a magnetic dipole in a constant magnetic field, it is the *Larmor frequency* of f_L, see Example 4. Read also Vlaardingerbroek [2], Webb [3], or Hashemi [4].

If we create a rotating magnetic field in space with a rotation frequency f close to the frequency f_L, we can expect a resonance phenomenon. The external excitation magnetic field must be perpendicular to the precession axis (i.e., to the constant magnetic field $\boldsymbol{B}_0$) to interact with a magnetic dipole that performs a precession movement. We create a rotating magnetic field using two mutually perpendicular pairs of coils, which are fed by currents with the same frequency and with a mutual phase shift of $\pi/2$ rad.

Figure 16 illustrates the situation where perpendicular pairs of coils are on the left. If z is the direction of the constant magnetic field $\boldsymbol{B}_0$ and hence the axis of the dipole precession, the x and y directions are perpendicular to the z-axis. One pair of coils creates the magnetic field of B_x in the x-axis direction, the other pair the field of B_y in the y-axis direction. The coil currents and thus the magnetic field components are phase-shifted by $\pi/2$ rad, and thus

$$B_x = B_1 \sin(\omega t + \psi), \text{and } B_y = B_1 \cos(\omega t + \psi).$$

Adding both components, we get the resulting $\boldsymbol{B}_1$ vector, which has a constant value of B_1 and rotates in the x-y plane with the ω angular frequency of the coil current. The right part of the figure shows the direction of the dipole precession

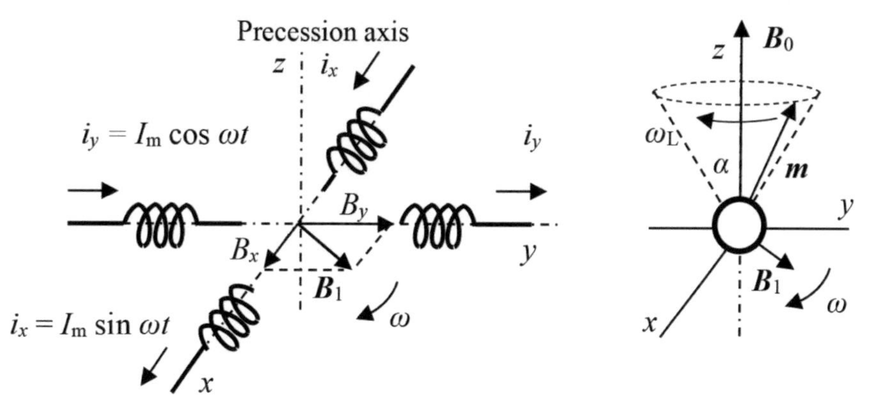

Figure 16.
Magnetic dipole in rotating magnetic field.

with the dipole moment of $\boldsymbol{m}$ and the direction of rotation of the rotating magnetic field.

Vector components of the $\boldsymbol{m}$ dipole moment are

$$m_z = m\cos\alpha, m_x = m\sin\alpha\sin(\omega_L t + \phi), \text{and } m_y = m\sin\alpha\cos(\omega_L t + \phi).$$

Magnetic dipole in the magnetic field $\boldsymbol{B}_0$ has potential energy

$$E_p = -\ \boldsymbol{m}\cdot\boldsymbol{B}_0 = -mB_0\cos\alpha. \tag{46}$$

If an external alternating magnetic field acts on the dipole, only the angle α can change at constant values of m and B_0. The following equation expresses the change of the potential energy dE_p of the dipole

$$dE_p = mB_0\sin\alpha\ d\alpha. \tag{47}$$

Power of external magnetic field torque is

$$P = \boldsymbol{M}\cdot\boldsymbol{\omega}_L = (\boldsymbol{m}\times\boldsymbol{B}_1)\cdot\boldsymbol{\omega}_L =$$
$$= mB_1\sin\alpha[\sin(\omega_L t + \phi)\cos(\omega t + \psi) - \cos(\omega_L t + \phi)\sin(\omega t + \psi)]\omega_L =$$
$$= mB_1\omega_L\sin\alpha\ \sin[(\omega_L - \omega)t + \phi - \psi]. \tag{48}$$

We can see that the power is time-varying for $\omega_L \neq \omega$ and the mean value of the power is zero. If $\omega_L = \omega$, the power has a time-invariant component, which reaches the maximum at $\varphi - \psi = \pi/2$ rad. We describe this phenomenon as *magnetic resonance*.

Then the work over the time dt is

$$\delta W = P\ dt = m\ B_1\ \omega_L\sin\alpha\ dt. \tag{49}$$

Comparing (47) and (49), we obtain for $dE_p = \delta W$

$$\frac{d\alpha}{dt} = \frac{B_1}{B_0}\omega_L = \gamma B_1. \tag{50}$$

As a result, the α angle of the 'precession funnel' varies uniformly in the magnetic resonance state with an angular velocity of $d\alpha/dt$, which depends on the amplitude of the induction of B_1 of the alternating magnetic field. These angle α changes are the periodic event, and therefore the magnetization of a substance changes periodically too. The magnetization inverts its value in the time

$$\tau_{180} = \frac{\pi}{\gamma B_1}, \tag{51}$$

or it is perpendicular to the initial direction in the time

$$\tau_{90} = \frac{\pi}{2\gamma B_1}, \text{and similar.} \tag{52}$$

It is typical for a forced oscillation of particles, and a forced precession of magnetic dipoles, that all particles oscillate synchronously with the same phase compared to the excitation signal.

1.3.5.2 FID signal origin

The paramagnetic material contains many magnetic dipoles randomly arranged due to particle thermal motion. Therefore, the resulting magnetic field of these dipoles is zero. If we insert the paramagnetic material into the $\boldsymbol{B}_0$ constant magnetic field, then the material magnetic dipoles partially arrange in the direction of the $\boldsymbol{B}_0$ vector. This behaviour better describes the magnetization vector ($\boldsymbol{M}_0 = \kappa\mu_0\boldsymbol{B}_0$), where the κ is the magnetic susceptibility of the substance. After switching on the $\boldsymbol{B}_1$ transverse alternating rotating magnetic field with an angular frequency $\omega = \omega_L$, a resonance occurs, which causes a coherent precession of the oriented magnetic dipoles. Let us apply the field $\boldsymbol{B}_1$ during the τ_{90} time. Then the $\boldsymbol{M}_0$ constant magnetization vector, parallel to the $\boldsymbol{B}_0$ vector, changes to the $\boldsymbol{M}$ vector, which has the same magnitude but rotates perpendicularly to the $\boldsymbol{B}_0$ with the angular frequency ω. The sample of a substance looks like a rotating magnet with a magnetic moment ($m^* = M_0V$), where V is the sample volume. If we place a detection coil perpendicularly to the axis of rotation, then the voltage induces in it is

$$u_{\text{FID}} \sim \frac{\mathrm{d}m^*}{\mathrm{d}t} \sim \omega_{\text{L}} M_0 \quad \sin \omega_{\text{L}} t. \tag{53}$$

Voltage induces in the coil only in the case of synchronous dipole precession, which results in rotating magnetization, and this can only happen if magnetic resonance conditions are met. For a given $\boldsymbol{B}_0$ and ω, the resonance occurs only for certain dipoles in the substance, which satisfy the condition $\omega = \omega_L = \gamma B_0$. Thus, by measuring the induced signal, the presence of magnetic dipoles with a corresponding gyromagnetic moment γ can be detected, and their concentration determined.

If we switch off the $\boldsymbol{B}_1$ excitation field, the periodic event begins to damp due to the interaction of the dipoles with the surrounding particles of the substance. The detected signal is, therefore, attenuated (**Figure 17**). This damped signal calls the FID signal (free induction decay). In biomedicine, the magnetic resonance uses protons (with the $\gamma = 2.68 \times 10^8\ \text{s}^{-1}\cdot\text{T}^{-1}$), which exist mainly as nuclei of hydrogen atoms and thus in water molecules.

The organic compounds, such as biological tissues, contain hydrogen atoms too. In specific cases, the magnetic resonance uses nuclei of other biogenic elements such as isotopes of carbon ^{13}C, fluorine ^{19}F, phosphorus ^{31}P, and so on (see **Table 1**, p. 8).

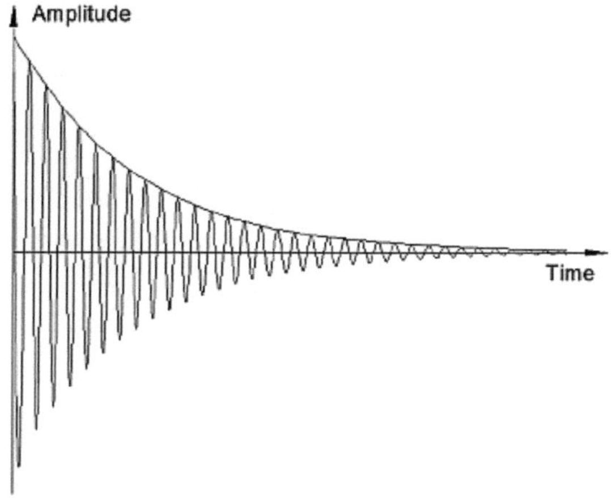

Figure 17.
FID signal after magnetic dipoles excitation.

1.3.5.3 Relaxation

Perpendicular magnetization is an imbalance caused by the external source of the alternating magnetic field $\boldsymbol{B}_1$. If the excitation force stops to act on the system, the aligned movement of the dipole array decays. From the viewpoint of the FID signal, the decay of the in-phase periodic precession movement at first occurs due to the inhomogeneity of the magnetic field $\boldsymbol{B}_0$, and due to the influence of surrounding dipoles, so-called spin-spin interaction. After switching-off the exciting magnetic field, the precision movement of the dipoles remains for a short time in a plane perpendicular to the $\boldsymbol{B}_0$ direction, but due to a small change in the local magnetic field, the precession of the single dipoles is out-phased, which results in an exponential decrease of the transverse magnetization, and thus an FID signal. This decrease characterises the time constant T_2. Its value is in the order of tenths of a second. The second slower mechanism of decay associates with the thermal relaxation of the imbalanced orientation of the magnetic dipoles and directs to the thermodynamic equilibrium of the dipoles, that is, to the equilibrium orientation of magnetization in the direction of the $\boldsymbol{B}_0$ vector. This process is approximately 10 times slower, and its time constant is denoted T_1.

Different substances, and thus tissues, have different values of relaxation times of T_1 and T_2. In medical applications, protons (nuclei of hydrogen) are mostly used as magnetic dipoles since the body contains many of the hydrogen atoms (especially as part of water molecules).

For illustration, see **Table 2**, which contains values of relaxation times T_1 and T_2 for water and some tissues, as well as the relative concentration of hydrogen atoms in tissues compared to the concentration in pure water.

Chemical analyses also use nuclei of other paramagnetic atoms as magnetic dipoles. Thus, we can investigate the content of specific atoms or substances in the samples by measuring the FID signal and the relaxation times.

1.3.5.4 Magnetic resonance imaging (MRI)

One of the applications of the magnetic resonance phenomenon is the *tomographic imaging* of the morphological structure of the organism. The method lies in the use of the detection of hydrogen atom nuclei, which are mainly contained in water and thus in soft tissues. Consequently, we can obtain a two-dimensional image of tissue structures by identifying different types of tissue (see **Figure 18**).

Using a relatively complicated device we call a *tomography*; it is possible to assign a specific T_1 and T_2 value or relative proton density PD to each point of the thin

Tissue	T_1 [ms]	T_2 [ms]	Relative concentration (^{1}H)
Water	4000	2000	1.00
Cerebrospinal fluid	2500	280	0.98
Edema	900	130	0.86
Grey matter	760	77	0.74
White matter	510	67	0.62
Muscle	900	50	0.50
Fat	250	60	1.00

Table 2.
Relaxation times and relative concentration of protons in water and selected tissues.

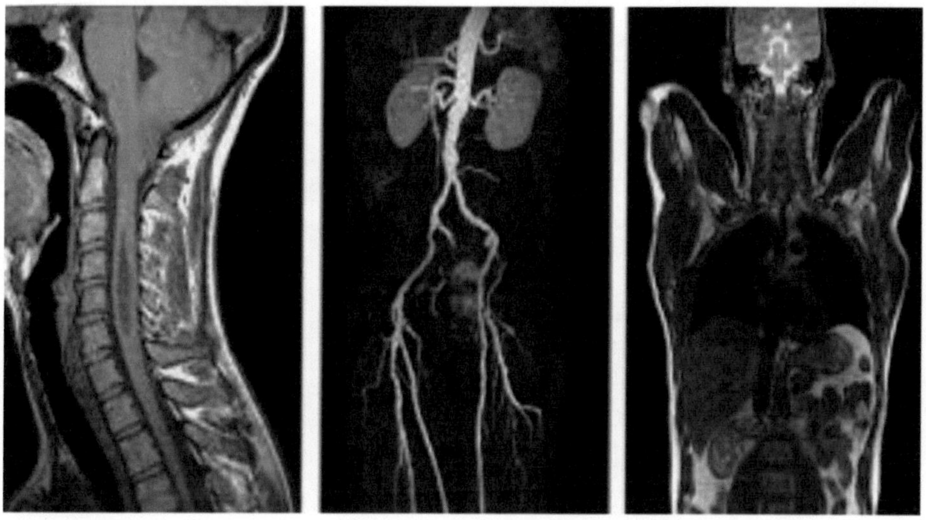

Figure 18.
MRI of the cervical spine, part of the vascular system, thorax.

transverse layer of the examined object (body) and thus to distinguish individual tissues. Different values of these quantities are assigned a certain level of grey colour when displayed on the device monitor (see **Figure 18**). In this way, we can obtain different images such as T1-image, T2-image, and PD image. Each of them has a different contrast concerning tissue differentiation and, thus, different advantages in medical diagnostics.

1.3.5.5 Magnetic resonance spectroscopy

The second application of magnetic resonance is *magnetic resonance spectroscopy* (MRS). By variation frequency ω, it is possible to select the type of atomic nucleus with the Larmor frequency of ω_L. Then, we identify the nucleus by the magnetic resonance FID signal at the frequency of $\omega = \omega_L$. The *magnetic field* $\boldsymbol{B}_0$ at the location of a given nucleus, and thus the Larmor frequency of ω_L, is slightly influenced by the magnetic field of the surrounding particles, such as electrons and other nuclei. The resonance frequency ω_L of the atom nucleus is thus slightly influenced by the chemical bonds where the magnetic dipoles (e.g., nuclei of hydrogen atoms) occur. By examining the spectrum of resonances, it is possible to identify individual hydrogen bonds in the sample under investigation, for example, O-H, C-H, C-H_2, C-H_3, N-H_2. Furthermore, we can identify the relevant organic substances (protein, enzyme, and metabolite) according to the measured resonance spectrum.

Figure 19 illustrates the organosilane spectrogram used in the manufacturing process of synthetic rubber. The horizontal axis is the offset of the resonant frequency in parts per million (ppm = 10^{-6}) relative to the reference frequency. The reference substance could be tetramethylsilane (TMS) or another proper substance. For example, hydrogen in the = CH_2 divalent group has a resonance frequency shifted by 1.3 ppm (A), in the -CH_3 monovalent group, up to 4.0 ppm (B). Each substance has a characteristic spectrogram according to which we can identify it, even at a very low concentration.

Magnetic resonance spectroscopy thus enables very sensitive biochemical diagnostics of different tissues or fluids and uses various biochemical markers to early diagnose a variety of diseases, such as epilepsy, Alzheimer's disease, Parkinson's

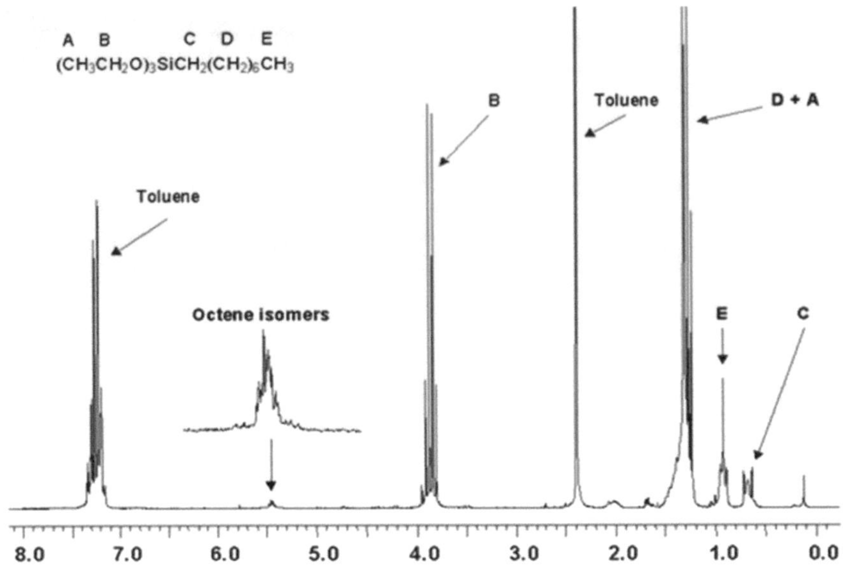

Figure 19.
Magnetic resonance spectrogram of organosilane.

disease, various cancers. Thus, magnetic resonance spectroscopy is a powerful diagnostic tool in medicine.

In specific cases, instead of hydrogen, the magnetic resonance spectroscopy uses the nuclei of other biogenic elements with an uncompensated magnetic moment such as ^{13}C, ^{19}F, ^{31}P. The MRS apparatus is quite demanding, and therefore, a special investigation of the content of other nuclei is used only rarely. Thus, the MRS uses preferably only ^{1}H (hydrogen-protons) for the determination of metabolite content, which in addition to MRI does not require additional devices and MRI and MRS images can be combined (see **Figure 20**). On the right side, it is an MRI

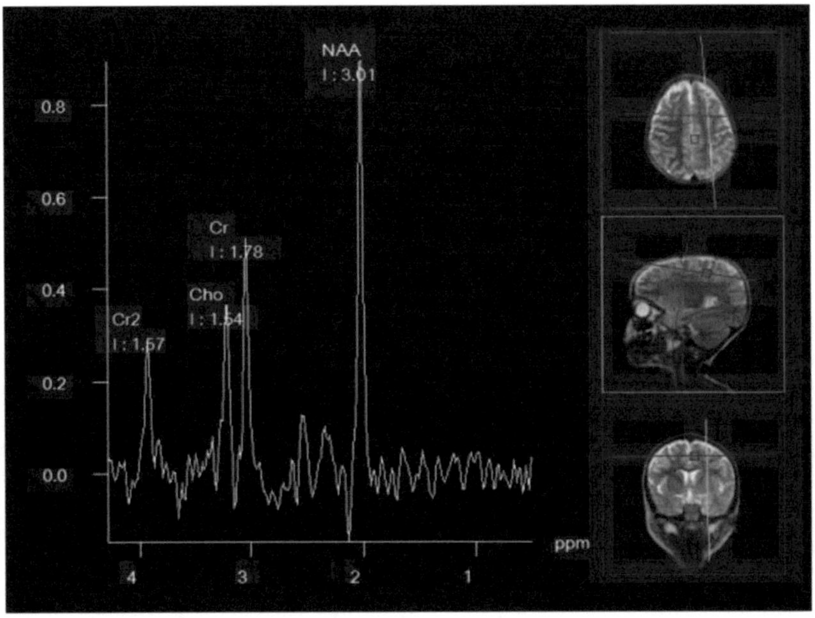

Figure 20.
Combination of MRS and MRI.

image with defined the specific location of analysis, on the left side is an MRS spectrogram of the substance at that location. From the spectral peaks typical for certain substances (here Cr-chromatin, Cho-choline, NAA-N-acetyl aspartate) and their size, it is possible to diagnose possible health disorders.

1.3.5.6 Magnetic resonance therapy

Magnetic resonance therapy (MRT) is a treatment method that uses targeted stimulation of specific structures by providing them with energy through magnetic resonance. During a resonant RF excitation pulse of the τ_{180} length, the alternating magnetic field supplies the dipole with energy [see Eq. (49)]. This energy is transferred only to the nucleus of the atoms that are in resonance with an alternating magnetic field. We can supply the energy of the electromagnetic field to specific parts of the structure that contain the resonant nucleus of the atoms. Thus, we can stimulate intracellular processes such as cell nucleus growth.

The method of magnetic resonance therapy is successfully used in the treatment of osteoarthritis and osteoporosis as we supply the energy to help cartilage and bone regeneration, as well as recovery for spinal pain following surgery (see **Figure 21**).

1.4 Oscillators

We are using various sources of periodic signals or motions, which are commonly called *oscillators*. Oscillators, mechanical or electrical, are systems with high Q-factor value and low losses having a frequency f_0 determined by the system parameters. However, each system always has, albeit small, losses that cause the oscillation to disappear at a time proportional to the quality factor [see Eq. (24)]. If the system is to oscillate continuously, we must balance its losses. This compensation consists of supplying energy equal to the losses in each period of oscillation, that is, the compensation process must be synchronous with the system's oscillations. We can achieve this by periodic power supply directly controlled by system oscillations, which means a *positive feedback method*. The classic example shows a child on a swing. If a child sits on a swing and the parent pushes it, it will swing for a while, but it will soon hang in a steady position. Children almost intuitively understand to keep the swing in motion. They must

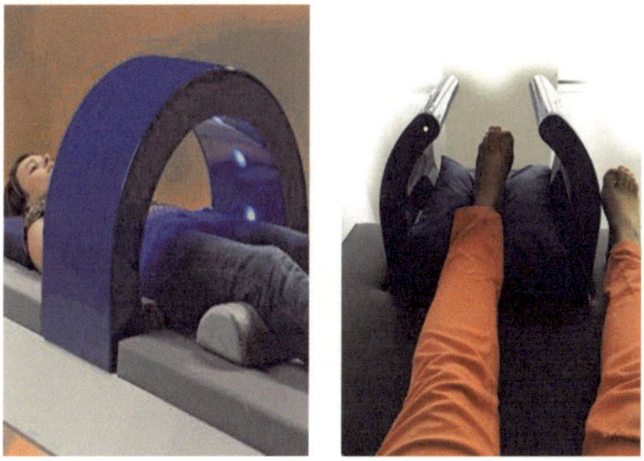

Figure 21.
MRT—Hip joints on the left, post-hip treatment on the right.

compensate for the loss of energy by properly digging their legs in one extreme position and kicking in the other, utilising the energy of their muscle activity to increase the potential energy twice within one oscillation slightly. The child performs this activity intuitively. Thus, the child's biological energy compensates for the energy losses of the swing.

Oscillators have a precisely defined frequency by their parameters. Therefore, we can use them as a reference time signal source. Thus, they represent the essential part of the clock (mechanical with pendulum, mechanical with the rotating flywheel on spiral spring, electrical with LC circuit, electrically controlled with crystal, atomically controlled with quantum transitions in caesium atoms). The electronic clock is a part of every computer and controls the operation of such components as the processor, data storage, and data exchange with peripherals.

1.4.1 Mechanical oscillator

A commonly known mechanical oscillator is a pendulum clock. **Figure 22** shows a pendulum (dashed line) and a zoomed positive feedback step mechanism. The step wheel with inclined teeth is driven through the gearing by a force *F* generated by a weight or a spring. In the picture, the pendulum moves to the right and the right inclined tooth 'b' pushes into the stop of the escapement and supports the right-hand rotation. After reaching the extreme position, the tooth is released to the right, and the wheel rotates so that the left step-stop rests on the left oblique tooth, which pushes into the stop of the escapement and supports the pendulum moving to the left. Thus, the inclined teeth of the wheel supply energy to the pendulum via a step mechanism. The wheel drive depends on the potential energy source of the weight or spring. The system is set up to maintain a stable pendulum operation.

There are many mechanical oscillators of analogous construction, for example, a flywheel on a spring in a mechanical wristwatch, a torsional pendulum of a decorative stand clock. The pendulum clock accuracy depends on the temperature regarding the thermal expansion of the mechanical parts. A special temperature-stabilised

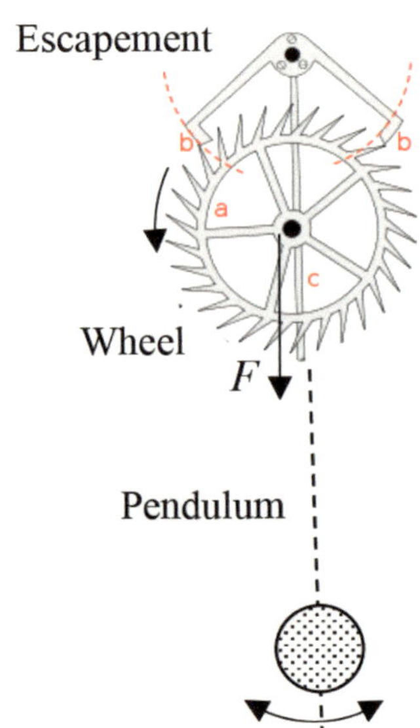

Figure 22.
Pendulum.

pendulum clock can achieve running stability of up to $\delta T/T_0 \approx 10^{-6}$ (1-second deviation in 12 days).

1.4.2 LC oscillator

The electric oscillators commonly use the LC circuit with the frequency of natural oscillations of $f_0 = \frac{1}{2\pi\sqrt{LC}}$. Due to the electrical resistance of the circuit, energy losses occur, which leads to oscillation damping. To cover energy losses and maintain the oscillations of the system, we must supply the LC circuit using a positive feedback method in connection with an amplifier. There are many LC circuit oscillators; **Figure 23** shows some examples.

These oscillators use a transistor amplifier connected with a common emitter that changes the signal phase by 180°. We must connect the output voltage of the oscillator to the input with the same phase, respectively, with offset by 2 × 180° = 360°. The input part is an LC oscillating circuit with a split capacitor: (a) Colpitts circuit, or a split inductor and (b) Hartley circuit. As shown in the figures, there is an opposite phase on split elements regarding the amplifier input and output. The (c) case shows the Meissner circuit, where phase reversal is achieved by inductive coupling with oppositely oriented windings. Figure (d) shows an example of an RC oscillator that does not use an LC circuit.

We achieve positive feedback by a three-stage RC phase shifter. The elements have a total phase shift of 3 × 60° = 180° at the desired oscillation frequency. Since the phase shifter is frequency-dependent, positive feedback occurs at only one frequency.

1.4.3 Crystal controlled oscillators

The applications demanding higher frequency stability consider the circuits mentioned above as unsatisfactory due to the used circuit elements. For example,

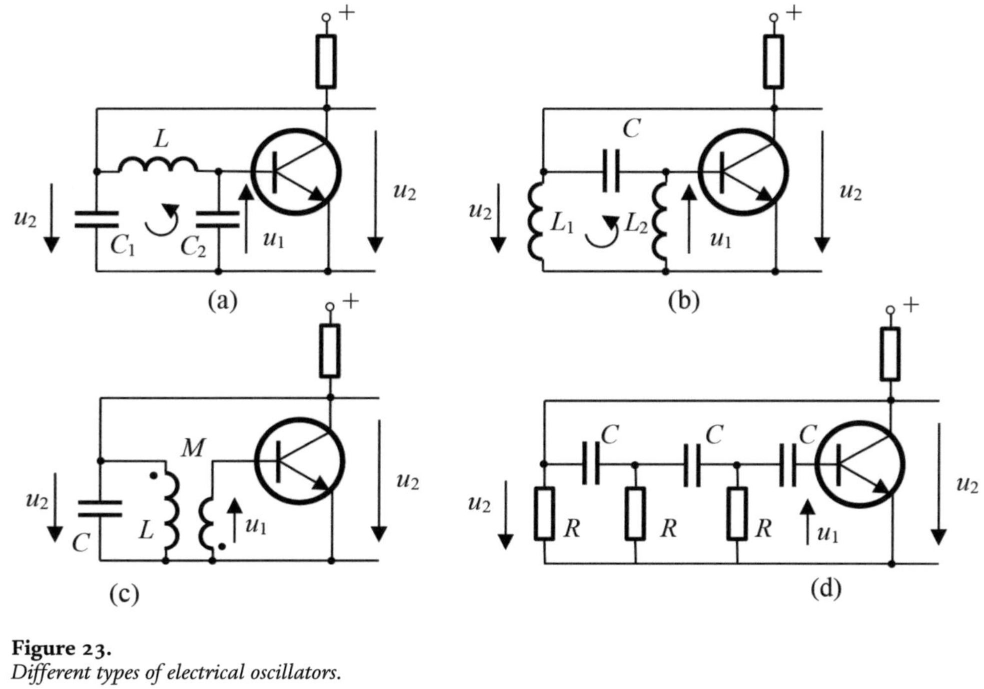

Figure 23.
Different types of electrical oscillators.

the inductors are highly temperature-dependent, or parasitic elements influence both the oscillator and amplifier circuits, and then voltage fluctuations, are applied. To suppress these parasitic effects, we are using piezoelectric crystals in the oscillating circuits instead of the inductors.

A piezoelectric crystal is an electromechanical oscillating system with a high Q-factor. This crystal is described by using the equivalent circuit diagram, as shown in **Figure 24(b)**. The inductance of the crystal depends on the mass of the crystal. The capacity corresponds to its rigidity and the resistance to the internal power losses. The capacity C_0 is the electrode capacity of $C_0 \gg C$. For the crystal as a reactance electrical circuit, the imaginary part of the complex impedance is important, and we can express it as follows:

$$X = \omega L \, \frac{\left(1 - \frac{1}{\omega^2 L C}\right)\left(1 + \frac{C}{C_0} - \omega^2 L C_0\right) - R^2 C_0}{\left(1 + \frac{C_0}{C} - \omega^2 L C_0\right)^2 + (\omega R C_0)^2}. \tag{54}$$

If we set the reactance equal to zero ($X = 0$), we can estimate the resonant frequency of the crystal. The reactance graph below (**Figure 25**) shows two resonant frequencies for the given values of the crystal (L = 100 μH, C = 100 pF, R = 1.0 Ω, C_0 = 10 nF). There is the f_s parallel and the f_p series

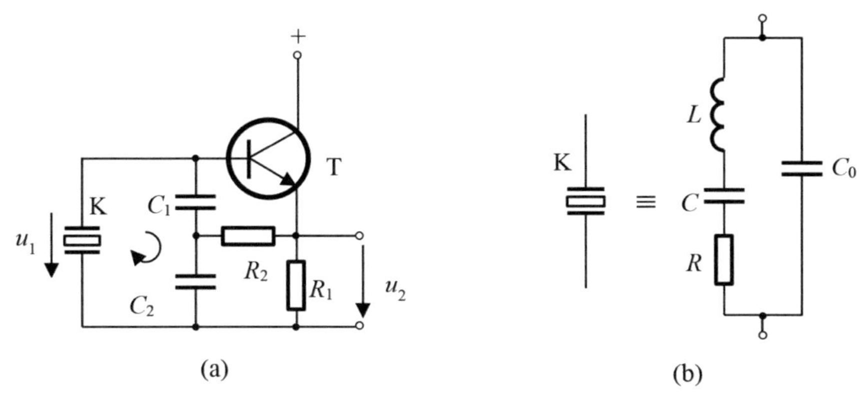

Figure 24.
Crystal controlled oscillator.

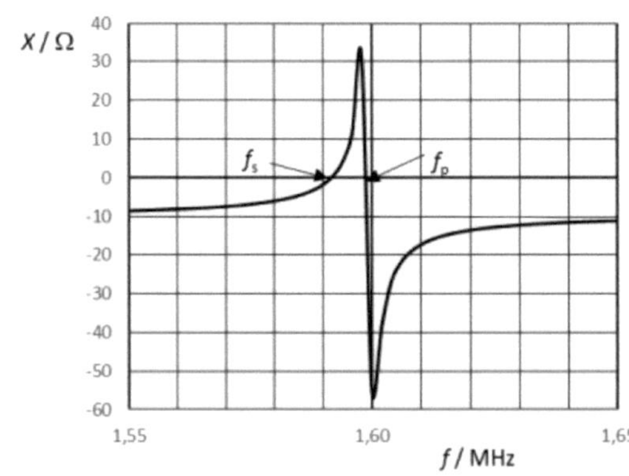

Figure 25.
Graph of the reactance X versus frequency f ot the crystal.

DOI: http://dx.doi.org/10.5772/intechopen.101649

resonances. The equivalent circuit with a high Q-factor has the resonant frequencies as follows:

$$f_s = \frac{1}{2\pi\sqrt{LC}}, \text{and } f_p = \frac{1}{2\pi\sqrt{LCC_0/(C + C_0)}}.$$

In our case, $f_s \approx 1.5916$ MHz and $f_p \approx 1.5994$ MHz. As shown in the reactance graph, we can see a narrow interval between the f_s and f_p when $X > 0$. This means that the crystal has an inductive character. The crystal is connected in the oscillating circuit as an inductor with a parallel split capacitor with C_1 and C_2 capacitances. Thus,

Figure 24(a) shows Pierce's circuit. The split capacitor is parallel connected to the C_0, and therefore, the interval between resonant frequencies gets narrower. Thus, the oscillator can oscillate in the very narrow frequency range, which ensures high stability of the oscillator frequency. We realise positive feedback by connecting non-inverting output through the R_2 resistor to the C_2 capacitor. On the other hand, we can tune the oscillator in the range of several Hz. If we need to tune the frequency in the broader range, we must change the crystal. The crystal-controlled oscillator has high stability in order of 10^{-9}, which means the time deviation of 1 s for 30 years. Achieving this stability, we use the thermostat to stabilise the temperature of the crystal. Due to the high-stability requirement, the computer clock uses only crystal-controlled oscillators as the clock pulse generator.

1.4.4 Multivibrators

In some cases, we require a harmonic signal for biomedical applications. There are diathermy, electrotherapy, sonography, or magnetic resonance. In other applications, we need to generate periodic, but non-harmonic voltages or currents. There are pacemakers or artificial lung ventilation. In these cases, we are using rectangular or sawtooth waveforms or short repetitive pacing pulses. The primary element of non-harmonic signal generators are multivibrators serving as sources of periodic rectangular pulses. Many mechanical and thermal devices switch between two states at regular intervals. There are electrical systems, which are the most important for biomedical applications. These systems serve as periodic and non-harmonic voltage sources. As an example, **Figure 26** shows the circuit of an astable flip-flop multivibrator.

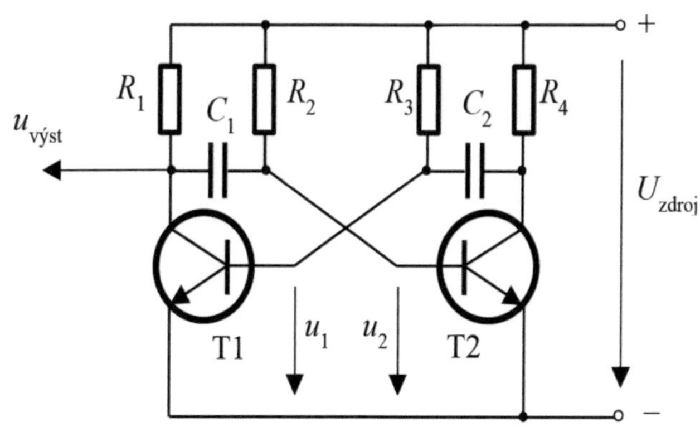

Figure 26.
Astable flip-flop circuit.

In the principle, the T1 transistor alternately switches between its ON/OFF states. If the T1 is open, the T2 is closed and vice versa. This process repeats periodically. The toggling period is given by time constants defined as R_2C_1 and R_3C_2. The output voltage is then rectangular. Connecting output to the differentiator circuit, we obtain short pulses, which can be used for the pacemakers. Using the integrator, we get a sawtooth waveform, which can be used for the generation of the linearly rising gradient field at magnetic resonance imaging.

Author details

Ivo Čáp*, Klára Čápová, Milan Smetana and Štefan Borik
Faculty of Electrical Engineering and Information Technology, University of Žilina, Slovakia

*Address all correspondence to: ivo.cap@fel.uniza.sk

References

[1] Halliday D, Resnick R, Walker J. Fundamentals of Physics. Hoboken NJ: John Wiley & Sons Inc.; 2008

[2] Vlaardingerbroek MT, Boer JA. Magnetic Resonance Imaging: Theory and Practice. Berlin, Heidelberg, New York:: Springer Science & Business Media; 2013

[3] Webb AG. Introduction to Biomedical Imaging. Hoboken NJ: John Wiley & Sons; 2017

[4] Hashemi RH, Bradley G, Lisanti CHJ. MRI: The Basics. Philadelphia PA: Lippincott Williams & Wilkins; 2011

Chapter 3

Coupled Oscillators

Ivo Čáp, Klára Čápová, Milan Smetana and Štefan Borik

1. Introduction

A wave is the propagation of oscillations in space through the coupling between individual oscillators. There is an obvious experiment to hit the right piano key, which sounds the tuning-fork tuned to the same frequency as the key we hit. Another example is breaking a fragile wine glass by the intense sound of the frequency that corresponds to the resonant frequency of the glass.

The crystal of the substance is formed by the regular arrangement of individual atoms, ions, or molecules that are bound together by electrical forces. Since the crystal keeps its form, it means that there are attractive forces between the particles. Each particle has its equilibrium position, which is given by the minimum potential energy in the force field of the surrounding particles. The particles oscillate around the equilibrium position concerning the homogeneity of the substance. Besides, the frequencies of the self-oscillations of all particles are the same. When one particle oscillates, energy transfers to the adjacent particle by resonance, and then the initial excitation travels through space. This excitation propagating is called the *wave*.

First, we show the oscillations of a system consisting of two or three particles. Then, we show the energy transfer between two particles and finally, the wave propagation in an infinite chain of the same oscillators.

1.1 Molecular vibration spectra

Radiation passing through the material medium vibrates the particles of the substance that are in resonance with the radiation. The particles then absorb the energy of the radiation, and thus, the radiation is attenuated. This phenomenon is used in spectroscopy to identify the particles with common properties in a specific medium.

1.1.1 The frequency of vibrations of the diatomic molecule

One of the oscillators of a gaseous environment is a molecule. The molecules consist of the individual atoms bound together. Thus, the system of bonded atoms represents an oscillator. The simplest is a diatomic molecule.

Consider a molecule in which two atoms with masses of m_1, m_2 are bound by the force $F = -k\,(r - r_0)$, where the k is the stiffness coefficient of the molecule, and the r_0 is the equilibrium distance of the centers of the atoms. If we denote r_1 and r_2 the coordinates of atoms, in the coordinate system of a straight line passing through the centers of atoms, the equations of motion of both atoms are.

$$m_1\ddot{r}_1 = -k\ \ (r_2 - r_1)\ \text{and}\ m_2\ddot{r}_2 = -k\ \ (r_1 - r_2).$$

Subtracting the equation, we get.

$$\ddot{r}_1 - \ddot{r}_2 = -\frac{k}{m_1}\ \ (r_2 - r_1) - \frac{k}{m_2}\ \ (r_2 - r_1),$$

IntechOpen

or

$$\ddot{r} = -\frac{k\,(m_1 + m_2)}{m_1 m_2}\,r. \tag{1}$$

The solution to the equation is a harmonic function of $r = r_m \sin \omega t$.
These are vibrations of a molecule with an angular frequency.

$$\omega = \sqrt{\frac{k}{m^*}}, \tag{2}$$

where $m^* = \frac{m_1 m_2}{m_1 + m_2}$ is the reduced mass of the particles.

The molecule, thus, represents a simple oscillating system.

If we apply an external periodic force, then we can achieve resonance when a molecule or array of molecules absorbs the energy. This phenomenon finds its place in spectroscopy. If we irradiate the gas consisting of the diatomic molecules with electromagnetic radiation, the resonance wavelengths are attenuated in the transmitted radiation.

Thus, we can determine the stiffness coefficient of the molecule by measuring the resonance frequency.

Example 1 The vibration frequency of some molecules.

Oxygen O_2: $m = 16 \times 1.67 \times 10^{-27}$ kg, $\mu = m/2$, $k = 1133$ N/m, hence $f = 46.3$ THz, wavelength in vacuum $\lambda = 6.47$ μm.

Nitrogen N_2: $m = 17 \times 1.67 \times 10^{-27}$ kg, $\mu = m/2$, $k = 2287$ N/m, hence $f = 63.9$ THz, wavelength in vacuum $\lambda = 4.70$ μm.

From this, we can see that the air in the atmosphere absorbs infrared radiation.

Example 2 Stiffness coefficient of the molecule.

The HCl molecule has the resonance frequency of $f = 86.7$ THz (wavelength 5.33 μm). For $m_H = 1.67 \times 10^{-27}$ kg and $m_{Cl} = 35 \times 1.67 \times 10^{-27}$ kg, $\mu = 1.62 \times 10^{-27}$ kg, we get the $k \approx 481$ N/m.

The NO molecule has the resonance frequency of $f = 56.3$ THz (wavelength 3.46 μm). For $m_N = 17 \times 1.67 \times 10^{-27}$ kg and $m_O = 16 \times 1.67 \times 10^{-27}$ kg, $\mu = 13.76 \times 10^{-27}$ kg, we get the $k \approx 1722$ N/m.

The CO molecule has the resonance frequency of $f = 66.3$ THz (wavelength 4.52 μm). Pre $m_C = 12 \times 1.67 \times 10^{-27}$ kg and $m_O = 16 \times 1.67 \times 10^{-27}$ kg, $\mu = 11.45 \times 10^{-27}$ kg, we get the $k \approx 1987$ N/m.

Example 3 Coupling stiffness coefficient.

The bonds of pairs of atoms in more complex molecules also show resonance character. The binding force and hence the frequency of the oscillations vary for different binding strengths, e.g., carbon bonds: -C $\equiv$ C- ($\lambda = 4.73$ μm), =C=C = ($\lambda = 5.90$ μm), $\equiv$C-C$\equiv$ ($\lambda = 9.48$ μm), heterogeneous bonds $\equiv$C-H ($\lambda = 3.00$ μm), -O-H ($\lambda = 2.80$ μm), -C $\equiv$ N ($\lambda = 4.40$ μm), =C=N- ($\lambda = 6.30$ μm).

1.1.2 Oscillations of multiatomic molecules

In the case of multiatomic molecules, vibrations of individual pairs of atoms, but also other collective stationary modes will occur. The spectrum of such molecules is more complex, and its theoretical calculation is complicated.

As a simple case, consider a CO_2 molecule that has a simple linear geometry. The O=C=O atoms are on one line, as opposed, e.g., to the two-dimensional H_2O molecule, in which the H-O-H atoms form a “V” structure with an opening angle of 104.5° and an O atom at the midpoint. Another example is the 3-dimensional

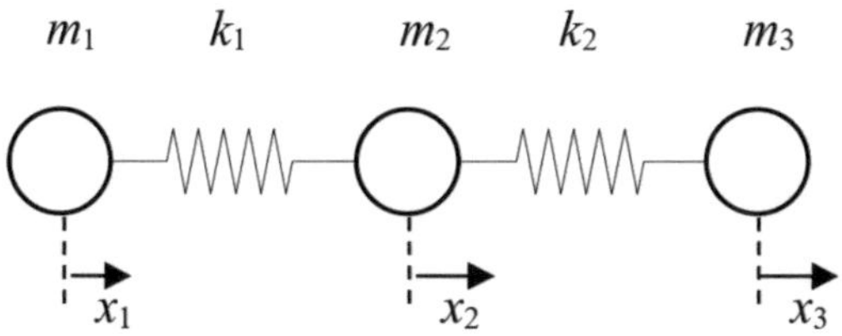

Figure 1.
Linear system of two bound particles.

molecule of NH_3. A similar linear structure has an N_2O molecule having the arrangement of $N \equiv N^+$-O^- or $N^- = N^+ = O$.

Consider the general case of a triple atom in a linear arrangement, see **Figure 1**. The equations of motion are.

$$\begin{aligned} m_1\ddot{x}_1 &= k_1 \ (x_2 - x_1), \\ m_2\ddot{x}_2 &= k_2 \ (x_3 - x_2) - k_1 (x_2 - x_1), \\ m_3\ddot{x}_3 &= -k_2 \ (x_3 - x_2). \end{aligned} \tag{3}$$

The stationary mode represents oscillations of the system in which all particles vibrate at the same frequency and constant amplitudes. If we use phasor symbolism, we get.

$$\mathbf{x}_1(t) = \mathbf{X}_1 \ \mathrm{e}^{\mathrm{j}\omega t}, \quad \mathbf{x}_2(t) = \mathbf{X}_2 \ \mathrm{e}^{\mathrm{j}\omega t}, \quad \mathbf{x}_3(t) = \mathbf{X}_3 \ \mathrm{e}^{\mathrm{j}\omega t}.$$

After substituting into differential equations, we get a system of algebraic equations.

$$\begin{pmatrix} -\omega^2 m_1 + k_1 & -k_1 & 0 \\ -k_1 & -\omega^2 m_2 + k_2 + k_1 & -k_2 \\ 0 & -k_2 & -\omega^2 m_3 + k_2 \end{pmatrix} \cdot \begin{pmatrix} \mathbf{X}_1 \\ \mathbf{X}_2 \\ \mathbf{X}_3 \end{pmatrix} = 0. \tag{4}$$

The condition of nontrivial solution is zero value of the system determinant (characteristic equation)

$$\left[\omega^4 - \omega^2\left(\frac{k_1}{m_1} + \frac{k_1 + k_2}{m_2} + \frac{k_2}{m_3}\right) + \left(\frac{m_1 + m_2 + m_3}{m_3 m_2 m_1}\right) k_1 k_2\right]\omega^2 = 0.$$

This is the equation of the third degree for ω^2.

The first solution is $\omega^2 = 0$ and $x_1 = x_2 = x_3$. It represents the translation of the molecule by uniform motion.

The other two solutions are the solution of the quadratic equation for ω^2

$$\omega^4 - \omega^2\left(\frac{k_1}{m_1} + \frac{k_1 + k_2}{m_2} + \frac{k_2}{m_3}\right) + \left(\frac{m_1 + m_2 + m_3}{m_3 m_2 m_1}\right) k_1 k_2 = 0,$$

which has two solutions.

$$\begin{aligned} \omega_{1,2}^2 = \frac{1}{2}\left(\frac{k_1}{m_1} + \frac{k_1 + k_2}{m_2} + \frac{k_2}{m_3}\right) \\ \pm\sqrt{\frac{1}{4}\left(\frac{k_1}{m_1} + \frac{k_1 + k_2}{m_2} + \frac{k_2}{m_3}\right)^2 - \left(\frac{m_1 + m_2 + m_3}{m_3 m_2 m_1}\right) \ k_1 k_2} \ . \end{aligned} \tag{5}$$

Example 4 The CO_2 molecule oscillations.

As an example, we will find the stationary mode frequencies of the linear molecule O=C=O (carbon dioxide), for which the $k_1 = k_2$ a $m_1 = m_3$. If we substitute it to the corresponding relation, we get.

$$\omega_{1,2}^2 = k_1 \left(\frac{1}{m_1} + \frac{1}{m_2}\right) \pm \frac{1}{m_2}, \tag{6}$$

from where $\omega_1 = \sqrt{k_1 \left(\frac{1}{m_1} + \frac{2}{m_2}\right)}$, and $\omega_2 = \sqrt{\frac{k_1}{m_1}}$.

f_1 = 40.92 THz (λ_1 = 7.33 μm), k_1 = 1766 N/m, f_2 = 78.35 THz (λ_2 = 3.83 μm).

The first oscillating mode with the angular frequency ω_1 represents the simultaneous movement of the outer atoms $x_1 = x_3$ and the movement of the central atom in the opposite direction. At the same time, the mass center remains at rest. In the second mode ω_2, the middle C atom is at rest, and the other O atoms oscillate against each other ($x_1 = -x_3$). In the CO_2 absorption spectrum, these absorption lines correspond to two wavelengths of λ_1 and λ_2.

In the case of two or three-dimensional molecules, there are several stationary modes. The complex structure of the spectrum of resonance frequencies is unique to each molecule and thus allows identifying the substance by measuring the resonance spectrum. This method represents spectral analysis. As can be seen from the above examples, the vibration modes have frequencies that belong to the region of infrared radiation (in the wavelength range from one to hundreds of μm).

Simple molecules of CO_2, SO_2, N_xO_y, and others, which enter the atmosphere as a result of human activity, absorb thermal radiation and create a *greenhouse effect*. These gases are so-called *greenhouse gases*.

The gases such as H_2, O_2, and N_2 have non-polar molecules. These molecules have zero dipole moment as opposed to the polar molecules of H_2O, CO_2, and others. Therefore, they interact very weakly with electromagnetic radiation, and they do not absorb the heat. Thus, the elementary atmospheric gases O_2, N_2 do not cause a greenhouse effect.

1.2 Energy transfer in the system of the coupled oscillators

As stated earlier, the nature of the wave is the propagation of oscillations in space. Let us consider a pair of coupled oscillators and then an extension to an infinite line chain of oscillators.

1.2.1 Two coupled oscillation systems

Consider a mechanical model of a pair of particles of an equal mass of the m bound to each other and stationary walls by springs with a stiffness of the k, **Figure 2**.

Suppose that particles can deviate from equilibrium positions in the longitudinal x-direction. Then, denote the displacements as x_1 and x_2. The following equations describe the motion of the particles:

$$m\,\ddot{x}_1 = k\,(x_2 - x_1) - k\,x_1 \qquad m\,\ddot{x}_2 = -\,k\,(x_2 - x_1) - k\,x_2, \tag{7}$$

or

$$\ddot{x}_1 = \omega_0^2\,(x_2 - x_1) - \omega_0^2\,x_1 \qquad \ddot{x}_2 = -\omega_0^2\,(x_2 - x_1) - \omega_0^2 x_2, \tag{8}$$

where $\omega_0^2 = k/m$.

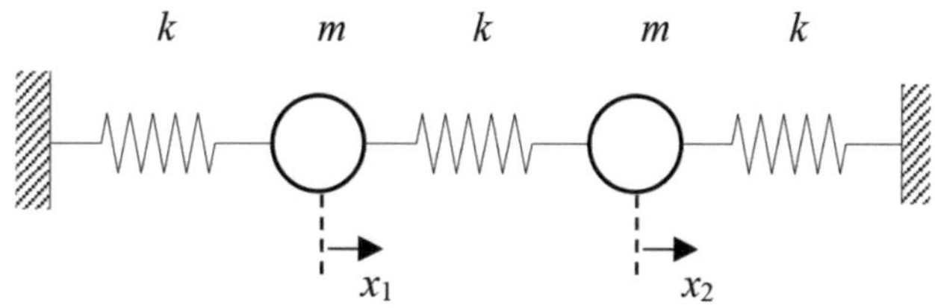

Figure 2.
System of coupled oscillators.

Consequently, we rewrite the equations to the form.

$$x_{1,2}^{(4)} + 4\omega_0^2 \ddot{x}_{1,2} + 3\ \omega_0^4 x_{1,2} = 0,$$

which has a harmonic solution

$$x_1 = A_{11} \sin(\omega_1 t + \alpha_{11}) + A_{12} \sin(\omega_2 t + \alpha_{12}) \tag{9}$$

$$x_2 = A_{21} \sin(\omega_1 t + \alpha_{21}) + A_{22} \sin(\omega_2 t + \alpha_{22}), \tag{10}$$

where $\omega_1 = \omega_0$, and $\omega_2 = \sqrt{3}\ \omega_0$.

The A_{ij} and α_{ij} are constants, which values are determined by the initial conditions such as displacements of the x_{10}, x_{20} and velocities of the v_{10}, v_{20} at the time of $t = 0$ and Eq. (8).

1.2.1.1 Stationary modes

Stationary oscillations are oscillations with a single frequency and a constant amplitude. There are two stationary modes in the system - one with a frequency of ω_1 and the other with a frequency of ω_2.

For the first mode, we have.

$$x_1 = A_{11}\ \sin(\omega_1 t + \alpha_{11}) \text{ and } x_2 = A_{21}\ \sin(\omega_1 t + \alpha_{21})$$

and after substituting to the (8), we get.

$$(2\omega_0^2 - \omega_1^2)\, x_1 = \omega_0^2 x_2 \text{ and thus, } x_1 = x_2. \tag{11}$$

The first stationary mode is characterized in that both particles vibrate with the same amplitude and the same phase, i.e., together.

The second stationary mode is then.

$$x_1 = A_{12}\ \sin(\omega_2 t + \alpha_{12}), \text{ and } x_2 = A_{22}\ \sin(\omega_2 t + \alpha_{22})$$

and after substituting into the (8), we get.

$$(2\omega_0^2 - \omega_2^2)\, x_1 = \omega_0^2 x_2 \text{ and thus, } x_1 = -x_2. \tag{12}$$

The second stationary mode characterizes two particles oscillating with the same amplitude but the opposite phase, which means opposite direction to each other.

Note: If the particles have an electric charge, then the dipole moment of the pair does not change at the mechanical oscillations of the first mode, while the second mode changes the electrical dipole moment of the pair. For this reason, the first oscillating mode only weakly interacts with the external EM field, while the second mode interacts with the EM *relatively strongly. The resonant excitation of mechanical oscillations by the EM field leads to the absorption of electromagnetic power, especially at the resonant frequency of ω_2, which is represented by a significant minimum in the spectral transmission characteristic of the substance.*

1.2.1.2 Stationary mode interference

Any movement of the described system is a superposition of stationary modes.

$$x_1 = A_1 \sin(\omega_1 t + \alpha_1) + A_2 \sin(\omega_2 t + \alpha_2)$$
$$x_2 = A_1 \sin(\omega_1 t + \alpha_1) - A_2 \sin(\omega_2 t + \alpha_2).$$

The oscillation character depends on the initial conditions such as the displacement of x_{10}, x_{20}, v_{10} a v_{20} and the particle velocities at the time $t = 0$.

As an example, we assume the case, when the first particle is shifted from the equilibrium and the second one is quiescent. The initial conditions are $x_{10} = x_m$, $x_{20} = 0$, $v_{10} = v_{20} = 0$. After substituting the initial conditions, we get.

$$x_{10} = A_1 \sin\alpha_1 + A_2 \sin\alpha_2 = x_m$$
$$v_{10} = \omega_1 A_1 \cos\alpha_1 + \omega_2 A_2 \cos\alpha_2 = 0$$
$$x_{20} = A_1 \sin\alpha_1 - A_2 \sin\alpha_2 = 0$$
$$v_{20} = \omega_1 A_1 \cos\alpha_1 - \omega_2 A_2 \cos\alpha_2 = 0\ ,$$

from where, we obtain amplitudes of $A_1 = A_2 = A = x_m/2$ and phases $\alpha_1 = \alpha_2 = \pi/2$ rad.

$$x_1 = A\ (\cos\omega_1 t + \cos\omega_2 t) = x_m \cos\left(\frac{\sqrt{3}-1}{2}\omega_0 t\right) \cos\left(\frac{\sqrt{3}+1}{2}\omega_0 t\right)$$
$$x_2 = A\ (\cos\omega_1 t - \cos\omega_2 t) = x_m \sin\left(\frac{\sqrt{3}-1}{2}\omega_0 t\right) \sin\left(\frac{\sqrt{3}+1}{2}\omega_0 t\right). \quad (13)$$

Time courses of displacements are in **Figure 3**.

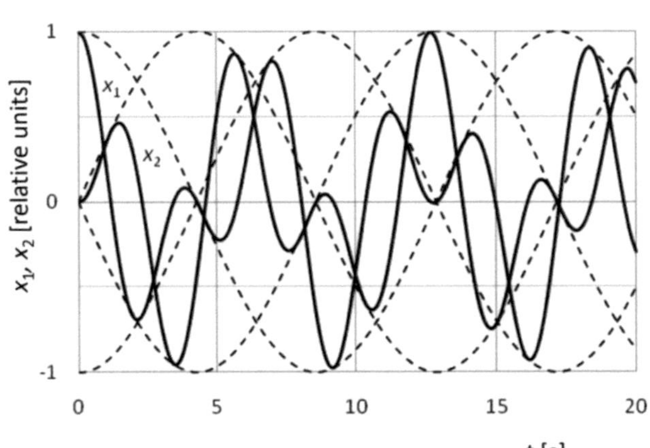

Figure 3.
Displacement of coupled oscillators for $\omega_o = 1\ rad \cdot s^{-1}$.

It is seen from relations (13) and **Figure 3** that oscillations are periodically transmitted from one body to another and backward. In the figure, the envelope curves of both oscillators are indicated by a dashed line. As a result of the coupling, there is a periodic exchange of energy between oscillators. At the time of $t = 0$ s, the first particle has the entire energy of the oscillations. On the other hand, in time of.

$$t_1 = \frac{2\pi}{\left(\sqrt{3}-1\right)\omega_0} \approx 8.6\ \mathrm{s}\ \left(\text{for } \omega_0 = 1.0\ \mathrm{s}^{-1}\right),$$

the whole energy is transferred to the second particle.

Example 2.5 Oscillation energy transfer rate.

Let us assume the aluminum ions from Example 1.5 have the angular frequency of $\omega_0 \approx 6.1 \times 10^{13}$ rad/s and a mutual distance $a \approx 2.8 \times 10^{-10}$ m. If we suppose the time of transfer $t_1 \approx 1.4 \times 10^{-13}$ s, the transfer rate is $v = a / t_1 \approx 2.0 \times 10^3$ m/s, which corresponds to the order of the ultrasound velocity in aluminum ($5.1 \times 10^3\ \mathrm{m{\cdot}s^{-1}}$).

As we see from a simple example, the energy of oscillations in a substance is transmitted due to mutual bonds, which are manifested externally as a coherent propagation of mechanical waves, e.g., sound and ultrasound, or incoherent heat propagation.

1.2.2 Propagation of oscillations in a long particle chain

Substances consist of a great number of less or more ordered fundamental particles, which can be molecules, atoms, or ions. Solids and liquids are formed by particles whose attraction to each other is sufficiently large to form a compact body. Each particle of solid or liquid substance has its equilibrium position, which is caused by the force of the surrounding particles. These forces are mainly electrical. The equilibrium position corresponds to the minimum potential energy, and around the minimum of the potential energy, each particle performs an oscillating movement. As a simplified crystal model, we will use an infinite chain of bound particles arranged in a single line.

1.2.2.1 Propagation of longitudinal oscillations along the chain

We see the line chain model in **Figure 4** suppose that at the beginning, only the leftmost particle is put into oscillating motion, and the remaining particles of the chain are quiescent. Let us further consider that an external time-dependent force keeps the extreme left particle in a steady oscillating motion with time dependence.

$$x_0(t) = x_{0\mathrm{m}} \sin \omega t. \tag{14}$$

The vibrations of the extreme left particle are gradually transferred to the other particles of the chain via bonds. After some time, all the particles of the system oscillate in harmonic oscillating motion with the same angular frequency of ω, but different amplitudes and different phases.

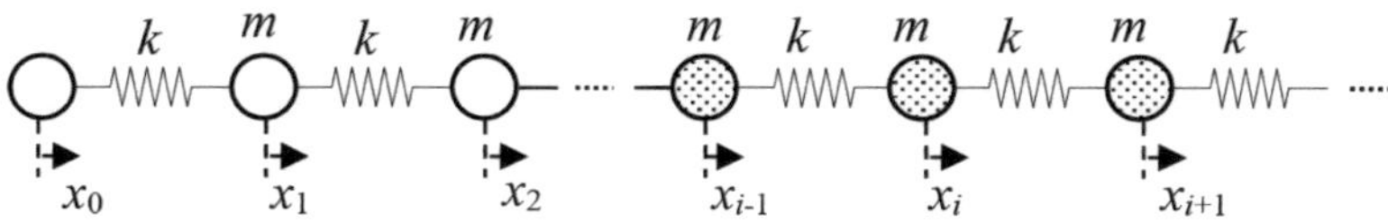

Figure 4.
Linear chain of coupled oscillators.

Consider three adjacent particles with indexes i - 1, i, i + 1, indicated by a dotted fill in the figure.

The equation of motion of the i-th particle has the form.

$$m\ddot{x}_i = -k(x_i - x_{i-1}) - k\ (x_i - x_{i+1}),\ \text{for}\ i > 0,$$

which can be expressed as.

$$\ddot{x}_i = -2\omega_0^2\ x_i + \omega_0^2\ x_{i-1} + \omega_0^2\ x_{i+1}, \tag{15}$$

where $\omega_0 = \sqrt{\frac{k}{m}}$.

If the particle chain is very long (theoretically infinite), then, the relationship between neighboring particles does not depend on i index.

We can use phasor annotation for the harmonic solution of the equation:

$$\mathbf{x}_i(t) = \mathbf{X}_i\,\mathrm{e}^{\mathrm{j}\omega t}.$$

Subsequently, we express the relationship between complex particle displacements by the constant using complex exponential form.

$$\frac{\mathbf{x}_{i+1}(t)}{\mathbf{x}_i(t)} = \mathrm{e}^{-\gamma},\ \text{resp.}\quad \mathbf{x}_{i+1}(t) = \mathbf{X}_i\,\mathrm{e}^{-\gamma}\,\mathrm{e}^{\mathrm{j}\omega t}, \tag{16}$$

where $\gamma = \beta + \mathrm{j}\,\alpha$.

Substituting to (15) we get.

$$2\omega_0^2 - \omega^2 = \omega_0^2\,(\mathrm{e}^{\gamma} + \mathrm{e}^{-\gamma}) = 2\omega_0^2\,\cosh\boldsymbol{\gamma},$$

and from there.

$$\cosh\boldsymbol{\gamma} = 1 - \frac{\omega^2}{2\ \omega_0^2}. \tag{17}$$

Let us consider $\cosh\gamma = \cosh\beta\cos\alpha + \mathrm{j}\sin\alpha\sinh\beta$. As right side of the (17) is real, the imaginary part of $\cosh\gamma$ is zero. Thus, we get $\sin\alpha = 0$ or $\sinh\beta = 0$.

In the case that $\sinh\beta = 0$, then $\beta = 0$, $\cosh\beta = 1$ and $\cosh\boldsymbol{\gamma} = \cos\alpha$:

$$\cos\alpha = 1 - \frac{\omega^2}{2\ \omega_0^2},\ \text{or}\ \tan\alpha = \frac{\omega}{\sqrt{2\ \omega_0^2 - \omega^2}}. \tag{18}$$

From $-1 \le \cos\alpha \le 1$, we get the corresponding interval of angular frequencies:

$$0 \le \omega \le \sqrt{2}\omega_0 = \omega_{\mathrm{m}}, \tag{19}$$

where $\omega_{\mathrm{m}} = \sqrt{\frac{2k}{m}}$ is the cut-off angular frequency.

From (16), we get $\mathbf{x}_{i+1}(t) = \mathbf{x}_i(t)\ \mathrm{e}^{-\mathrm{j}\alpha}$ and thus, for amplitudes $x_{i+1} = x_i$.

All particles oscillate with the same amplitude, but the neighboring particles have different phase shift α of their oscillations. Thus, there is propagating *the undamped traveling harmonic wave* along the chain.

The phase shift α corresponds to a time shift of $\Delta t = \alpha / \omega$. If the distance between the adjacent particles is a, the phase velocity is

$$v = \frac{a}{\Delta t} = \frac{a}{\alpha}\ \ \omega = \frac{\omega\ a}{\arctan\ \frac{\omega}{\sqrt{\omega_{\mathrm{m}}^2 - \omega^2}}}. \tag{20}$$

For small angular frequencies $\omega << \omega_{\mathrm{m}}$, we can use an approximation for $x << 1$, and thus, $v_0 \approx a\ \ \omega_{\mathrm{m}} = a\sqrt{\frac{2k}{m}} = a\,\omega_0\,\sqrt{2}$.

The low-frequency waves propagate along the chain having a constant phase velocity of v_0.

In the case of $\omega > \omega_{\mathrm{m}}$, then $\cosh \gamma < -1$. As comes from $\cosh x \geq 1$, we can fulfill (17), if $\sin a = 0$ and $\cos a = -1$.

The (17) gets then.

$$\cosh \beta = \frac{\omega^2}{2\ \omega_0^2} - 1, \text{and } \alpha = \pi \text{ rad}. \tag{21}$$

The relationship between the displacements of two adjacent particles has the form.

$$x_{i+1} = -x_i\ \ \mathrm{e}^{-\beta}. \tag{22}$$

The adjacent particles oscillate with opposite phases and the amplitude of the oscillation exponentially decreases along the chain. Thus, the *exponentially damped standing wave* is arising in the chain.

1.2.2.2 Wave energy transfer in chain of particles

To investigate oscillation propagation along the particle chain, it is important to observe the transfer of energy in this bound system. Let us assume that an external source generates oscillations according to (14). We denote these particle oscillations as x_0.

For subcritical frequencies $\omega < \omega_{\mathrm{k}}$, the power of the source is.

$$\begin{aligned} P &= F v_0 \\ &= k\ \ (x_0 - x_1)\ \ \omega x_0\ \cos \omega t = k\,\omega x_0^2 \cos \omega t[\,\sin\,\omega t -\ \sin\,(\omega t - a)] \\ &= \omega \frac{k x_{0\mathrm{m}}^2}{2}\,[(1 -\ \cos a\,)\,\sin 2\,\omega t +\ \sin a(1 +\ \cos 2\,\omega t)\,] \end{aligned}$$

The power has time-dependent parts and constant parts. The constant part represents a steady energy flow.

$$\langle P \rangle = \omega \frac{k x_{0\mathrm{m}}^2}{2}\ \ \sin a = \frac{\sqrt{km}}{2}\ \sqrt{1 - \left(\frac{\omega}{2\,\omega_0}\right)^2}\ \ \omega^2\ x_{0\,\mathrm{m}}^2. \tag{23}$$

At angular frequencies of $\omega < \omega_{\mathrm{m}}$, the chain can transfer energy without any losses.

In the case of supercritical angular frequencies of $\omega > \omega_{\mathrm{k}}$, the power is.

$$\begin{aligned} P &= F v_0 \\ &= k(x_0 - x_1)\ \ \omega x_0\ \cos \omega t = k\,\omega x_{0\mathrm{m}}^2 \cos \omega t \sin \omega t\left(1 + e^{-b}\right) \\ &= \omega \frac{k x_{0\mathrm{m}}^2}{2}\left(1 + e^{-b}\right) \sin 2\,\omega t. \end{aligned} \tag{24}$$

We can see that the power mean value is $\langle P \rangle = 0$. At supercritical frequencies of $\omega > \omega_m$, the chain cannot transfer energy, and thus, the power of the source is reactive.

1.2.2.3 Heat transfer in substances

A substance consists of many particles (atoms, ions, molecules) interacting with each other. If any of them oscillate, the oscillations spread to the surrounding medium, and energy is transmitted. If the surface particles of the body vibrate coherently (together with the same phase), the wave propagates through the medium as described in paragraph 1.2.2.1. In this way, a coherent wave arises in the medium. However, if the particles vibrate randomly (uncoordinated), there is also energy transfer, but the disturbance propagation process is not a coherent wave. Such transfer of energy from higher energy particles to lower energy particles is called thermal transfer. Since the energy of the particles is related to the temperature at a given location of the substance, we observe the transfer of energy from the higher temperature locations to the lower temperature locations. This phenomenon is called heat conduction in the substance. The interaction of particles in different substances varies, and therefore some substances conduct heat better (thermal conductors), others worse (thermal insulators). The power density is proportional to the temperature gradient.

$$\frac{P}{S} = -\lambda \frac{\partial T}{\partial x}, \tag{25}$$

where the λ is the specific thermal conductivity of the substance.

High thermal conductivity is typical for substances consisting of an ordered structure of small particles, especially metals. In contrast, disordered structures and substances consisting of large molecules (glass, plastics, etc.) are mostly thermal insulators. E.g., pure metal is a good conductor of heat, but steel, which contains many different impurities and structure failures, has a significantly lower thermal conductivity. As an example, compare an aluminum spoon and a stainless-steel spoon immersed in a hot tea - the aluminum end is soon hot, but the stainless-steel end remains cool.

1.2.3 Oscillation's propagation in a long LC chain

The electrical system analogous to the long chain of bound particles is a chain consisting of a homogeneous series of LC segments. The harmonic voltage $u_0 = U_0 \sin \omega t$ is connected to the input, **Figure 5**.

If a chain is very long (theoretically infinite), its properties do not change when we add another segment to it. If the input impedance is **Z**, it does not change by adding an LC segment to the beginning, **Figure 6**.

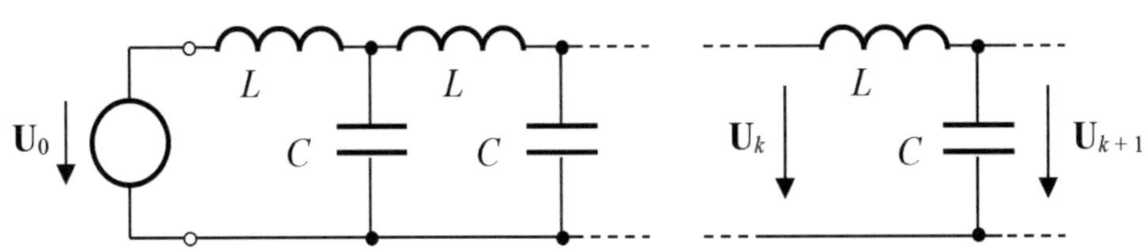

Figure 5.
Long-chain of identical LC segments.

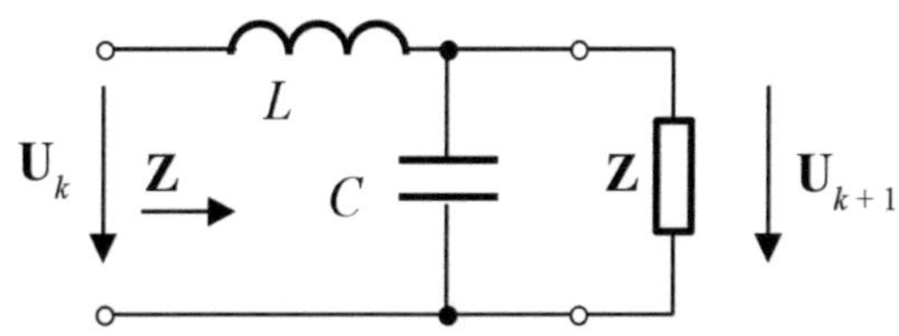

Figure 6.
Equivalent circuit using the total impedance of Z.

$$\mathbf{Z} = \mathrm{j}\omega L + \frac{\mathbf{Z}\ \frac{1}{\mathrm{j}\omega C}}{\mathbf{Z}\ + \frac{1}{\mathrm{j}\omega C}}. \tag{26}$$

Then we get $\mathbf{Z} = \frac{\mathrm{j}\omega L}{2} + \sqrt{\frac{L}{C} - \left(\frac{\omega L}{2}\right)^2}$, while $|\mathbf{Z}| = \sqrt{\frac{L}{C}} = R$.
Complex voltage transfer of the **Z** loaded segment is then.

$$\mathbf{A}_k = \frac{\mathbf{U}_{k+1}}{\mathbf{U}_k} = \frac{\mathbf{Z}}{\mathbf{Z}\ (1 - \omega^2 CL) + \mathrm{j}\omega L} = \frac{\sqrt{\frac{L}{C} - \left(\frac{\omega L}{2}\right)^2} - \frac{\mathrm{j}\omega L}{2}}{\sqrt{\frac{L}{C} - \left(\frac{\omega L}{2}\right)^2} + \frac{\mathrm{j}\omega L}{2}}. \tag{27}$$

If we define a cut-off angular frequency of ω_{m} and characteristic resistance of R_0 as,

$$\omega_{\mathrm{m}} = \frac{2}{\sqrt{LC}}, \text{and } R_0 = \sqrt{\frac{L}{C}}, \tag{28}$$

then, we can express the impedance of the chain and complex voltage transfer as.

$$\mathbf{Z} = R_0\left(\sqrt{1 - \frac{\omega^2}{\omega_{\mathrm{m}}^2}} + \mathrm{j}\frac{\omega}{\omega_{\mathrm{m}}}\right), \text{and } \mathbf{A}_k = \frac{\sqrt{1 - \left(\frac{\omega}{\omega_{\mathrm{m}}}\right)^2} - \mathrm{j}\frac{\omega}{\omega_{\mathrm{m}}}}{\sqrt{1 - \left(\frac{\omega}{\omega_{\mathrm{m}}}\right)^2} + \mathrm{j}\frac{\omega}{\omega_{\mathrm{m}}}}. \tag{29}$$

If $\omega < \omega_{\mathrm{m}}$ (low-frequency oscillations), the absolute value of voltage transfer and voltage phase shift on one segment are.

$$|\mathbf{A}_k| = 1, \text{and } \varphi_k = -2\ \arctan\frac{\omega}{\sqrt{\omega_{\mathrm{m}}^2 - \omega^2}}. \tag{30}$$

The voltage of the n-th segment in chain is then.

$$u_n\ (t) = U_0\ \sin\ (\omega t + n\ \varphi_k). \tag{31}$$

It follows from this result that the voltage amplitude along the chain remains constant and the phase shift gradually increases: $\varphi_n = n\ \varphi_k$. Assuming harmonic excitation at the input, *the harmonic undamped wave* propagates along the chain.

If we know the segment length d and we express the phase difference as $\varphi_k = \omega\ \Delta t$, then, we can determine the velocity of the phase propagation (phase velocity of the wave):

$$v = \frac{d}{\Delta t} = \frac{d}{-\varphi_k/\omega} = \frac{\omega\ d}{2\arctan\frac{\omega}{\sqrt{\omega_{\mathrm{m}}^2 - \omega^2}}}. \tag{32}$$

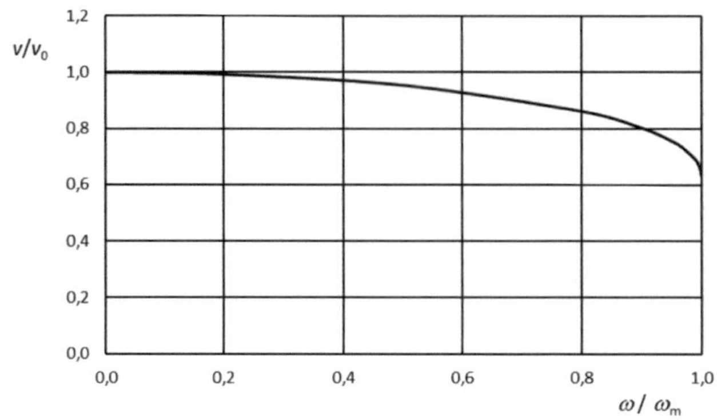

Figure 7.
The v/v$_o$ *normalized velocity as a function of normalized angular frequency of* ω/ω$_m$.

For very low frequencies of excitation $\omega << \omega_{\mathrm{m}}$ (taken an approximation arctan $x \approx x$ for $x << 1$), the velocity is constant and equals

$$v_0 \approx \frac{d}{2}\omega_m = \frac{d}{\sqrt{LC}}. \tag{33}$$

For frequencies $\omega \rightarrow \omega_{\mathrm{m}}$ the velocity $v \rightarrow \dfrac{\omega d}{\pi}$.

Normalized dependency of velocity v versus angular frequency ω is in **Figure** 7.

Low frequency oscillations having the angular frequency of $\omega << \omega_{\mathrm{m}}$ propagate along the chain as an *undamped harmonic wave* with constant velocity of v_0, for $\omega \rightarrow \omega_{\mathrm{m}}$ the velocity decreases to the v_{m}.

At $\omega > \omega_{\mathrm{m}}$ we get.

$$\mathbf{Z} = \mathrm{j}\ R_0\ \left(\sqrt{\frac{\omega^2}{\omega_{\mathrm{m}}^2} - 1} + \frac{\omega}{\omega_{\mathrm{m}}}\right), \text{and } \mathbf{A}_k = -\frac{\frac{\omega}{\omega_{\mathrm{m}}} - \sqrt{\left(\frac{\omega}{\omega_{\mathrm{m}}}\right)^2 - 1}}{\frac{\omega}{\omega_{\mathrm{m}}} + \sqrt{\left(\frac{\omega}{\omega_{\mathrm{m}}}\right)^2 - 1}} = -b. \tag{34}$$

Absolute value of voltage transfer is$A_k = b = \ \mathrm{e}^{-\beta} < 1$, while $\beta = -\ln b > 0$.

The impedance has inductive character (reactive character). Voltage transfer is less than one, which means that the voltage along the chain exponentially decreases.

$$u_n(t) = -U_0\ e^{-n\beta}\ \sin \omega t. \tag{35}$$

Since the complex voltage transfer is a negative real number, adjacent segments oscillate with the opposite phase, but the phase constant of the segment does not change. It is, therefore, a *damped standing wave*.

When a harmonic voltage source is connected to the chain, its complex power supplied to the chain is.

$$\mathbf{S} = \mathbf{U}_0 \cdot \mathbf{I}^* = \frac{U_0^2}{\mathbf{Z}^*} = \frac{U_0^2}{R}\left(\sqrt{1 - \frac{\omega^2}{\omega_{\mathrm{m}}^2}} - \mathrm{j}\frac{\omega}{\omega_{\mathrm{m}}}\right) = P\ +\ \mathrm{j}\ Q.$$

For frequencies $\omega < \omega_{\mathrm{m}}$ the complex power of source consists of the active power part of P and the reactive part of Q.

$$P = \frac{U_0^2}{R}\sqrt{1 - \frac{\omega^2}{\omega_\mathrm{m}^2}}, \text{and } Q = \frac{U_0^2}{R}\frac{\omega}{\omega_m}. \tag{36}$$

Thus, the chain transfers the power (permanently draws energy from the source).

For frequencies $\omega > \omega_\mathrm{m}$.

$$P = 0, \text{and } Q = \frac{U_0^2}{R}\left(\sqrt{\frac{\omega^2}{\omega_m^2} - 1} - \frac{\omega}{\omega_m}\right). \tag{37}$$

The chain is unable to transmit energy. The power source is only reactive, i.e., the mean value of the energy supplied by the source into the chain is zero.

We can see from these two cases that the oscillating events of mechanical and electrical are analogous, and thus there is electro-mechanical duality. One of the practical possibilities of using this feature is to model mechanical systems using electrical circuits. In the field of biomedicine, we can consider an example of blood flow modeling in blood vessels using electrical circuits [1].

Author details

Ivo Čáp*, Klára Čápová, Milan Smetana and Štefan Borik
Faculty of Electrical Engineering and Information Technology, University of Žilina, Slovakia

*Address all correspondence to: ivo.cap@fel.uniza.sk

References

[1] Čáp I., Čápová K. Electromagnetic modelling of mechanical processes - blood flow in wessels. In: JASEM studies in applied electromagnetics and mechanics 13, Tokyo 2009

Chapter 4

Mechanical Waves

Ivo Čáp, Klára Čápová, Milan Smetana and Štefan Borik

1. Introduction

One of the physical phenomena used in medical diagnostics and therapy is ultrasound. We know, for example, ultrasonography, ultrasonic lithotripsy, ultrasonic massages. One of the basic communication channels of humans is sound. The human body is also affected by infrasound. To understand the basic principles of these phenomena, we explain here the origin, properties, and detection of mechanical waves in a matter.

Every continuous medium consists of individual particles (atoms and molecules) that interact with each other. If we do not perceive the microscopic structure, we only see the resulting continuous substance—a *continuum.* The forces of interaction among microscopic particles are observed from outside as macroscopic forces of a different character. The first group represents elastic forces, connected with elastic deformation, which disappears when the force ceases to act. These forces have a *conservative character*, which means they do not cause any heat losses. Elastic forces occur in solids and liquids. Among the elastic forces can be included gas pressure forces if the deformation of the gaseous body is adiabatic (without thermal exchange). The application of the elastic forces is a condition for the transmission of mechanical waves.

Besides, there act the forces connected with losses of mechanical energy in substances, related to plastic deformation, irradiation, heating, etc. These forces are non-conservative and cause the damping of mechanical waves.

1.1 Propagation of longitudinal deformation in an elastic material

Consider a semi-infinite homogeneous elastic medium with a planar surface. On this surface, we cause mechanical deformation by force with area density $f_0\ (t)$ perpendicular to the surface. This deformation is described by the time function $u_0\ (t)$ of the surface displacement perpendicular to the surface. The deformation propagates in the medium due to its elasticity in the direction of the *z-axis* perpendicular to the surface. The displacement of the medium particles is a function $u\ (z, t)$ of the coordinate z and time t, **Figure 1**. Suppose that surface deformation is the same over the entire surface of the medium and does not depend on transversal x and y coordinates. Therefore, even the propagating deformation does not depend on the transverse coordinates and represents a *plane wave*.

In the medium, we define an elementary cylinder with an axis perpendicular to the surface, the cross-section S, and length $\mathrm{d}z$. When compiling the physical model of wave propagation, we replace individual particles of a substance by volume elements with a volume $\mathrm{d}V = S\,\mathrm{d}z$, where $\mathrm{d}z$ is the length of the cylindrical element. The mass of the element is $\mathrm{d}m = \rho\,\mathrm{d}V$, where ρ is the density of the medium. A discrete spring model of the previous chapter, we replace with the elastic forces F acting on the given element from left and right. During the movement, the mass element is also subjected

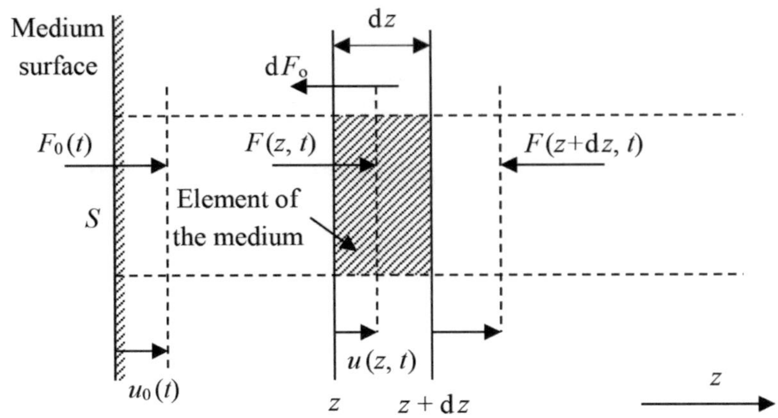

Figure 1.
Dynamics of the volume element of the elastic medium.

to internal friction, which is represented by a resistive force d F_o dependent on the speed of the element movement.

Due to the propagation of the deformation of the medium, the bases of the elements move in the longitudinal direction z. The deflection of the given cross-section with the coordinate z from the balanced position is denoted as $u\ (z, t)$.

The motion of an element is described by the equation of mechanical motion

$$dm\ a = F(z,t) - F(z + dz,t) - dF_o, \tag{1}$$

where $a = \frac{\partial^2 u\ (z,t)}{\partial t^2}$ is the acceleration of the element.

The compressive forces F cause a linear deformation of the element, which is described by Hooke's law for tensile stress

$$\sigma = k\ \varepsilon = \frac{F}{S} = k\ \frac{u(z,t) - u(z + dz,t)}{dz}, \tag{2}$$

where σ is the tensile stress, k is the coefficient of elasticity of the environment and ε is the relative compression of the element.

The resistive force usually has the character of a viscous resistance, which is characterised by a linear dependence on the speed of movement of the element. The bulk density of this force is

$$\frac{dF_o}{dV} = -r\ \frac{\partial u(z,t)}{\partial t}, \tag{3}$$

Where $v = \frac{\partial u(z,t)}{\partial t}$ is the speed of movement of the element and r is the coefficient of resistance of the medium.

We express slight differences ΔF a Δu using their gradient

$$F(z,t) - F(z + dz,t) = -\frac{\partial F}{\partial z}\ dz, \quad u(z,t) - u(z + dz,t) = -\frac{\partial u}{\partial z}\ dz.$$

The compressive forces F cause a linear deformation of the element, which is described by Hooke's law for tensile stress, then takes the form

$$\sigma = -k\ \frac{\partial u(z,t)}{\partial z} \tag{4}$$

and represents the tensile (mechanical) stress in the deformed medium caused by the propagation of the mechanical deformation.

The motion of an element is described by the equation of mechanical motion (1), which thus has the form

$$\rho\,\frac{\partial^2 u(z,t)}{\partial t^2} = k\,\frac{\partial^2 u(z,t)}{\partial z^2} - r\,\frac{\partial u\,(z,t)}{\partial t},$$

or

$$\frac{\partial^2 u\ \ (z,t)}{\partial z^2} - \frac{r}{k}\,\frac{\partial u\,(z,t)}{\partial t} - \frac{\rho}{k}\,\frac{\partial^2 u\ \ (z,t)}{\partial t^2} = 0. \tag{5}$$

The dynamics of motion of the elements of a continuous elastic medium being described by this partial differential equation.

1.1.1 Longitudinal mechanical waves in a lossless elastic material

The space–time distribution of oscillations of particles (volume elements) of the medium is obtained by solving the differential Eq. (5) under specific initial and boundary conditions.

Let us first consider a simple case of oscillation propagation in a medium with negligible losses (ideal elastic medium). Eq. (5) is simplified by omitting the mean term for $r = 0$. The differential equation takes the form

$$\frac{1}{c^2}\,\frac{\partial^2 u\ \ (z,t)}{\partial t^2} = \frac{\partial^2 u\ \ (z,t)}{\partial z^2}, \tag{6}$$

where $c^2 = \frac{k}{\rho}$.

The solution of this equation is a function

$$u(z,t) = f(z \pm ct), \tag{7}$$

which we can be convinced by direct substitution into the Eq. (6).

The shape of the function f is shown in **Figure 2**.

The elements of the medium oscillate around their equilibrium positions and their movement is described by the displacement u from the equilibrium position.

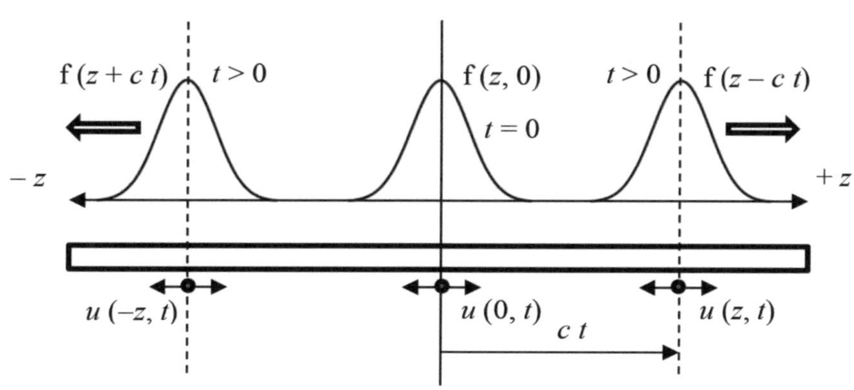

Figure 2.
Wave propagation in the medium.

The distribution of the displacement in the medium at the beginning ($t = 0$) is shown by the function f $(z, 0)$—*an initial deformation* (source of deformation). At time $t > 0$ the waveform is shifted along the z-axis by a length $\pm c\,t$. For a solution with a sign $(-)$, the shift is to the right, for a sign $(+)$ to the left, if the medium allows it. The initial deformation thus propagates along the z-axis to both sides at a speed $\Delta z/t = c$ without attenuation and distortion. Thus, a *mechanical wave* occurs that propagates in the medium at the speed, see relation [Eq. (6)],

$$c = \sqrt{\frac{k}{\rho}}. \qquad (8)$$

Such a wave both transmits the energy associated with the oscillations of the elements of the substance and transmits information. If we enter a certain disturbance (source signal) at one end of the rod with length L, this disturbance is transmitted with a delay L/c to the other end, where it can be detected by a suitable detection device.

If the medium is solid, the elastic constant k has the meaning of the modulus of elasticity E, and the speed of propagation of the longitudinal wave is $c = \sqrt{\frac{E}{\rho}}$.

Example 1 Propagation of longitudinal mechanical wave in steel.

Steel, as well as other flexible solids, allows the propagation of longitudinal mechanical waves, for example, ultrasound. For modulus of elasticity value $E = 200$ GPa and density $\rho = 7.8 \times 10^3$ kg·m^{-3} the propagation speed is $c \approx 5.1 \times 10^3$ m·s^{-1}.

In other solids, the speed of longitudinal ultrasound is usually lower, around $(3 \div 5) \times 10^3$ m·s^{-1}.

1.1.2 Transverse mechanical waves in an elastic medium

In the previous part, we solved an example of the propagation of *longitudinal* deformation in an elastic medium. This section shows how the *transversal* (*shear*) deformation propagates in an elastic medium. The situation is shown in **Figure 3**. The medium is deformed so that the displacement u of its elements is perpendicular to the direction of propagation z.

Eq. (1) remains valid without change. The only difference is that the longitudinal deformation is replaced by shearing strain, and then Eq. (2) gets the form

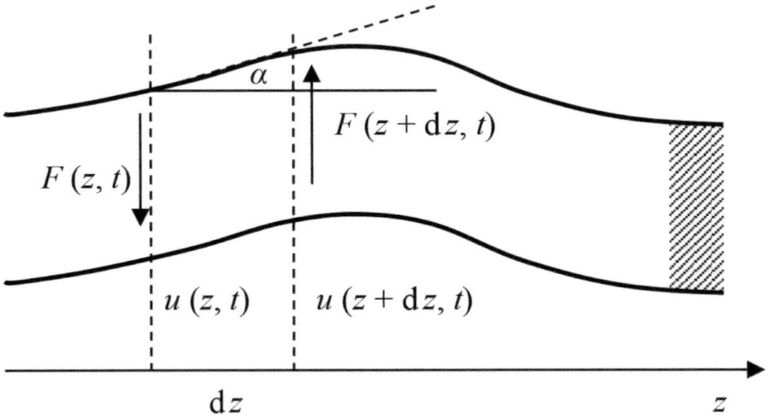

Figure 3.
Propagation of shear deformation in a material.

$$\frac{F}{S} = -G\frac{u(z+dz,t) - u(z,t|)}{dz}. \tag{9}$$

where G is the shear modulus of a given medium.

The deformation of the medium associated with the propagating wave causes shear stress in the elastic environment

$$\tau = -G\ \frac{\partial u(z,t)}{\partial z}. \tag{10}$$

If the wave is undamped or weakly damped, the transverse wave propagates in the medium at a speed

$$c = \sqrt{\frac{G}{\rho}}. \tag{11}$$

Example 2 Propagation of transverse mechanical wave in steel.

Shear modulus of steel is G = (79 ÷ 89) GPa and density ρ = 7.8 × 10^3 kg·m^{-3}. For the value of G = 80 GPa, according to Eq. (11), the speed of the wave is $c \approx 3200$ m·s^{-1}.

Because applies to solid materials $E/3 < G < E/2$, transverse wave propagation speed is 60% ÷ 70% of the longitudinal wave speed, for example, for steel $c_\mathrm{L} \approx 5.1$ km·s^{-1}, $c_\mathrm{T} \approx 3.2$ km·s^{-1}.

As is clear from the physical origin of the wave, the transverse wave *cannot* propagate in liquid and gaseous media, as these media cannot be deformed by shear stress (G = 0). When shear is applied in a liquid medium, creep occurs, and the transverse stress has a highly viscous (lossy) character. A transverse wave can only propagate in *elastic solid materials*.

1.1.3 Propagation of mechanical waves along an elastic string

Another example of a common cause of wave motion is the propagation of transverse excitation along an elastic flexible string.

A string element with a mass dm moves under the effect of the tensile forces of the string, **Figure 4**. The longitudinal motion equation has the form

$$\mathrm{d}m\ \ a_z = F\ \ (z + dz, t)\ \ \cos\ \alpha(z + dz, t) - F\ \ (z,t)\ \ \cos\ \alpha(z,t)$$

and in the transverse direction

$$\mathrm{d}m\ \ a_y = F\ \ (z + \mathrm{d}z, t)\ \ \sin\ \alpha(z + \mathrm{d}z, t) - F\ \ (z,t)\ \ \sin\ \alpha(z,t).$$

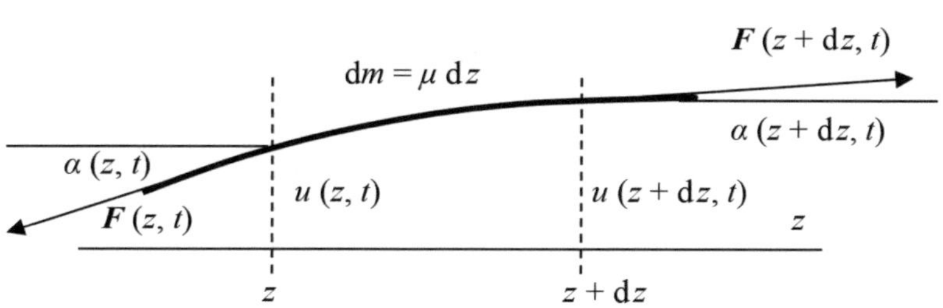

Figure 4.
Transverse movement of a section of a string.

For very small deviations, it is valid: $\cos\alpha \approx 1$ and $a_z \approx 0$.
From the first equation we get

$$F\,(z + \mathrm{d}z, t) \approx F\,(z, t) = F.$$

The fibre is stretched with the same force F along its entire length.

For small angles α is valid $\sin\alpha \approx \tan\alpha = \dfrac{\partial u}{\partial z}$. The second equation thus takes the form

$$\mathrm{d}m\,\frac{\partial^2 u}{\partial t^2} = F\left[\frac{\partial u\,(z + dz, t)}{\partial z} - \frac{\partial u\,(z, t)}{\partial z}\right] = F\frac{\partial^2 u\,(z, t)}{\partial z^2}\mathrm{d}z$$

If we express the mass of the element $\mathrm{d}m = \mu\,\mathrm{d}z$, where μ is the line mass density of the string, the equation gets the form of a wave equation

$$\frac{\partial^2 u(z, t)}{\partial z^2} - \frac{\mu}{F}\frac{\partial^2 u}{\partial t^2} = 0,$$

where $c = \sqrt{\frac{F}{\mu}}$ is the speed of propagation of the transverse wave along the string.

The speed of the wave can be changed by changing the line mass density μ and the force F that stretches the string. As we will show later, the speed c determines the oscillation frequency of a string with a finite length l, for example, the strings of a musical instrument, and as we know, the pitch can be changed by a tuning pin that changes the tensioning force, and the strings for lower tones are thicker than the strings for higher tones.

The *vocal cords* work on the principle of string oscillation. The length of the vocal cords varies between men and women and changes with age. Therefore, women and children have higher voices (higher frequencies) and men have deeper voices (lower frequencies). The person can control the mechanical tension of the vocal cords by means of the fine muscles of the larynx, and thus change the height of the emitted sound. This ability is used for singing.

1.1.4 Mechanical waves in gases

Compression wave propagation takes place in gases. If the pressure increases at a certain point, the change of the pressure gradually propagates through the gas. As the pressure change process is very fast, the adiabatic process is applied (without heat exchange)

$$p\,V^{\kappa} = p_0\;V_0^{\kappa}, \tag{12}$$

where κ is the adiabatic constant (for air $\kappa = 1.4$).
If the volume changes according to **Figure 1**, we get

$$V = V_0 + S\;[u\;\;(z + \mathrm{d}z, t) - u(z, t)] = S\,\mathrm{d}z + S\;\frac{\partial u}{\partial z}\;\mathrm{d}z = \left[1 + \frac{\partial u}{\partial z}\right]\;S\,\mathrm{d}z.$$

Substituting into Eq. (12) we have

$$p = p_0\;\frac{1}{\left(1 + \frac{\partial u}{\partial z}\right)^{\kappa}} \approx p_0\;\left(1 - \kappa\frac{\partial u}{\partial z}\right),$$

and the pressure change is

$$\Delta p = -p_0 \kappa \frac{\partial u}{\partial z}. \tag{13}$$

The gas elasticity constant for adiabatic waves is then $k = \kappa p_0$.
Force on the element is

$$\mathrm{d}F = S[p(z,t) - p(z + \mathrm{d}z, t)] = -S \frac{\partial p}{\partial z} \; \mathrm{d}z.$$

The equation of motion has the form

$$\rho \frac{\partial^2 u}{\partial t^2} = \kappa p_0 \frac{\partial^2 u}{\partial z^2}.$$

It is the wave equation of a wave with a speed

$$c = \sqrt{\frac{\kappa p_0}{\rho}}.$$

Example 3 Sound propagation in the air.

The sound propagates well in the air and thanks to this fact we can communicate and perceive sounds from the surroundings. Under normal conditions (pressure p_0 = 101 kPa, temperature t = 20°C or T = 293.15 K) is according to the gas state equation for molar mass M_m = 29 × 10^{-3} kg·mol^{-1} and gas constant R = 8.314 J·K^{-1}·mol^{-1} air density $\rho = \frac{p_0 M_\mathrm{m}}{RT} \approx 1.20$ kg·m^{-3}. For the air adiabatic constant, κ = 1.4 is the speed of sound propagation in the air $c = \sqrt{\frac{\kappa R T}{M_\mathrm{m}}} \approx 340$ m·s^{-1}.

As we can see from the theoretical result, the speed of sound in the air does not depend on the air pressure, but only on the thermodynamic temperature T. At the temperature t = 40°C is $c \approx 355$ m·s^{-1} and at the temperature t = −10°C is $c \approx 325$ m·s^{-1}. Usually, we do not notice this difference, but it is significantly manifested, for example, when tuning wind instruments. The speed of sound propagation is manifested, for example, by the delay of the sound thunder after the lightning during a storm or by the reverberation or echo when the sound reflects from an obstacle.

1.1.5 Mechanical waves in liquids

Liquids represent a fluid medium in which there is zero shear elasticity. Therefore, liquids *do not transmit* transverse mechanical waves. The mechanical stress thus has a longitudinal orientation and causes a change in the volume (compression) of the liquid. If we consider a plane wave in which deformation occurs only in one direction z, the deformation can be described by the relation

$$p = -\frac{1}{\gamma} \frac{\partial u(z,t)}{\partial z},$$

where γ is the compressibility of the liquid.

The speed of propagation of a mechanical wave in a liquid is $c = \sqrt{\frac{1}{\rho \gamma}}$.

For water with values γ = 4.8 × 10^{-10} Pa^{-1} and ρ = 1.0 × 10^3 kg·m^{-3} we have the speed of sound (ultrasound) $c \approx 1.44 \times 10^3$ m·s^{-1}.

Material	Density kg·m^{-3}	Phase velocity m·s^{-1}	Specific attenuation dB/(m·MHz)	Acoustic resistance ×10^6 kg·m^4·s^{-1}
Air at 20°C	340	1.2	—	0.0004
Water	1000	1480	0.22	1.48
Bone	1975	3476	690	7.38
Blood	1060	1570	20	1.68
Brain	1040	1560	60	1.62
Fat	950	1478	48	1.40
Breast	1020	1510	75	1.54
Muscle	1050	1547	109	1.62
Tendon	1100	1670	470	1.84
Myocardium	1060	1576	52	1.67
Lungs	1060	1595	50	1.69

Source: http://www.science.mcmaster.ca/medphys/images/files/courses/772/Ultrasound/Pressure_attenuation_for_tissues_and_materials.pdf.

Table 1.
Characteristic acoustic parameters of selected substances and tissues at frequency $f_0 = 1$ *MHz.*

As the soft tissues of the human body have high water content (up to 70%), their mechanical properties are close to water. In such tissues, only ultrasound with longitudinal polarisation propagates and the propagation speed does not differ very much from the value for water, see **Table 1**.

1.1.6 Wave polarisation

As shown in the previous section, the waves propagate in space at a speed c. The individual particles or volume elements of the medium oscillate around their equilibrium positions, but they do not propagate in space together with the wave. The particles can oscillate in different directions with respect to the direction of wave propagation. The direction of oscillation of the particles is called the *polarisation of the wave*. One of the basic polarizations is *longitudinal polarisation*, where the particles oscillate in the same direction as the direction of the wave propagation. Typical examples are in paragraphs 1.1.5 or 1.1.4. The second basic polarisation is the *transverse polarisation*, where the particles oscillate in a direction perpendicular to the direction of the wave propagation. If the direction of oscillation does not change, we speak of *linear polarisation*. An example is a transverse wave in a solid medium, paragraph 1.1.2, or on an elastic string, paragraph 1.1.3. By suitable excitation, it is also possible to generate a harmonic wave with transverse polarisation, in which the displacement vector follows an ellipse in the transverse plane or a circle—*elliptical* and *circular* transverse polarisation. Such polarisation arises from the superposition of two waves with linear polarisation in mutually perpendicular directions, perpendicular to the propagation direction, and with a phase shift of $\pi/2$ rad. In addition, waves with combined transverse and longitudinal polarisation can be generated, when the total displacement of the particles is a superposition of the displacements in the longitudinal and transverse directions. A typical example is waves on the water surface. The Rayleigh surface wave is elliptically polarised in a plane perpendicular to the material surface and parallel to the direction of wave propagation (particles on the material surface describe an ellipse in a plane perpendicular to the surface and parallel to the direction of wave propagation).

Material	Speed of wave c [$m \bullet s^{-1}$]		
Polarisation	**Longitudinal**	**Transversal**	**Elliptical**
Steel	5100	3200	
Concrete	3000	2000	
Water	1440	—	
Air (100 kPa, 32°F)	340	—	
Seismic Rayleigh waves	—	—	3000
Tsunami waves on the open seas	—	—	30
Guitar string—chamber A	—	500	
Vacuum	—	—	

Table 2.
Mechanical waves speed in selected media.

Table 2 shows some typical values of wave propagation speed with different polarizations in different materials. In fact, the values have a considerable variance for different conditions—the values given are only indicative for creating a basic representation. In fluids (liquids and gases), mechanical waves with transverse polarisation cannot propagate, and in a vacuum, the mechanical wave cannot propagate at all.

1.2 Mechanical behaviour of mechanical waves

1.2.1 Particle displacement and particle velocity

As shown, the elements (particles) of the medium oscillate around their equilibrium positions. The first of the quantities describing their motion is the particle displacement $\boldsymbol{u}_a(\boldsymbol{r}, t)$. In general, it is a vector quantity that is a function of the position $\boldsymbol{r}$ and time t.

The movement of medium elements is described by *particle velocity* $\boldsymbol{v}_a = \partial \boldsymbol{u}_a / \partial t$. It is the velocity of oscillating motion of particles.

The particle velocity $\boldsymbol{v}_a$ is not related to the speed c of the wave. While the particle velocity $\boldsymbol{v}_a$ is a function of position $\boldsymbol{r}$ and time t, the propagation speed c is constant and depends only on the properties of the medium.

1.2.2 Acoustic pressure and acoustic power

The waves are accompanied by local deformation of the elastic medium. As shown in the analysis of the propagation of individual types of waves, for example, Eqs. (4), (10), or (13), mechanical stress or pressure, are directly proportional to the gradient of the particle displacement and their magnitude can be expressed by a quantity of *acoustic pressure*

$$p_a = \rho \; c^2 \; \frac{\partial u_a(z, t)}{\partial z}, \qquad (14)$$

where z is the coordinate in the direction of wave propagation and t is time.

As a result of this acoustic pressure, the strength limit of the material may be exceeded and thus the material is destroyed, or cavitation (formation of vacuum bubbles) may occur in the liquid. These phenomena are used in ultrasonic cleaning of objects, for example, fine mechanics, surgical instruments, in which the particles of impurities are separated from the cleaned body by the action of ultrasound. The action of intense ultrasound also achieves the spraying of liquids, which use, for example, ultrasonic humidifiers. In technical practice, ultrasonic drills, and cutters suitable for working especially of hard and brittle materials such as ceramics, glass, and porcelain, are used.

In medicine, intensive ultrasound is used in *ultrasound lithotripsy*—the destruction of kidney stones, bladder stones, or gallstones. The ultrasonic wave of power ultrasound device using an acoustic lens (condenser) is focused on the place with the stone. The effect of a series of ultrasonic pulses (tens to thousands of pulses with a repetition frequency of several Hz) crushes the stone into the form of sand, which is then washed away by the urinary or bile ducts.

The device shown in **Figure 5** is used for extracorporeal lithotripsy (ultrasound device is outside of the patient body). It also contains an X-ray positioning device, which precisely targets the location of the stone. Due to the very different acoustic impedance of the stone and the surrounding tissue, the ultrasonic pulse will not cause tissue damage. The main advantage is that the procedure is *non-invasive*.

Intracorporal lithotripsy is also currently used. In **Figure 6** is a device that allows lithotripsy by ultrasonic or pneumatic pulse. The thin metallic probe transmitting the ultrasound is introduced through a body orifice (urinary) or a small body cut, tightly to the stone, and large and hard stones are disrupted by intense pressure or pneumatic shock waves with the energy of up to 100 mJ. An ultrasonic probe with a pulse power of up to 150 W and a frequency of approximately 25 kHz crashes the stone and removes soft stones and residues after crushing. This method is very

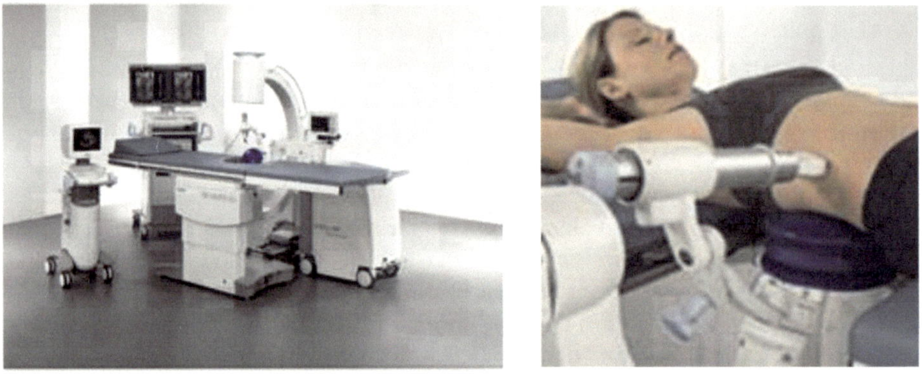

Figure 5.
Extracorporeal lithotripsy.

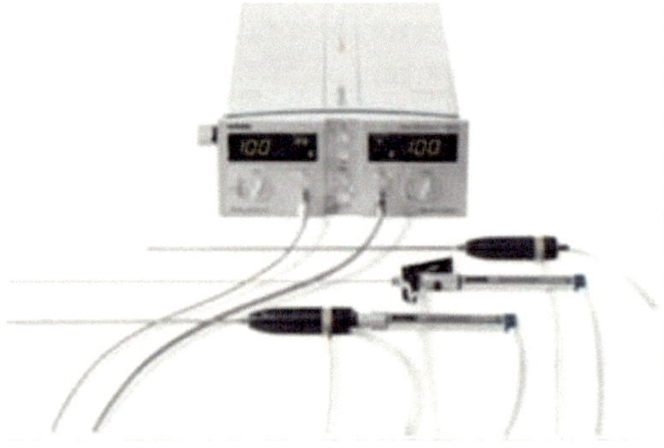

Figure 6.
Intracorporal lithotripter.

effective, relatively patient-friendly, and requires only minimal surgery to create an incision for the probe.

Another application is in ophthalmic surgery in the process of phacoemulsification. Ultrasound converts the eye lens into an emulsion, which is then aspirated. After this removal of the lens, a new artificial lens is implemented.

Cavitation using intensive ultrasound is also used by cavitation ultrasonic liposuction. Ultrasound disrupts the membranes of fat cells, whereby the liquid contents of the cells enter the intercellular space and from there are washed away by the lymphatic system. It serves for the non-invasive removal of local fat and cellulite and serves to strengthen the subcutaneous muscles.

The exertion of acoustic pressure on moving particles of the medium represents mechanical power, which expresses the *acoustic power density* (power per unit of transverse area)

$$\pi_\mathrm{a} = -p_\mathrm{a}\ v_\mathrm{a} = -\rho c^2\ \frac{\partial u_\mathrm{a}}{\partial z}\ \frac{\partial u_\mathrm{a}}{\partial t}. \tag{15}$$

This power is supplied to the mechanical wave by a wave source, and the power propagates in the medium along with the wave. In this way, the mechanical wave can be used to transfer energy, for example, by ultrasonic heating of the tissue. In medical ultrasound applications, for example, in ultrasonic sonography, care must be taken to limit the power used to avoid burns, especially on the surface layers of the body. Mean value of acoustic power

$$I = \langle \pi_\mathrm{a} \rangle = -\rho c^2\ \left\langle \frac{\partial u_\mathrm{a}}{\partial z}\ \frac{\partial u_\mathrm{a}}{\partial t} \right\rangle \tag{16}$$

represents the *wave intensity*.

The *wave intensity* is decisive in the formation of auditory perception. The sound volume is directly proportional to the log I (logarithm of intensity).

In biomedicine, the power of a focused ultrasound beam is used to destroy a target tissue in the focal point (usually a tumour) by 'burning' it. Ultrasonic ablation controlled by magnetic resonance is used, for example, for non-invasive removal of uterine fibroids. Magnetic resonance imaging serves to accurately target the site of the tumour into which the ultrasound beam is focused.

Ultrasound with a frequency of about 20 kHz uses an *ultrasonic scalpel* in surgery. Its application causes the cutting surface to heat to a temperature of 50–100°C, which causes coagulation of soft tissues during cutting and reduces bleeding from small vessels.

Ultrasound therapy is used, for example, in tissue regeneration, promoting the formation of new cells, stimulating blood flow to the tissue, etc. It is used in the treatment of joints, supports the dissolution of fibroblasts, the formation of collagen, reduces tension in the tissue, has an analgesic and anti-inflammatory effect, and positively stimulates wound healing after injuries. It is also used in dermatology and cosmetics.

1.3 Plane harmonic mechanical wave

The function f (z, t), see Eq. (7), was not specified in more detail and can have a very diverse course. There may exist pulse waves, for example, lithotripsy uses a series of high-energy ultrasound pulses, or various modulated waves are used to transmit information, for example, human voice, or a series of pulses in the digital transmission of information. A special case represents a harmonic wave, which is generated by a source with harmonic time dependence. Harmonic waves are often used, for example, in medical diagnostics. We know that any course of the periodic function f (z, t) can be considered as a superposition of harmonic waves, using the Fourier transform. The analysis of harmonic waves is, therefore, of considerable theoretical and practical importance. We will especially appreciate the harmonic dependence of the waves in cases of more complex transmission properties of the medium, for example, propagation of waves in a lossy or dispersive medium.

1.3.1 Harmonic mechanical waves

Harmonic waves are generated by a source of harmonic oscillations on the surface of the transmission medium. We express the particle displacement on the surface ($z = 0$) by a harmonic function

$$u(0,t) = U_0 \sin \omega t.$$

The symbolic-complex method is preferably used to solve time-harmonically dependent functions. In linear systems, all steady-state harmonic response functions have the same time dependence.

$$\mathrm{f}(z \pm ct) = \mathrm{F}(z)\ \mathrm{e}^{\mathrm{j}\omega t},\ \ \text{e.g.,}\ \mathbf{u}(z,t) = \mathbf{U}(z)\ \mathrm{e}^{\mathrm{j}\omega t},$$

where **u** is a complex particle displacement and **U** is its complex amplitude (phasor).

The differential Eq. (5), including the damping element, takes the form

$$\frac{\mathrm{d}^2\mathbf{U}(z)}{\mathrm{d}z^2} + \left(\frac{\omega^2}{c^2} - \mathrm{j}\omega\eta\right)\mathbf{U}(z) = 0, \tag{17}$$

Where $\eta = r/E$ is the coefficient of losses due to internal friction in the medium. We got a regular differential equation that has an exponential solution

$$\mathbf{u}(z) = \mathbf{U}_0\ \mathrm{e}^{\pm \mathrm{j}\ \mathbf{k}z}, \text{and thus } \mathbf{u}(z,t) = \mathbf{U}_0\ \mathrm{e}^{\mathrm{j}(\omega t \pm\ \mathbf{k}z)}, \tag{18}$$

where

$$\mathbf{k} = \sqrt{\frac{\omega^2}{c^2} - \mathrm{j}\omega\eta} = \alpha + \mathrm{j}\beta \text{ is a } \textit{complex wave number}. \tag{19}$$

From relation [Eq. (19)] we determine the components of the complex wavenumber

$$\alpha = \frac{\omega}{\sqrt{2}c}\sqrt{1 + \sqrt{1 + \left(\frac{\eta c^2}{\omega}\right)^2}}, \tag{20}$$

$$\beta = \frac{\omega}{\sqrt{2}c}\sqrt{-1 + \sqrt{1 + \left(\frac{\eta c^2}{\omega}\right)^2}}. \tag{21}$$

For low-loss medium is valid $\frac{\eta c^2}{\omega} << 1$, or for angular frequency $\omega >> \eta c^2$, we will use simplification $\sqrt{1+x} \approx 1 + \frac{1}{2}x$ for $x < < 1$ and adjust the coefficients to a simplified form.

$$\alpha \approx \frac{\omega}{c}, \text{ and } \beta \approx \frac{1}{2}\eta c.$$

Using the components of a complex wavenumber, we get a complex deflection form, which is a linear combination of both solutions, (Eq. 18),

$$\mathbf{u}(z,t) = \mathbf{U}_{01}\,\mathrm{e}^{-\beta z}\ \mathrm{e}^{\mathrm{j}(\omega t - \alpha z)} + \mathbf{U}_{02}\,\mathrm{e}^{\beta z}\ \mathrm{e}^{\mathrm{j}(\omega t + \alpha z)},$$

or real form of the equation

$$u(z,t) = U_{01}\,\mathrm{e}^{-\beta z}\ \sin(\omega t - \alpha z\ + \psi_1) + U_{02}\,\mathrm{e}^{\beta z}\ \sin(\omega t + \alpha z\ + \psi_2).$$

The first wave function describes an exponentially damped wave propagating in the z-axis direction, the second is an exponentially damped wave propagating in the opposite direction z.

The real component of a complex wave number is the *wave attenuation coefficient*, which provides information about the *effective wave propagation length*

$$\delta = 1/\beta, \tag{22}$$

which indicates the distance over which the amplitude of the particle displacement drops to $1/\mathrm{e} \approx 37\%$ of the initial amplitude at the surface.

The harmonic component of the wave function is a periodic function with a period of 2π rad. The expression in parentheses is the phase of the wave, ψ is the phase constant. At z = constant, the function is periodic in time with period T. The reciprocal value of the period is the frequency $f = 1/T$.

For t = constant, the function is periodic in space with a period λ, which is called the *wavelength*.

For the temporal and spatial periods of the wave we have

$$T = \frac{2\pi}{\omega} \text{ and } \lambda = \frac{2\pi}{\alpha}. \tag{23}$$

A certain place of medium with a constant wave phase $\omega\, t \pm \alpha\, z + \psi$ = const. travels with time. For the time $\Delta\, t$, the place of the constant phase is shifted by $\Delta\, z$, while for zero phase change, we have $\omega\, \Delta\, t \pm \alpha\, \Delta\, z = 0$, from where

$$c = \frac{\omega}{\alpha} = \frac{\mp\Delta z}{\Delta t} \quad \text{or } \lambda = \frac{c}{f}. \tag{24}$$

The quantity c is the *phase velocity* of the harmonic wave.

The attenuation of ultrasound relates to various physical mechanisms as the intrinsic viscosity, dispersion on inhomogeneities, turbulent losses in gases, etc. The individual influences are frequency dependent, which is described by the frequency dependence of the attenuation coefficient β. It can be approximated by the power dependence $\beta = \beta_0\ (f/f_0)^\kappa$, where f_0 is the reference frequency and κ a suitable approximation factor. Medical sonography uses ultrasound in the frequency range of units up to tens of MHz. Viscous losses predominate for most tissues in this frequency range, in which a linear approximation ($\kappa = 1$) is satisfactory. A few typical values are in **Table 1**. The values in the table, valid for biological tissues, are only indicative; they may differ for tissues of the same species from different sources. For fat or bone, the variety is especially great. For water and tissues, the attenuation coefficient increases approximately in direct proportion to frequency. For air, however, the dependence is more progressive ($\kappa \to 2$) due to another mechanism of wave energy loss, among which turbulent losses dominate.

For air, the characteristic values are β = 0.22 dB·m^{-1}/22 dB·m^{-1}/236 dB·m^{-1} for frequencies 1 MHz/10 MHz/33 MHz.

Ultrasound attenuation is significant at the imaging of internal organs using sonography. Since the ultrasound beam reflected from a given organ is used for imaging, the level of the received signal depends on the depth of the organ under the body surface and thus of the total attenuation. The frequency of the ultrasound, therefore, is adopted to the possibilities of signal detection. Frequencies above 10 MHz are used for ophthalmic sonography. In the sonography of obese patients, a lower frequency of about 2 MHz is chosen to reduce the signal attenuation.

1.3.2 Particle displacement and particle velocity of a harmonic wave

Consider a wave with harmonic time dependence with a complex particle displacement

$$\mathbf{u}_a(z,t) = \mathbf{U}_0 \ e^{j(\omega t - kz)}. \tag{25}$$

The direction of the phasor $\mathbf{U_0}$ of the surface particle displacement with respect to the direction of wave propagation determines the direction of polarisation of the wave.

Complex particle velocity is

$$\mathbf{v}_a(z,t) = \frac{\partial \mathbf{u}_a(z,t)}{\partial t} = j\omega \mathbf{U}_0 \ e^{j(\omega t - kz)} = j\omega \ \mathbf{u}_a(z,t). \tag{26}$$

The particle velocity is also described by a complex harmonic function and its phase shift relative to the particle displacement is $\pi/2$ rad.

1.3.3 Acoustic pressure and acoustic power of a harmonic wave

Following the relation [Eq. (14)], we express the acoustic pressure of a harmonic wave

$$\mathbf{p}_a(z,t) = -\rho c^2 \ \frac{\partial \mathbf{u}_a(z,t)}{\partial z} = j\mathbf{k} \ \rho c^2 \ \mathbf{U}_0 \ e^{j(\omega t - kz)} = j\mathbf{k} \ \rho c^2 \mathbf{u}_a(z,t).$$

Acoustic pressure is related to particle displacement and particle velocity

$$\mathbf{p}_a(z,t) = j\mathbf{k} \ \rho c^2 \mathbf{u}_a(z,t) = \mathbf{k} \ \frac{\rho c^2}{\omega} \ \mathbf{v}_a(z,t). \tag{27}$$

The ratio of acoustic pressure and particle velocity is one of the characteristic wave properties of the medium and is called *acoustic impedance*

$$\mathbf{Z}_a = \frac{\mathbf{p}_a}{\mathbf{v}_a} = \frac{\rho c^2}{\omega} \ \mathrm{k} = \rho c \sqrt{1 - j \ \frac{\eta c^2}{\omega}} = R_a + j \ X_a. \tag{28}$$

The complex acoustic impedance has a real component *acoustic resistance* and an imaginary component *acoustic reactance*.

For low loss or lossless medium, $\frac{\eta c^2}{\omega} < < 1$ an approximate relationship is valid

$$\mathbf{Z}_\mathrm{a} = \rho c \ \sqrt{1 - \mathrm{j} \ \frac{\eta c^2}{\omega}} \approx \rho c \ \left(1 - \mathrm{j} \ \frac{\eta c^2}{2\omega}\right).$$

Acoustic resistance and acoustic reactance are

$$R_\mathrm{a} = \frac{\rho c^2}{\omega} \ \alpha = \rho c, \text{ and } X_\mathrm{a} = -\mathrm{j} \ \frac{\eta c^2}{2\omega} \ \rho c = -\mathrm{j} \ \frac{\eta c^2}{2 \ \omega} R_\mathrm{a}. \tag{29}$$

The acoustic properties of selected substances and tissues are in **Table 1**.
The complex power density, see Eq. (15), is expressed by the relation

$$\boldsymbol{\pi}_\mathrm{a} = \mathbf{p}_\mathrm{a} \mathbf{v}_\mathrm{a}^* = \mathbf{k} \ \omega \rho c^2 \mathbf{u}_\mathrm{a}(z,t) \ \mathbf{u}_\mathrm{a}^* (z,t) = \omega^2 \frac{\rho c^2}{\omega} \mathbf{k} \ u_\mathrm{am}^2 = \mathbf{Z}_\mathrm{a} \ v_\mathrm{am}^2 = \frac{1}{\mathbf{Z}_\mathrm{a}^*} \ p_\mathrm{am}^2. \tag{30}$$

The real part represents an active power, the imaginary part a reactive power of the wave. The energy transfer by a wave is expressed by the mean value of the active component of the complex power. It is the *acoustic flux intensity* of the harmonic wave

$$I = R_\mathrm{a} \ \frac{v_\mathrm{am}^2}{2} = R_\mathrm{a} \ v_\mathrm{aef}^2 = \frac{p_\mathrm{aef}^2}{R_\mathrm{a}}, \tag{31}$$

where $v_\mathrm{aef} = \frac{v_\mathrm{am}}{\sqrt{2}}$, and $p_\mathrm{aef} = \frac{p_\mathrm{am}}{\sqrt{2}}$ are the effective values of particle velocity and acoustic pressure.

The acoustic wave intensity in the medium decreases exponentially after the formula

$$I = R_\mathrm{a} \ \frac{v_\mathrm{am0}^2}{2} \ \mathrm{e}^{-2\beta z} = I_0 \ \mathrm{e}^{-2\beta z}.$$

Attenuation is the result of the conversion of acoustic wave energy into heat. The volume density of the heat created by the attenuation of a wave passing the medium and causing its heating is

$$q = -\frac{\partial I}{\partial z} = 2\beta \ I_0 \ \mathrm{e}^{-2\beta z} = q_0 \ \mathrm{e}^{-2\beta z},$$

where $q_0 = 2\beta I_0 [\mathrm{W \cdot m^{-3}}]$ is the heat density at the surface (at the wave source).

The highest heat density is in the surface layer of the medium with a thickness of $\delta/2$ (half the effective wave propagation length).

Ultrasound is used in medicine to heat the surface layers of tissues. The thickness of the heated layer can be adjusted by changing the frequency of the ultrasound. Warming the tissue increases blood flow and supports regeneration processes, the breakdown of muscle metabolites, etc. Focused ultrasound is also used for hyperthermia and tissue ablation, for example, in the brain in the treatment of Parkinson's disease. The mechanical pressure, induced by the ultrasonic wave, is also used in *sonophoresis*, which is the support of drug transport into muscles and tendons through the skin. In dermatology, sonophoresis is used to transport cosmetics or pharmaceuticals, such as hyaluronic acid, various proteins, and moisturisers. Ultrasound massage increases blood flow, and thus oxygenation of the skin tissue reduces fatigue of cellular structures and partially breaks down subcutaneous fat.

1.4 Wave reflection and dispersion

In a homogeneous medium, the wave proceeds in one direction as a *travelling wave*. If inhomogeneity occurs in the path of the wave (body, change of substance properties, etc.), the wave is reflected or dispersed. Sound reflection is known as echo or reverberation. We speak of *wave reflection* if the dimensions of the reflecting area are significantly larger than the wavelength of the wave, for example, sound reflection from room walls or in nature from a rock wall or water surface. If the dimensions of the inhomogeneity are comparable or less than the wavelength, the usual imagination cannot be used, and diffraction on the inhomogeneities must be considered. In such a case, we speak of *wave dispersion* at dispersing centres, for example, scattering of ultrasound on blood erythrocytes.

1.4.1 Reflection of the wave from a planar interface

1.4.1.1 Laws of reflection and refraction

The reflection of waves from the raged interface is complicated. To explain the phenomenon, we use a simple case of wave reflection from the planar interface of two homogeneous media.

To display the propagation of the waves, we use a geometric representation of the rays (**Figure 7**). In a homogeneous medium, the rays are lines, in a non-homogeneous medium, the rays are curves.

The laws of reflection and refraction are satisfied with the reflection of waves from the interface and the transition through it. For the angle of incidence α, angle of reflection α' and refractive angle β, relative to the normal to the interface (**Figure 7**), are valid following formulas

$$\alpha' = \alpha, \text{ and } \sin\beta = \frac{c_2}{c_1}\sin\alpha, \tag{32}$$

where c_1 and c_2 are the speeds of waves in both media.

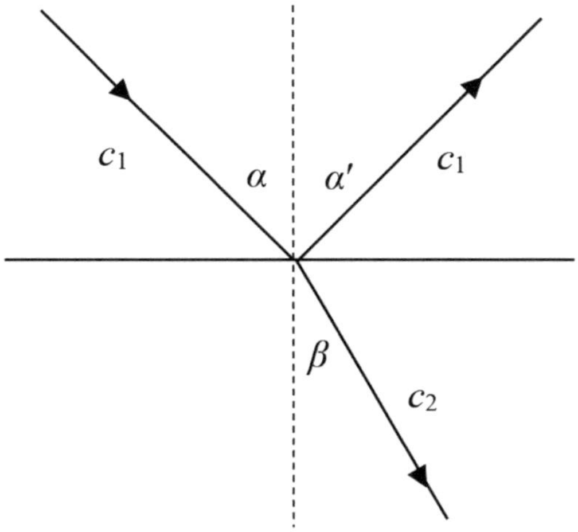

Figure 7.
Reflection and refraction of the wave at the interface of two media.

1.4.1.2 Total reflection

If the wave passes from a medium with a lower speed to a medium with a higher speed, for example, $c_2 > c_1$, there are angles of incidence for which is

$$\sin\beta = \frac{c_2}{c_1}\sin\alpha > 1, \text{or } \sin\alpha > \frac{c_1}{c_2} = \sin\alpha_m. \tag{33}$$

Since $\sin\beta \leq 1$, for $\alpha > \alpha_m$ there cannot occur transition of the wave to the second medium, and there is a complete (*total*) *reflection*. The angle α_m is called the *limiting angle of total reflection*.

Example 4 Total sound reflection at the water/air interface.

The sound propagates in the air at a speed of approximately $c_1 = 340\ \text{m}\cdot\text{s}^{-1}$, and in water at a speed of $c_2 = 1440\ \text{m}\cdot\text{s}^{-1}$. The edge angle α_m of total reflection is $\alpha_m \approx 14°$, according to Eq. (33). The sound that hits from the air the surface of the water at angle $\alpha > 14°$ will not penetrate under the water level.

1.4.1.3 Energy transfer of wave across the interface

To assess the intensity of the reflected wave and the wave penetrating the second medium, we will use the case of the perpendicular impact of the wave on the interface to simplify the calculations (**Figure 8**).

Consider the perpendicular incidence of a longitudinally polarised wave at the interface of two media with acoustic impedances $\mathbf{Z}_1$ and $\mathbf{Z}_2$. In the first medium propagate the incident wave (i - incident), and the reflected wave (r - reflected). In the second medium, only the penetrating wave (t - transmitted) propagates.

The total sound pressure at the left and right interfaces is the same

$$\mathbf{p}_i + \mathbf{p}_r = \mathbf{p}_t,$$

the particle velocity at the interface must be the same from the left and the right

$$\mathbf{v}_i + \mathbf{v}_r = \mathbf{v}_t.$$

According to Eq. (28), there is $\mathbf{p}_i = \mathbf{Z}_1\,\mathbf{v}_i$, $\mathbf{p}_r = -\mathbf{Z}_1\,\mathbf{v}_r$ and $\mathbf{p}_t = \mathbf{Z}_2\,\mathbf{v}_t$, and after substitution and editing we get

$$\begin{aligned} \mathbf{v}_t &= \frac{2\mathbf{Z}_1}{\mathbf{Z}_1 + \mathbf{Z}_2}\mathbf{v}_i & \mathbf{p}_t &= \frac{2\mathbf{Z}_2}{\mathbf{Z}_1 + \mathbf{Z}_2}\mathbf{p}_i \\ \mathbf{v}_r &= \frac{\mathbf{Z}_1 - \mathbf{Z}_2}{\mathbf{Z}_1 + \mathbf{Z}_2}\mathbf{v}_i & \mathbf{p}_r &= \frac{\mathbf{Z}_2 - \mathbf{Z}_1}{\mathbf{Z}_1 + \mathbf{Z}_2}\mathbf{p}_i\ . \end{aligned} \tag{34}$$

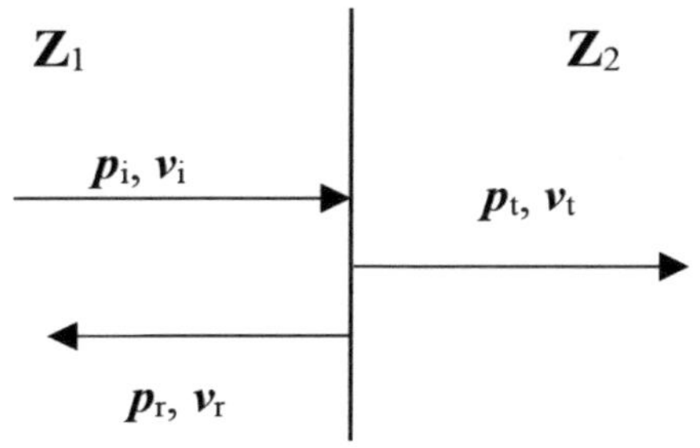

Figure 8.
Reflection of the wave from the interface and transition of the wave across the interface.

Since the impedances are generally complex quantities, the corresponding wave quantities are also complex - phasors.

In the case of a wave incident perpendicularly to the interface, the intensities of the passing and reflected waves are

$$I_{\mathrm{r}} = \left|\frac{\mathbf{Z}_2 - \mathbf{Z}_1}{\mathbf{Z}_1 + \mathbf{Z}_2}\right|^2 I_{\mathrm{i}}, \quad I_{\mathrm{t}} = I_{\mathrm{i}} - I_{\mathrm{r}} = \frac{4\,\mathrm{Re}\left\{\mathbf{Z}_1 \mathbf{Z}_2^*\right\}}{\left|\mathbf{Z}_1 + \mathbf{Z}_2\right|^2} I_{\mathrm{i}}, \tag{35}$$

where $I_{\mathrm{i}} = \mathrm{Re}\left\{\mathbf{p}_{\mathrm{i}} \mathbf{v}_{\mathrm{i}}^*\right\}$, $I_{\mathrm{r}} = \mathrm{Re}\left\{\mathbf{p}_{\mathrm{r}} \mathbf{v}_{\mathrm{r}}^*\right\}$ and $I_{\mathrm{t}} = \mathrm{Re}\left\{\mathbf{p}_{\mathrm{t}} \mathbf{v}_{\mathrm{t}}^*\right\}$ are the intensities of the incident, reflected, and penetrating wave, respectively.

The result shows that the reflection of the wave from the interface occurs only in the case of a change in acoustic impedance. If the magnitude of the impedance ratio is several orders of magnitude, there is a practically total reflection (with the same or opposite phase).

The principle of wave reflection is used to investigate the structure of bodies. In nature, the reflection of sound is observed as an echo. The use of reflected ultrasound, for example, bats, flaw detectors, or sonar works on the principle of reflection from the inhomogeneous medium. In medicine, ultrasonography works on the principle of ultrasound reflection. Ultrasound is transmitted by a probe into the body, and the signal reflected from individual organs is received. Mirror reflection takes place from the planar interfaces. The flat surface of the reflecting body needs not to be perfectly smooth. If the surface is rough, and the irregularities are considerably smaller than the wavelength of the wave, the surface behaves as planar. If the irregularities are randomly distributed and larger than the wavelength, the waves are reflected in different directions concerning the surface plane. It is called *diffuse reflection* and *diffuse dispersion*. If the diffuse dispersion is ideal, the waves are scattered, in all directions. An example of diffuse reflection is the reflection of sound from a ragged wall of a room or a waving water level. An example of diffuse dispersion is, for example, sound dispersion from broken walls in a music hall.

1.4.1.4 Transmission of wave through an acoustic layer

A significant case represents the transition of a wave through an acoustic layer. The wave propagation through a layer is proper for impedance matching, the formation of reflective or non-reflective layers, or acoustic resonators. The simple model illustrates (**Figure 9**), which utilises a perpendicular wave impact on the plane-parallel acoustic layer.

The conditions on the interfaces are described in the previous paragraph.

$$\mathbf{p}_{\mathrm{i}} + \mathbf{p}_{\mathrm{r1}} = \mathbf{p}_{\mathrm{t1}} + \mathbf{p}_{\mathrm{r21}} \qquad \mathbf{p}_{\mathrm{t12}} + \mathbf{p}_{\mathrm{r2}} = \mathbf{p}_{\mathrm{t3}}$$

$$\mathbf{v}_{\mathrm{i}} + \mathbf{v}_{\mathrm{r1}} = \mathbf{v}_{\mathrm{t1}} + \mathbf{v}_{\mathrm{r21}} \qquad \mathbf{v}_{\mathrm{t12}} + \mathbf{v}_{\mathrm{r2}} = \mathbf{v}_{\mathrm{t3}},$$

where

$$\mathbf{p}_{\mathrm{i}} = \mathbf{Z}_1 + \mathbf{v}_{\mathrm{i}}, \qquad \mathbf{p}_{\mathrm{r1}} = -\mathbf{Z}_1\mathbf{v}_{\mathrm{r1}}, \mathbf{p}_{\mathrm{t1}} = \mathbf{Z}_2\mathbf{v}_{\mathrm{t1}}, \qquad \mathbf{p}_{\mathrm{r21}} = -\mathbf{Z}_2\mathbf{v}_{\mathrm{r21}}, \mathbf{p}_{\mathrm{t12}} = \mathbf{Z}_2\mathbf{v}_{\mathrm{t12}},$$

$$\mathbf{p}_{\mathrm{t3}} = \mathbf{Z}_3\mathbf{v}_{\mathrm{t3}}, \qquad \mathbf{p}_{\mathrm{t12}} = \mathbf{p}_{\mathrm{t1}}\ \mathrm{e}^{-\mathrm{j}\mathbf{k}d}, \qquad \mathbf{p}_{\mathrm{r21}} = \mathbf{p}_{\mathrm{r2}}\ \mathrm{e}^{-\mathrm{j}\mathbf{k}d},$$

$$\mathbf{v}_{\mathrm{t12}} = \mathbf{v}_{\mathrm{t1}}\ \mathrm{e}^{-\mathrm{j}\mathbf{k}d}, \qquad \mathbf{v}_{\mathrm{r21}} = \mathbf{v}_{\mathrm{r2}}\ \mathrm{e}^{-\mathrm{j}\mathbf{k}d}.$$

After substituting and editing, we get relationships for complex transition and reflection coefficients

$$\mathbf{t} = \frac{\mathbf{v}_{t3}}{\mathbf{v}_i} = \frac{4Z_1Z_2}{(Z_1 + Z_2)(Z_2 + Z_3)\ e^{j\mathbf{k}d} + (Z_2 - Z_1)(Z_3 - Z_2)e^{-j\mathbf{k}d}} \tag{36}$$

$$\mathbf{r} = \frac{\mathbf{v}_{r1}}{\mathbf{v}_i} = \frac{(Z_1 - Z_2)(Z_3 + Z_2)e^{j\mathbf{k}d} + (Z_1 + Z_2)(Z_2 - Z_3)e^{-j\mathbf{k}d}}{(Z_1 + Z_2)(Z_2 + Z_3)\ e^{j\mathbf{k}d} + (Z_1 - Z_2)(Z_2 - Z_3)e^{-j\mathbf{k}d}}. \tag{37}$$

The complex amplification **a** of the acoustic wave inside the layer describes the ratio of the particle velocity on the input surface inside the layer and the resulting particle velocity on the outside surface of the layer from the side of the wave source

$$\mathbf{a} = \frac{\mathbf{v}_{t1}}{\mathbf{v}_i + \mathbf{v}_r} = \frac{(Z_2 + Z_3)}{(Z_2 + Z_3) + (Z_2 - Z_3)e^{-j2\mathbf{k}d}}. \tag{38}$$

The input impedance of the layer is

$$Z_{in} = \frac{\mathbf{p}_i + \mathbf{p}_{r1}}{\mathbf{v}_i + \mathbf{v}_{r1}} = Z_1 \frac{\mathbf{v}_i - \mathbf{v}_{r1}}{\mathbf{v}_i + \mathbf{v}_{r1}} = \frac{Z_2 + Z_3 - (Z_2 - Z_3)\,e^{-j2\mathbf{k}d}}{Z_2 + Z_3 + (Z_2 - Z_3)\,e^{-j2\mathbf{k}d}}\ Z_2. \tag{39}$$

From the Eqs. (37) and (39), we get the relation for the reflection factor

$$\mathbf{r} = \frac{Z_1 - Z_{in}}{Z_1 + Z_{in}}.$$

As can be seen from the resulting relations, the quantities **r**, **t**, **a**, and Z_{in} depend on the thickness d of the layer and of the phase thickness $k\ d$.

We will identify two extreme cases:

For the case (+) is $k\ d = \pi$ rad, $d = \lambda/2$, and $e^{jkd} = e^{j\pi} = -1$, we have

$$\mathbf{a}^+ = \frac{Z_2 + Z_3}{2Z_2}, \qquad Z_{in}^+ = Z_3, \tag{40}$$

$$\mathbf{r}^+ = \frac{Z_1 - Z_3}{Z_1 + Z_3}, \qquad \mathbf{t}^+ = -\frac{2Z_1}{Z_1 + Z_3}. \tag{41}$$

For the case (−) is $k\ d = \pi/2$ rad, $d = \lambda/4$, and $e^{jkd} = j$.

$$a^- = \frac{Z_2 + Z_3}{2Z_3}, \qquad Z_{in}^- = Z_3\left(\frac{Z_2}{Z_3}\right)^2, \tag{42}$$

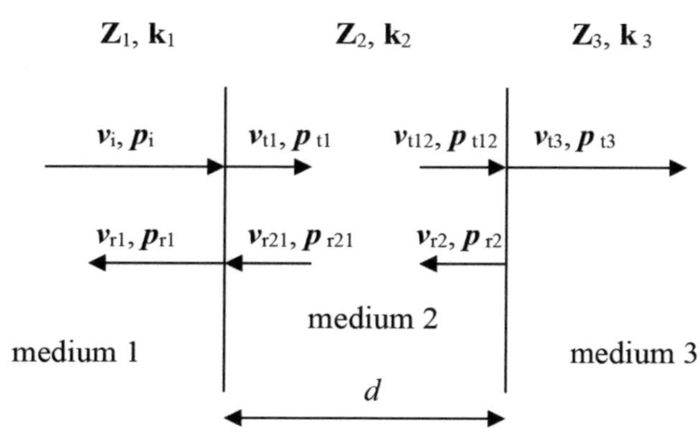

Figure 9.
Transition of wave through an acoustic layer.

$$\mathbf{r}^- = \frac{\mathbf{Z}_1\mathbf{Z}_3 - \mathbf{Z}_2\mathbf{Z}_2}{\mathbf{Z}_1\mathbf{Z}_3 + \mathbf{Z}_2\mathbf{Z}_2}, \qquad \mathbf{t}^- = -j\,\frac{2\mathbf{Z}_1\mathbf{Z}_2}{\mathbf{Z}_1\mathbf{Z}_3 + \mathbf{Z}_2\mathbf{Z}_2}. \tag{43}$$

For $\mathbf{Z}_2 \ll \mathbf{Z}_3$ is $\mathbf{a}^+ \gg 1$, it means in the layer, the acoustic field is considerably amplified in the first case (+). This is the *half-wave resonator*, for example, air layer limited by rigid walls (room with concrete walls) or some musical wind instruments.

A room without dispersion elements (bare parallel walls) is a half-wave resonator (for d = 12 m is λ = 24 m and $f \approx$ 14 Hz). A very gentle vibration of the walls, caused by, for example, traffic or a rotating machine in the cellar, results in a resonantly greatly amplified infrasound, which is not audible but harms humans.

If $Z_2 \gg Z_3$ an amplification occurs in the second case ($-$), $\mathbf{a}^- \gg 1$. This is the *quarter-wave resonator*. An example is a solid plate placed in water or air, for example, a piezoelectric transducer generating ultrasound into soft tissue during ultrasonography. The ear canal in the outer ear also acts as a quarter-wave resonator: length $l \sim$ 25 mm, $\lambda \approx$ 10 cm, $f \approx$ 3.3 kHz—this frequency is best perceived by the ear due to resonant amplification (see **Figure 12**, p. 31).

Next, we see that the layer transforms the impedance from the value Z_3 to Z_{in}. When the structure meets impedances $Z_1 \neq Z_3$, the waves are reflected at their interface. If we insert the layer between them with the proper thickness so that the impedances are $Z_{in} = Z_1$ and $Z_{out} = Z_3$, there are no reflections, and the *non-reflective matching* occurs. From Eq. (43) follows that non-reflective matching occurs by inserting a layer with a thickness $\lambda/4$ and impedance $\mathbf{Z}_2 = \sqrt{\mathbf{Z}_1\mathbf{Z}_3}$.

The layer acts as an *impedance transformer*. The transformer can be single or multi-layered, where the impedance transformation (impedance matching) takes place gradually in finer steps—*a stepped transformer*. It can also be continuous, where the impedance changes continuously along with the transformer. A typical example is a funnel transformer that was mounted on historical gramophones to transfer the sound from a phonograph needlepoint into space. The funnel-shaped are some wind instruments with embouchure like a trumpet, French horn, or speakers, alarm siren, etc. An inverted funnel transformer is used for listening, for example, an older funnel stethoscope. A similar principle also utilises a modern stethoscope (see **Figure 10**).

The auricle of the outer ear also acts as an adjusting element (sometimes we increase its effect by placing the palm to the ear) (see **Figure 10**).

The acoustic transformer is also used as a power concentrator (**Figure 10(a)**). If we generate a wave with intensity $I_1 = P/S_1$ on the area S_1 of the source side of the funnel, then the power propagates through the funnel without reflection to the other end. The output intensity is $I_2 = P/S_2$. It increases the intensity (and the acoustic pressure), $I_2 = I_1\,(S_1/S_2)$. The output of the concentrator can serve as a working tool, for example, a drill for very hard and brittle materials, or a tool for surface treatment and engraving of hard bodies (glass, ceramics, crystals), etc.

1.4.2 Wave dispersion

When there are small objects compared to the wavelength in the transmission path, the previous idea of reflection from a large area is not applicable. In this case, we consider a wave reflection on the elements of the object surface and the subsequent superposition on elementary reflected waves. It is the diffraction of waves. This phenomenon is called *wave dispersion*. The dispersion theory is relatively complicated, but for small particles with radius R, for which applies the condition $(2\,\pi\,R/\lambda) \ll 1$, where λ is the wavelength of the wave, the intensity I of the wave dispersed by the angle ϑ related to the original direction of propagation of the wave expresses the Rayleigh relation

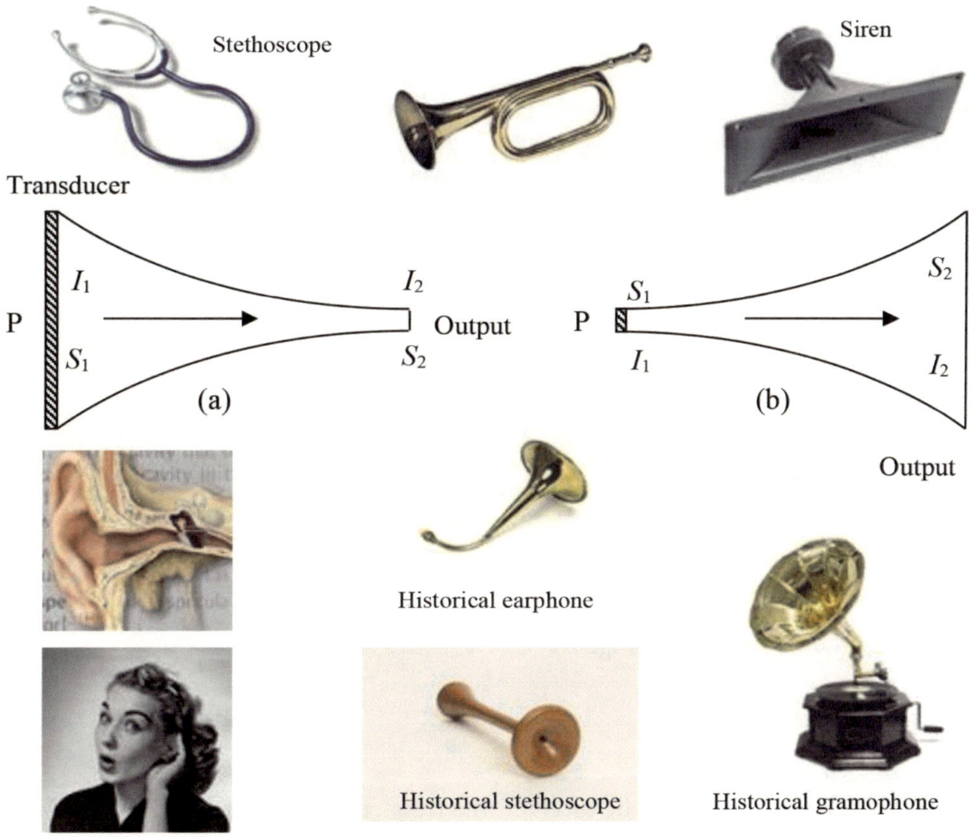

Figure 10.
Several methods of acoustic impedance matching used in sound transmission and reception, (a) sound amplification, (b) sound matching to the open air.

$$I = I_0\, k\, R^2 \left(\frac{R}{\lambda}\right)^4 \left(1 + \cos^2 \vartheta\right) \frac{1}{r^2}, \tag{44}$$

where k is the proportionality constant that depends on the particle concentration, ϑ angle of dispersion, r distance from the dispersing particle, and I_0 intensity of the incident wave.

It follows from Rayleigh's relationship that small particles disperse waves in all directions $\vartheta \in (0, \pi)$ rad. The intensity of the dispersed wave depends on the concentration of the particles.

Dispersion of ultrasound with a frequency of about 15 MHz (wavelength of about 100 μm) by red blood cells with a diameter of about 10 μm is used to imaging and measure the speed of blood movement using the Doppler effect.

Ultrasound dispersed on small particles is also used in ultrasonography in the examination of cavities using a contrast medium, which is a liquid with small (micron) particles or microscopic bubbles whose size is smaller than the wavelength of the wave.

1.5 Doppler effect

Several significant applications are related to the *Doppler effect*, which is manifested by a change of the frequency of the detected waves when the source and receiver are in relative motion.

1.5.1 Moving source and static receiver

If the transmitter (source) moves towards the stationary receiver, during time T_0 of one wave period transmitted by the source, the distance between the source and receiver changes by $\Delta l = v\, T_0 \cos\alpha$, where v is the velocity of the source and α the angle between the direction of the vector of source velocity and connecting line source-receiver. The beginning of the wave period comes to the receiver at the speed c of the wave for a time $t_1 = l/c$. The end of the period comes in the time $t_2 = T_0 + (l - v\, T \cos\alpha)/c$. The receiver thus records the time between the end and the beginning of the period $T = t_2 - t_1 = T_0 - T\, v \cos\alpha/c$. It means that the received wave period is

$$T = \frac{T_0}{1 + \frac{v}{c}\cos\alpha}.$$

The receiver thus records the frequency of the incoming wave $f = 1/T$

$$f = f_0\left(1 + \frac{v}{c}\cos\alpha\right). \tag{45}$$

The relative frequency change is

$$\frac{\Delta f}{f_0} = \frac{v}{c}\cos\alpha. \tag{46}$$

As the source approaches the receiver, the frequency increases. If it moves away, the frequency decreases. If the source moves perpendicularly to the source-receiver line, the frequency does not change. By measuring the change in frequency, the velocity $v \cos\alpha$ of the receiver relative to the source can be measured.

1.5.2 Static source and moving receiver

Now, the source moves towards a stationary receiver at speed $u \cos\beta$, where β is the angle between the velocity vector $\boldsymbol{u}$ and the connecting line source-receiver. If the source sends the beginning of the period T_0 of the wave, it comes to the receiver in time $t_1 = l/c$. Before sending the end of the period, the source moves to the receiver by $T_0\, u \cos\beta$. The end of the period goes to the receiver in time $t_2 = (l - T_0\, u \cos\beta)/c$. The time between receiving the end and the beginning of the period is $T = T_0 + t_2 - t_1$

$$T = T_0 + \frac{l - T_0 u \cos\beta}{c} - \frac{l}{c} = T_0\left(1 - \frac{u}{c}\cos\beta\right).$$

The frequency of the received wave is as follows

$$f = \frac{f_0}{1 - \frac{u}{c}\cos\beta}. \tag{47}$$

The relative frequency change is

$$\frac{\Delta f}{f_0} = \frac{\frac{u}{c}\cos\beta}{1 - \frac{u}{c}\cos\beta}, \quad \text{for } u \ll c \text{ we have } \frac{\Delta f}{f_0} \approx \frac{u}{c}\cos\beta. \tag{48}$$

If the source approaches the receiver, the received frequency increases, if the receiver moves away, the received frequency decreases. The frequency of the received wave changes only if the distance between the source and receiver changes. If the source moves perpendicularly to the source-receiver connecting line, the received frequency remains the same as that of the source. From the change of received frequency, it is possible to determine the speed $u \cos\beta$ of the source relative to the receiver.

1.5.3 Wave reflection from a moving object

Let us consider the source of the wave with frequency f_0 propagating towards an object moving in direction of the connecting line at speed $u \cos\beta$. Frequency f_1 of the wave caught by the moving object is given by the Eq. (47). The wave with frequency f_1 reflects from the object back to the source. The object now represents a moving transmitter with the speed $u \cos\beta$ and the source a stationary receiver. The frequency f_1 changes to f according to Eq. (45). The frequency of the received reflected wave is thus

$$f = \frac{f_1}{1 - \frac{u}{c}\cos\beta} = f_0 \frac{1 + \frac{u}{c}\cos\beta}{1 - \frac{u}{c}\cos\beta},$$

for $u \ll c$ we have $f \approx f_0\left(1 + 2\frac{u}{c}\cos\beta\right)$ or $\frac{\Delta f}{f_0} \approx 2\frac{u}{c}\cos\beta$.

The relative change of the wave frequency is thus directly proportional to the speed of the object approaching or moving away from the acoustic wave source.

Other acoustic devices utilise the Doppler principle, for example, SONAR (sound navigation and ranging) for the identification of moving objects under the sea level (submarines, flocks of fish), or when using electromagnetic waves to measure the speed of road vehicles, flying aircraft, clouds, etc.

In biomedicine, the Doppler effect is mainly used in ultrasonography, or to measure the velocity of blood flow in blood vessels. Doppler effect is a common phenomenon of all waves irrespective of their physical nature.

Example 5 LIDAR.

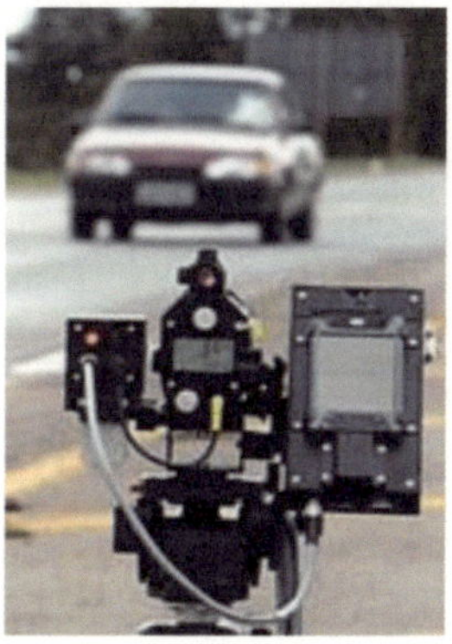

LIDAR (Light Radar) is a device that uses the EM waves of a laser beam reflected from a monitored object. RADAR has a wide range of uses, for example, in air traffic, meteorology, etc. LIDAR is used, for example, to control speed in road transport. Older types used microwave radiation; today's modern devices use optical waves. A narrow beam (3 mrad) of radiation with a wavelength of 905 nm (infrared radiation) is transmitted towards the vehicle in pulses of length τ = 30 ns.

From a vehicle distance of 1 km, the pulse returns in 6.7 μs. Due to the Doppler effect, at the speed of the vehicle, $u = 50$ km/s, period T_0 between pulses changes by $\Delta T/T_0 \approx 10^{-7}$. At the repetition period, $T_0 = 1$ ms and sending of $N = 500$ pulses is the measurement time $t = 0.5$ s. During this time is the total Doppler shift $\Delta t = t$ $(\Delta T/T_0) \approx 50$ ns. This shift can be safely evaluated using digital analysis. The laser beam is precisely pointed on the oncoming vehicle, up to about 1 km (normally 300 m). The measured speed is documented, and with built-in binoculars or a photo camera, the vehicle is addressable.

The same principle is used by meteorological radars, which use EM waves of the wavelength of 2–10 cm (microwaves). The result is, for example, maps of clouds movement and precipitation. The radar can also distinguish the type of precipitation (rain, snow).

1.6 Spectral bands of mechanical waves

The effects and practical use of mechanical waves depend on their frequency. The frequency bands of mechanical waves are defined concerning the frequency band of sound audible by the human ear. For a healthy hearing organ, an audible sound interval is 20 Hz–20 kHz. The music reference tone is *chamber A* with a frequency of $f = 440$ Hz, which is also the fundamental tone of the human voice. It is the tone according to which tune musical instruments. The technical reference frequency is 1 kHz. The human ear is most sensitive to a frequency range of approximately 300 Hz–5.5 kHz with a maximum sensitivity at about 3 kHz.

Single-frequency or *monochromatic* sound is a harmonic one with only one frequency. Most sounds are *multi-frequency or polychromatic* ones, which means that they contain waves with more frequencies. If the sound frequency spectrum is continuous, then we speak about *sound noise*. If the sound spectrum is discrete and composed of the fundamental frequency and higher harmonic components, the sound is called *tone*. The fundamental frequency determines the *pitch of tone* and content of the higher harmonics *colour of tone* (*timbre*). If one plays a tone of the same pitch on different instruments, it sounds different on each of them. The difference is in the colour of the tone, it means the content of higher harmonics.

Sound affects the human psyche. The relaxing effects of classical music or, conversely, the excitatory effects of aggressive forms of music are known. These effects are used in sound therapy, sometimes to manipulate masses of people.

The hearing organs of various animals differ and have a different frequency range of sensitivity. For example, the dog hears a sound frequency range of 40 Hz–40 kHz, like a horse. Elephants, on the contrary, perceive vibrations with a frequency of up to 16 Hz. The bats perceive ultrasound with a frequency of up to 150 kHz.

Waves with a frequency $f < 20$ Hz are not heard by humans but can be perceived as mechanical vibrations. Waves with these frequencies are called *infrasound*. The wavelengths of infrasound in the air are $\lambda > 17$ m. It is comparable with the dimensions of building structures. Infrasound occurs in halls, offices, and living spaces. Low-frequency vibrations produce the operation of various rotating machines, traffic, or seismic processes. Infrasound has a significant effect on humans, mostly negative with long-term exposure. It can lead to mental disorders and reduced immunity, which is an open path to secondary diseases. Controlling the level of infrasound in living and working areas is an important task of hygienic inspection.

The influence of low-frequency infrasound on the human psyche is used to create specific moods. A typical example is the deep tones of organ pipes, which are supposed to evoke a deeper spiritual experience in cathedrals. On the contrary, the deep tones with high intensity at discotheques intend to put participants into a trance.

Waves with a frequency $f > 20$ kHz are not heard by humans and represent *ultrasound* (US). Due to a wide spectrum of ultrasound, some bands have a special name, for example, 100 kHz US, MHz US, *hypersound* ($f > 1$ GHz), etc. Ultrasound is used in medical diagnostics—ultrasonography (2–20 MHz), or in physical ultrasound therapy—massage, warming of muscles and tendons (about 1 MHz), ultrasound lithotripsy (crushing kidney, bladder, or gallstones by a series of intense ultrasound pulses 25–30 kHz), etc.

The MHz-US probe can be inserted into a vessel using a catheter to dissolve the thrombus by ultrasound support of the thrombolytic drugs.

An important application is transdermal sonophoresis (drug transfer through the top layer of the skin), in which the barrier of the top layer of the skin (*stratum corneum*) to the transfer of large organic drug molecules with a relative molecular weight greater than 500 is overcome by ultrasound of frequency of 150 kHz.

1.7 Sources and detectors of mechanical waves

There is a direct interaction between the oscillations of the particles and the wave. Particle oscillations (dynamic deformation of the medium) are a source of the wave. On the other hand, waves in the medium cause oscillations of particles. It represents the principle of generation and detection of mechanical waves (sound, infrasound, and ultrasound).

A mechanical wave is generated by any time-varying (dynamic) deformation of the elastic or quasi-elastic medium. The sources can be divided according to the physical principle or according to the properties of the waves. According to the physical principle, they can be mechanical, thermal, electro-dynamic, optical, etc. The sources are coherent or incoherent, or from the geometric point of view: dot, line, surface, specially structured, etc. In this part, the sources of mechanical waves are discussed in terms of physical principles. To create a wave in a medium, the initial disturbance of the medium is necessary. According to the mechanism of this disturbance, we know the following sources of mechanical waves, regardless of the time course or geometric structure of the generated field of particle displacement.

In the following section, on the contrary, we describe the physical principles of mechanical wave detection. The wave cause oscillations that can be detected mechanically, electro-dynamically, optically, etc. Accordingly, we distinguish among diverse ways of detection of mechanical waves (infrasound, sound, and ultrasound).

1.7.1 Mechanical sources of mechanical waves

The mechanical excitation of mechanical waves occurs during mechanical excitation of the surface by an external force. A classic example is the collision of two rigid bodies, for example, the impact of a hammer on the anvil. In this way, for example, the sound of musical instruments such as piano or drums is generated. The impact sound is incoherent, but using a resonator, a coherent harmonic component (appropriate tone) can be selected from a wide range of sounds.

The excitation of mechanical waves also occurs due to friction. Sometimes we hear the whistling of vehicle brakes or the sound of a wheel rubbing against the road during heavy braking. Children know the sound of 'whistling chalk' on the blackboard, which also results from friction between the chalk and the blackboard. Regarding musical instruments, it is about creating sound in string instruments by rubbing the bow against a string. The vibration of the body can also occur by the friction of the flowing gas. Such oscillates the tongue of reed musical instruments, for example, clarinet or saxophone. We observe this principle even when sound is produced in the *vocal cords*. The air flowing through the vocal cord openings, their flexible walls oscillate, generating sound. By changing the tension in the vocal cords, the pitch of the generated tone is controlled. Mechanical wave also occurs due to the turbulent flow of a liquid or gas. In laminar flow, the movement of the individual particles of the medium is smooth and there is no excitation of the disturbances. Laminar flow is also called *silent flow* (e.g., water flowing in a smooth straight trough). However, in the case of eddy (vortex) flow, due to the irregular movement of individual elements of the fluid, mechanical excitations occur. They generate mechanical waves propagating inside and outside the medium. The turbulence arises in fluid when passing a sharp obstacle (bypassing water around stones in a stream). We know, for example, the excitation of the sound in the bottle by blowing on her throat. This principle is used by musical instruments such as various flutes.

Turbulent flow occurs in the tube when the critical value of the Reynolds number is exceeded. This number gives the formula $Re = d\, v\, \rho/\eta$ (d is tube diameter, v flow rate, ρ density, η fluid viscosity) and describes the ratio between viscous and dynamic resistance. The critical value, about $Re \sim 2300$, determines the critical flow rate of the fluid at which the flow changes from laminar to turbulent. In the case of a low-density gas, this velocity is low, and therefore, we hear hissing when blowing through narrowed lips. This method of sound excitation occurs when playing the trumpet. As turbulence arises during the flow of air through the respiratory organs, the flow of air in the trachea is heard using a *stethoscope*. Medical doctors use this phenomenon for the diagnosis of respiratory disease.

There is also turbulent blood flow in the cardiovascular system, audible with a stethoscope. Typical is, for example, examining the heart by listening to the murmur of blood passing through the valves, or the flow of blood in the aorta. Besides the heart and aorta, the flow in healthy vessels is laminar (quiet). However, turbulence can occur when any obstacle occurs. In this way, the arising sound can discover thrombus in a vessel or sclerotic or pressure narrowing an artery. Medical diagnostics use this phenomenon in the *auscultation method of measuring blood pressure*. The inflatable cuff constricts the artery and thus the flow of blood through the place of constriction vanishes or gets turbulent. One can hear it using a stethoscope. The sounds accompanying the turbulent flow are called *Korotkoff sounds*. They occur when the cuff press ranges from *diastolic* to *systolic* blood pressure. By measuring the pressure in the cuff and listening to the Korotkoff sounds of flowing blood, one determines the values of both limit pressures.

The principle of mechanical excitation of oscillations and mechanical detection of sound use the human hearing organ. The membrane represented by the eardrum oscillates due to the pressure modulation of the air (sound waves). Fine auditory bones (hammer, anvil, and stirrups) in the middle ear transmit the oscillations to the detection system of the inner ear (*cochlea*—snail).

1.7.2 Thermic sound excitation

Thermic excitation of mechanical waves arises due to the thermal expansion of the medium during a sudden change of temperature. If a place heats up quickly, it expands due to thermal expansion, causing the medium particles to move. This movement represents excitation, which then propagates like a mechanical wave due to the elasticity of the medium. Depending on the frequency, it is infrasound, sound, or ultrasound. In practice, we observe this phenomenon, for example, in electric discharges in gases. An electric discharge causes a sudden heating of the gas at the point of discharge and thus its expansion. The resulting sound is audible as a crack accompanying the discharge, for example, crackling the very high voltage insulators—400 kV, or thunder accompanying lightning during a storm. This sound is a non-coherent wave. However, there are also coherent spark sources in which the waves are excited by a pulse generator with regularly repeating sparks.

Thermal excitation can also be achieved by absorbing light radiation. In practice, the excitation of mechanical waves by power pulsed laser radiation is used. If the focused high-power laser beam impacts a certain place on or below the surface of the body, the medium absorbs the radiation, and thus it is locally heated. By the action of a laser beam with pulse modulation, it is possible to excite in the exposed body a mechanical wave with a frequency equal to the repetition rate of the pulse modulation. This phenomenon uses, for example, *photoacoustic tomography* (PAT) or *photoacoustic microscopy* (PAM).

In medical practice, *laser laparoscopic lithotripsy* uses the photoacoustic excitation of power ultrasound. The laser radiation propagates by an optical fibre to the surface of a kidney, bladder, or gall stone. Series of power optical pulses excites an ultrasound with intensity, at which the acoustic pressure exceeds the edge strength of the material. In such a way, the stone is mechanically broken into small pieces, which are then naturally washed out of the relevant organ. The advantage of this procedure is that it is only slightly invasive. It requires only small cuts for laparoscopic probes. The targeting of the laser pulse to the stone is more accurate and easier compared to extracorporeal ultrasound lithotripsy.

1.7.3 Electrodynamic sources and detectors of mechanical waves

Electrodynamic sources (speakers) and sound detectors (microphones) use the interaction between a moving conductor and a magnet in whose magnetic field it moves. A force $\mathrm{d}\boldsymbol{F} = I\,\boldsymbol{d\,l} \times \boldsymbol{B}$ exerts on the element $\boldsymbol{d\,l}$ of the length of the conductor in the magnetic field of magnetic induction $\boldsymbol{B}$, and through which passes the electric current I. The conductor has a shape of a cylindrical coil that moves in the direction of its axis. Changes of the current cause changes of the force $\boldsymbol{F}$, and thus a change of the coil acceleration. If a membrane is attached to the coil, the movement of the coil cause movement of the membrane. Its oscillations then generate a mechanical wave (sound). Electrodynamic loudspeakers have various configurations. They appear in radio and TV receivers, audio sets, headphones, etc. Their advantage is the high fidelity of the transformation of the electrical signal into sound. Electrodynamic loudspeakers provide a wide range of power from μW to kW and a great dimensional variability from tiny electroacoustic transducers with dimensions of the order of 1 mm to large loudspeakers with dimensions of about 1 m for generating intensive sound or infrasound.

If the coil is forced to move in the magnetic field of the magnet, or if the magnet moves inside the coil, an electric voltage induces in the coil according to Faraday's law, $u = \mathrm{d}\Phi/\mathrm{d}t$, where Φ is the magnetic flux of the coil. The movement of the coil follows the movement of the connected mechanical part of the system, which oscillates due to the alternating pressure of the incident sound wave. In such an arrangement, electrodynamic microphone, or electrodynamic phonograph pickups are constructed. In the case of a microphone, the sound wave drives the membrane connected with the coil, and thus the acoustic wave is transformed into an electric signal.

Electrodynamic microphones enable precise recording of sound in a very wide frequency range from infrasound to low-frequency ultrasound (tens of kHz). In addition to their normal use in sound technology, they are also used to measure the level of 'acoustic pollution' of the environment, especially in the field of infrasound, which negatively affects the quality of the environment. Similarly, an ultrasound that is inaudible to the human ear can be sensed. Sensitive microphones are also used in the detection of ultrasound, used, for example, by bats or dolphins for spatial orientation.

From a technical point of view, a moving coil system is mainly used in loudspeakers (sound sources), while detectors use a moving magnet and fixed coil arrangement.

If current flows through the coil, the turns of the winding are attracted to each other. During the flowing of alternating current or current pulses, the coil vibrates and generates sound. For example, exciting coils in a magnetic resonance device are very noisy, which is a negative aspect of the MRI investigation.

1.7.4 Electrostatic source and detector of mechanical waves

The electrostatic loudspeaker uses the dependence of the force between two parallel electrodes of a capacitor on the electrical voltage between them. If one electrode is fixed and the other is a fine movable membrane, the effect of the time-varying voltage causes deflection of the membrane. In this way, the membrane oscillations generate a mechanical wave in the surrounding medium. This type of speaker is suitable only for special purposes, for example, as simple sound indicators.

Electrostatic microphones are used more often. The incident mechanical wave deflects the movable flexible electrode (membrane) of the capacitor and changes the capacitance of the capacitor. Keeping the voltage constant, it modulates the current $i = u \, \mathrm{d}C/\mathrm{d}t$ passing the capacitor. This current represents the output electrical signal. Electrostatic microphones have a balanced frequency response, high sensitivity, and low distortion. They are utilised in studio technology and for precise acoustic measurements.

1.7.5 Magnetostrictive transducer

Magnetostriction is observed in ferromagnetic materials. The external magnetic field changes the orientation of the spontaneous magnetization domains, which is accompanied by a small change in the size of the material sample. In the direction of the magnetic field, the sample dilates in the direction perpendicular to the magnetic field contracts. The alternating magnetic field generated by the current coil, the rod of ferromagnetic material is in, causes the rod to oscillate. The oscillations are transmitted by acoustic coupling to the surrounding environment. The mainly used ferromagnetic material is nickel and its alloys.

Magnetostrictive transducers are used as ultrasound sources in a wide frequency range, or as actuators in automation.

There exists also an inverse magnetoelastic phenomenon. The mechanical deformation of a ferromagnetic rod changes its magnetization. It results in induced voltage in the coil wound around the ferromagnetic rod.

Magnetostrictive transducers are not used in medicine.

1.7.6 Piezoelectric transducer

Piezoelectric transducers are important technical sources and detectors of mechanical waves with lots of applications. The principle is based on a direct or inverse piezoelectric effect. The piezoelectric transducer consists of a plate of piezoelectric material with deposited metallic electrodes, like a parallel-plate capacitor. After connecting the voltage to the electrodes and raising an electric field in the piezoelectric plate, the thickness of the plate changes (inverse piezoelectric effect). By applying a time-varying voltage, the plate mechanically vibrates and generates a mechanical wave in the surrounding medium. Most applications of the piezoelectric transducers are *ultrasound sources*. The transducer efficiency increases mechanical resonance. The thickness of the plate is then $\lambda/2$ (half-wavelength resonator), where λ is the wavelength of the ultrasound in the plate at a given frequency. At a thickness of under 1 mm, the resonant frequency is above 1 MHz. Piezoelectric transducers are advantageous for generating and detecting mechanical waves in a frequency range from Hz to tens of GHz.

In the case of mechanical deformation of the plate, for example, by compression, an electric voltage appears directly between the electrodes in direct proportion to the relative change in thickness (direct *piezoelectric effect*). When a mechanical wave hits the transducer, it mechanically oscillates and thus deforms over time. An electrical voltage appears between the electrodes with a time dependence corresponding to the time dependence of the deformation. The piezoelectric transducer thus serves as an *ultrasound detector*. In practice, one transducer is often used as a wave generator and a wave detector with a time separation of transmission and receiving modes (single-probe pulse method).

The piezoelectric phenomenon occurs in some types of anisotropic crystals, for example, SiO_2, $LiNbO_3$, etc. In technical practice are cheaper piezoelectric ceramics Pb (Zr_xTi_{1-x}) O_3, referred to as PZT (lead zirconium titanate) ceramics, or organic piezoelectric foils, for example, polyvinylidene dihydrochloride (PVDF). Ceramics or organic foils can be easily shaped during production and allow to make various structured transducers. A great advantage of piezoelectric transducers is their very small size, if necessary. It is possible to incorporate them directly into microchips as part of electronic integrated circuits. Structured piezoelectric probes can be composed of piezoelectric segments. It is used, for example, in *ultrasonographic* medical instruments. Organic films are mainly used as low-power ultrasound generators or sensitive ultrasound detectors. Ceramic transducers, on the other hand, can generate acoustic power of up to 10^7 W•m^{-2} at frequencies of tens of kHz. Intensive ultrasound is used, for example, in ultrasonic cleaners, ultrasonic machining, ultrasonic welding, etc.

Medicine utilises ultrasound very widely. In addition to ultrasonography, which is an important diagnostic tool, ultrasound is used in sonophoresis (incorporation of nutrients or drugs into the skin), deep micro-massage, lipolysis (fat dissolution), deep heating, removal of dental plaque, etc. Intensive ultrasound uses lithotripsy (crushing of kidney, bladder, or gall stones) or ultrasonic scalpels.

1.8 Perception of sound by human hearing

Sound represents periodic fluctuations of air pressure. The eardrum hitting a sound wave oscillates. The oscillations are transmitted through a system of fine bones (*hammer, anvil, stirrup*) to the entrance of the ear canal of the inner ear (*snail*), oval window (**Figure 11(a)**). It represents the entrance of the sound channel in the inner snail and generates a wave propagating inside the snail. Along with the snail, there are nerve endings. The nerve fibres getting out of them, create the auditory nerve. It transmits a signal to the auditory centre in the brain, where auditory perception arises. The auditory organ distinguishes not only the intensity of the sound but also the pitch (frequency) of the tone. **Figure 11(b)** schematically shows the snail and the places of maximum sensitivity to different frequencies of sound. **Figure 11(c)** shows the width of the widening snail sound channel from the *cochlear base* (left) to the *cochlear apex* (right).

The snail channel is a complex acoustic resonator in which the maxima of oscillations with different frequencies are at different places along the channel, as

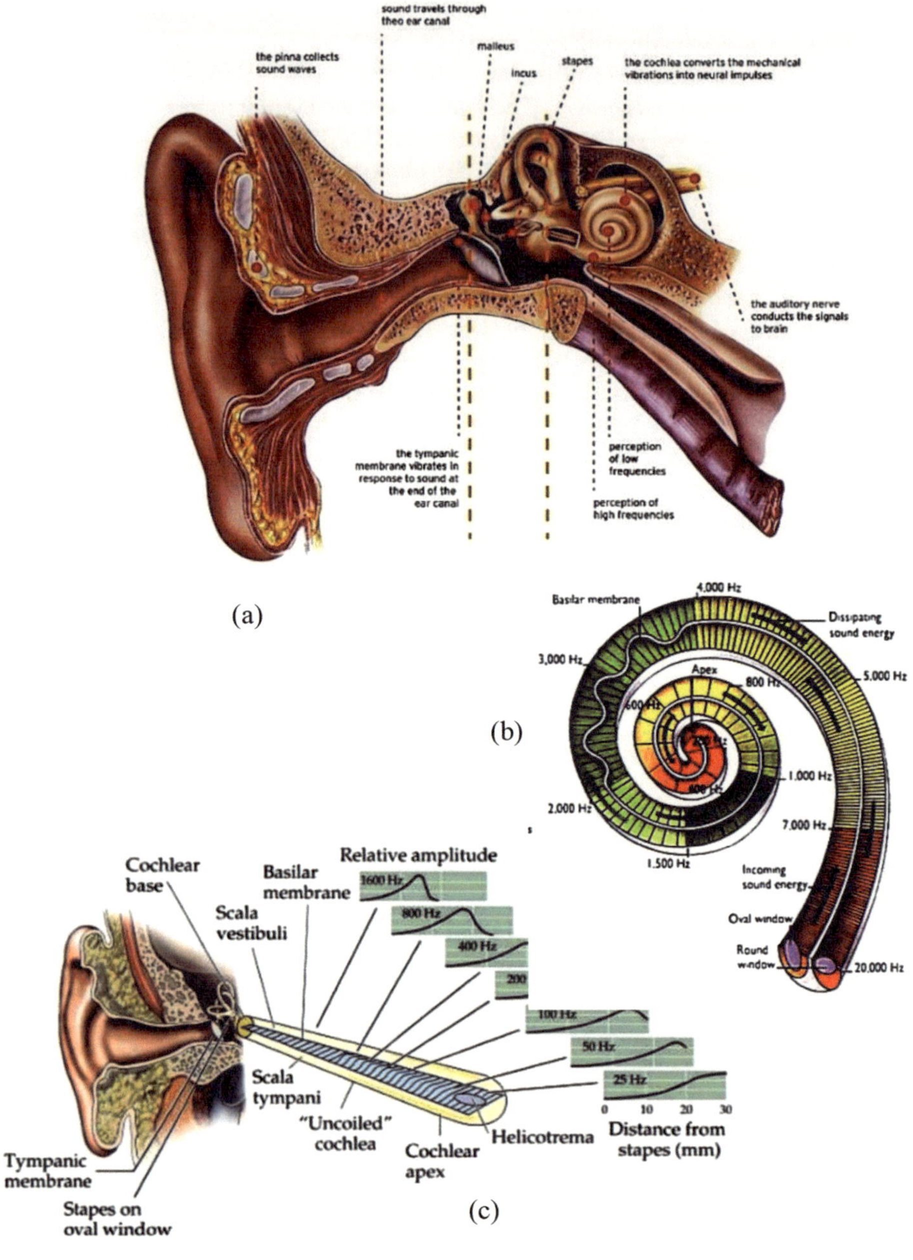

Figure 11.
Human ear apparatus involve: (a) human ear structure, (b) the sound detecting snail, (c) uncoiled cochlea with points of sensitivity to different frequences.

indicated in **Figure 11(b)** and **(c)**. The snail expands from the oval window, which increases the resonant wavelength and thus decreases the resonant frequency. Since the sound attenuation increases with frequency, the smallest transverse dimension is at the beginning (high tones) and the largest at the end (deep tones). The nerve endings on the perimeter of the snail are sensitive to resonant vibrations at given locations. Each nerve fibre thus transmits a different frequency. The snail is a complex frequency analyser of sound. Bundle of nerve fibres—*cochlear nerve*, transmits stimuli to the auditory centre in the brain. In this way, we perceive different tones.

A certain minimum of wave intensity is required for nerve excitation. In a healthy ear, the minimum sound pressure at the eardrum required for perception of the sound at a frequency of 1 kHz is on average p_0 = 20 μPa. In the air with an impedance of $Z \approx 400$ kg • m^{-2} • s^{-1} it corresponds to the acoustic intensity $I_0 \approx 1$ pW • m^{-2} (10^{-12} W • m^{-2}). This value at 1 kHz determines the *threshold of audibility*.

The sound perception of the human auditory organ is a *logarithmic* function of the sound intensity. It provides its enormous range of perception. Therefore, a *logarithmic acoustic intensity level* I_{dB} (in dB-decibels) is used to evaluate the sound level. It is given by the relation

$$I_{\text{dB}} = 10 \log \frac{I}{I_0}.$$

Typical values of the sound intensity level are given in **Table 3**.

Intensive sound threatens the ear not only by its intensity but also by the time of its action. For example, noise with the intensity level of 80 dB damages the cells of the ear when exposed for more than 8 hours, of the level of 90 dB for only 1 hour, and the level of 120 dB for only 10–16 seconds. Sound of the level of 140 dB and above, damages cells of the ear immediately, and the changes are irreversible. Damage of the cells often accompanies 'phantom' sound (tinnitus), such as humming or whistling in the ear. Sound of an intensity level $I_{\text{dB}} > 120$ dB is accompanied by pain. The intensity level of 120 dB, means I = 1 W·m^{-2}, therefore, determines the *threshold of pain*. Sound with an intensity level $I_{\text{dB}} > 150$ dB paralyses a person, causing unconsciousness or even death.

A person evaluates sound subjectively by its perception by an auditory organ. One perceives the sound with the same intensity differently at different frequencies. The measure of sound perception is *loudness*. The loudness H of the sound of a given frequency is equal to the intensity I of the sound of a frequency of 1 kHz with the same subjective impression. The *level of loudness (volume)* is defined similarly to the level of intensity I_{dB} by a logarithmic relationship

$$H_{\text{dB}}(f) = 10 \log \frac{H}{H_0},$$

where $H_0 = H_0(f)$ is the *threshold of audibility* at the sound frequency f. The unit of measure of the loudness level H_{dB} is Ph (Phon). A graphical representation of the loudness level spectrum is in **Figure 12**. The lowest curve corresponds to the

Sound	Intensity level [dB]
Audibility threshold	0
Leaf murmur	10
Whispering	30
Loud call	60
Scream, symphonic orchestra	80
Rock concert, disco	110
Jet aircraft take-off, from the distance of 1 m	120
Pain threshold	120
Firecracker, flash grenade	170

Table 3.
Sound energy flux density level of typical sounds.

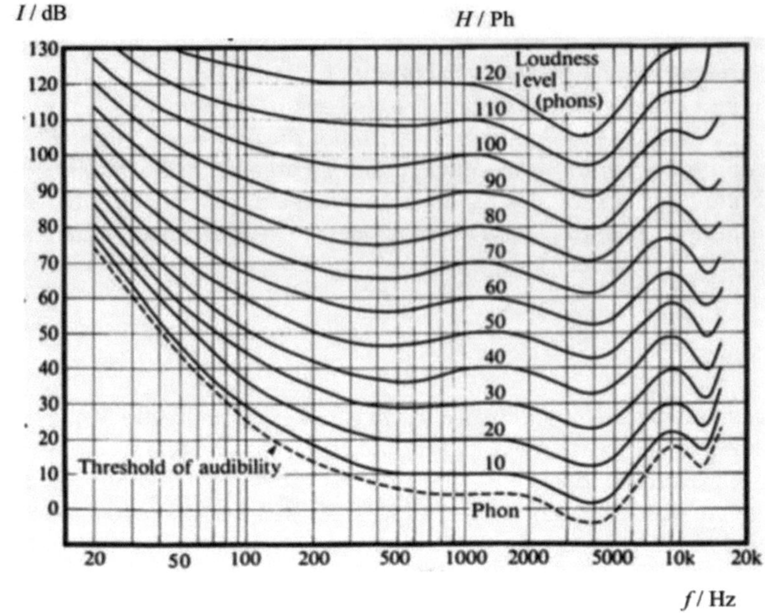

Figure 12.
Loudness level spectrum (Study library: https://studylib.net/doc/5632183/lecture14).

threshold value H_0 as a function of the sound frequency f. It was determined experimentally as the average value of the data from many tested subjects with normal hearing.

The thick lines correspond to the constant loudness with the values marked on the middle scale (at 1 kHz the values of loudness level are the same as the intensity level on the right scale). The threshold of audibility is lowest at around 3 kHz and increases towards extreme sound frequencies. We hear sound with a frequency of 30 Hz only at an intensity level of around 60 dB. The graph is standardised and corresponds to the average hearing organ of a healthy young person. With increasing age, the ability to hear sound generally decreases, mostly at extreme frequencies.

The volume is also affected by the external auditory canal and the auricle. The auricle is an acoustic transformer that adjusts the ambient impedance to the impedance of the external auditory canal. The effect of the ear can be supported by its effective enlargement using the palm or a funnel, **Figure 12**.

The auditory meatus is a $\lambda/4$ resonator, which amplifies the sound around the resonant frequency. With its length of approximately 2.5 cm and sound speed of 340 m/s, the resonant frequency is $f_r \approx 3.4$ kHz. In **Figure 13**, we can see the minimum of curves in the vicinity of this frequency. We also see that at low loudness, the sensitivity to bass and treble significantly reduces. If you want to ‘enjoy’ the entire frequency range of a song while listening to music, we need to choose a loudness level of around 80 dB. To understand the spoken word, it is also necessary to capture the edge frequencies of the spectrum, which also leads to the requirement to speak loudly enough.

1.9 Medical diagnostics using sound and ultrasound

1.9.1 Audiometry

The diagnostic method of *audiometry* deals with the investigation of the spectral sensitivity of the auditory organ of individual people, **Figure 13**. The patient is in an

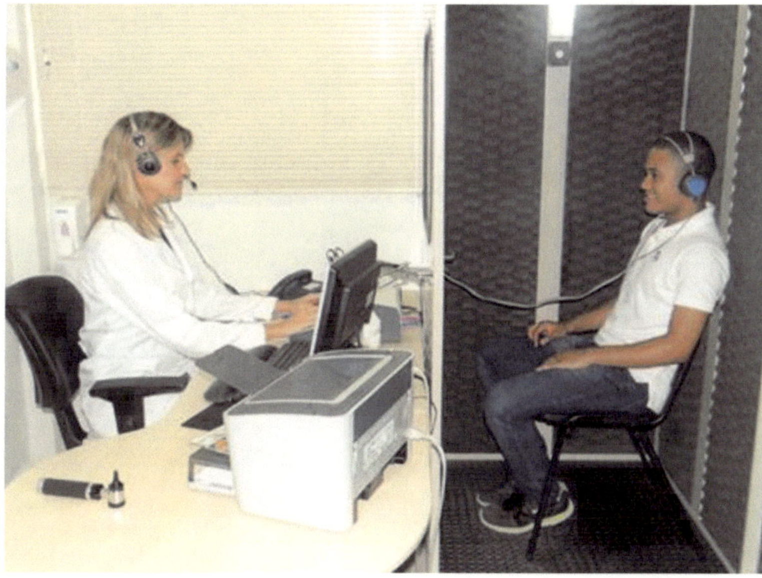

Figure 13.
Audiometric chamber.

acoustically isolated chamber and from the technician (left) receives into the headphones sound with different frequencies and gradually increasing intensity. The patient signals the moment when he begins to hear a sound. The line of resulting lowest levels of the sound intensities versus frequency is an *audiogram*.

The sound propagates to the inner ear (snail) through the eardrum or a skull bone, **Figure 14**. The air-conduction hearing test is performed using headphones, bone-conduction by placing the transducer directly on the bone behind the ear. The audiogram shows measurements by air (solid curve) and bone (dashed curve). The audiograms on the right show the airway for the right (red curve) and the left (blue curve) ear. The yellow area shows the intensity and frequency typical for hearing individual sounds of speech. The healthy hearing audiogram (above) provides a comfortable understanding of speech. The audiogram of hearing loss (below) shows hearing that is unable to understand speech—to distinguish the sounds.

Hearing correction is enabled by various instruments, see **Figure 15**. We often observe that for improving the hearing perception, we tend to put the palm to the ear (left picture). In old films from the 1920s, we can see listening to 'funnels'. Today, hearing loss is solved by electronic listening aids inserted into the ear canal, the picture on the right.

1.9.2 Auscultation

The classical method of examining body sounds is listening—*auscultation*. The method utilises sounds (murmurs) which produce a turbulent flow of fluids (liquids and gases) in the cardiovascular or respiratory system. For example, the murmurs of the blood flow through the heart valves or aorta are audible through the walls of the chest. By listening to them, the doctor can assess the normal functioning of the heart or its disorders. Murmurs also arise due to the obstacles (stenosis, thrombus, etc.) in vessels. By listening to these murmurs, it is possible to identify problem areas. Similarly, auscultation of sounds that produces air flowing through the trachea and bronchial tubes allows investigating respiratory diseases. Another case is an examination of a foetus in the body of a mother. Various sound concentrators

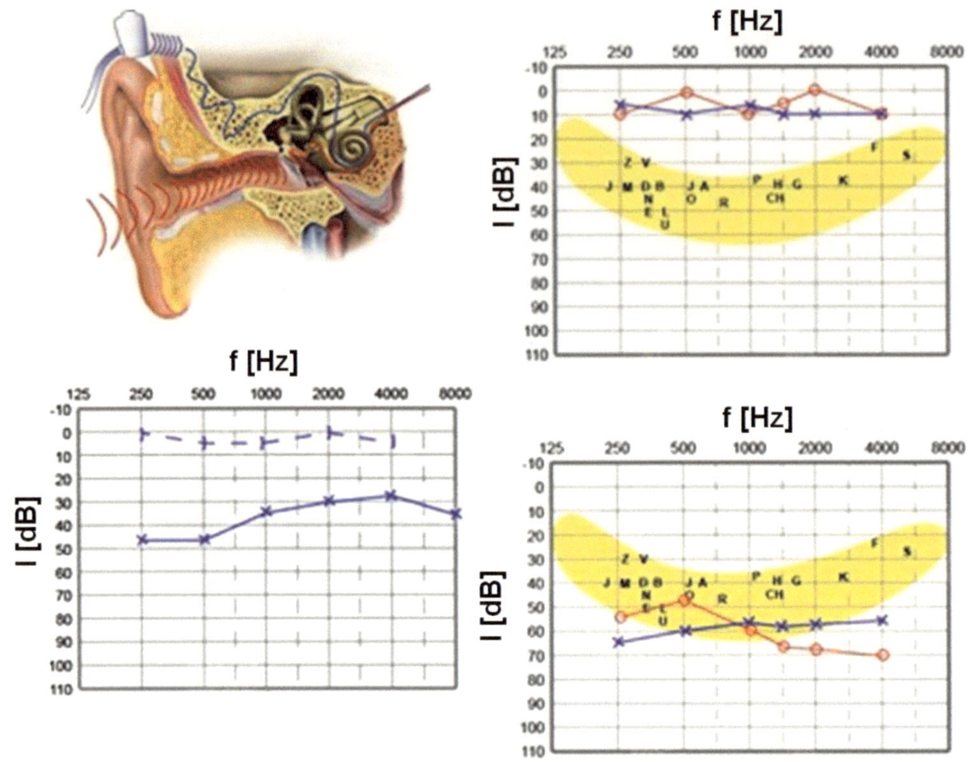

Figure 14.
Audiogram and its evaluation.

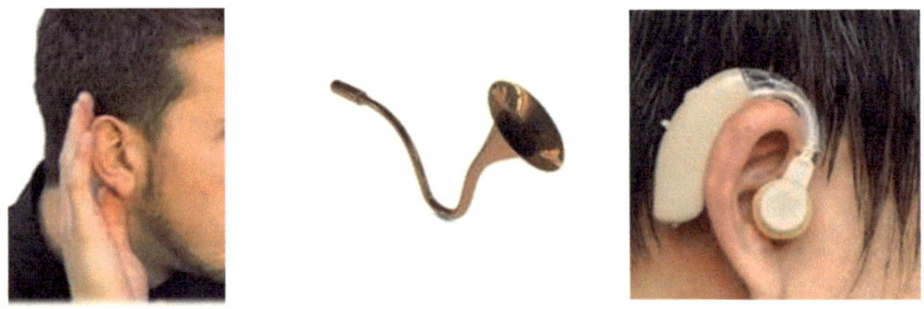

Figure 15.
Hearing aids.

help to amplify the murmurs. The historical tool was a funnel. Modern medicine utilises a *stethoscope*.

Obstruction as a source of murmurs can also be the narrowing of the vessel by the application of lateral pressure. This uses the auscultation method of measuring blood pressure, **Figure 16**. The cuff around the limb is inflated with a balloon to a pressure higher than the systolic one. The pressure stops flowing blood in the artery, and no sound is heard in the stethoscope applied under the cuff. If the pressure in the cuff drops below the systolic (SYS) one after the cuff slow deflating, blood begins to flow through the constricted artery. The flow is turbulent and is accompanied by murmurs—*Korotkov's sounds* (*Nikolay Korotkov 1874 - 1937*), heard in a stethoscope. The volume of the murmurs at first increases to its maximum value and then gradually decreases. The murmur disappears when the pressure drops to the diastolic (DIA) one, and the blood flow becomes laminar (silent). The doctor monitors the pressure in the cuff with a connected pressure gauge, and at the

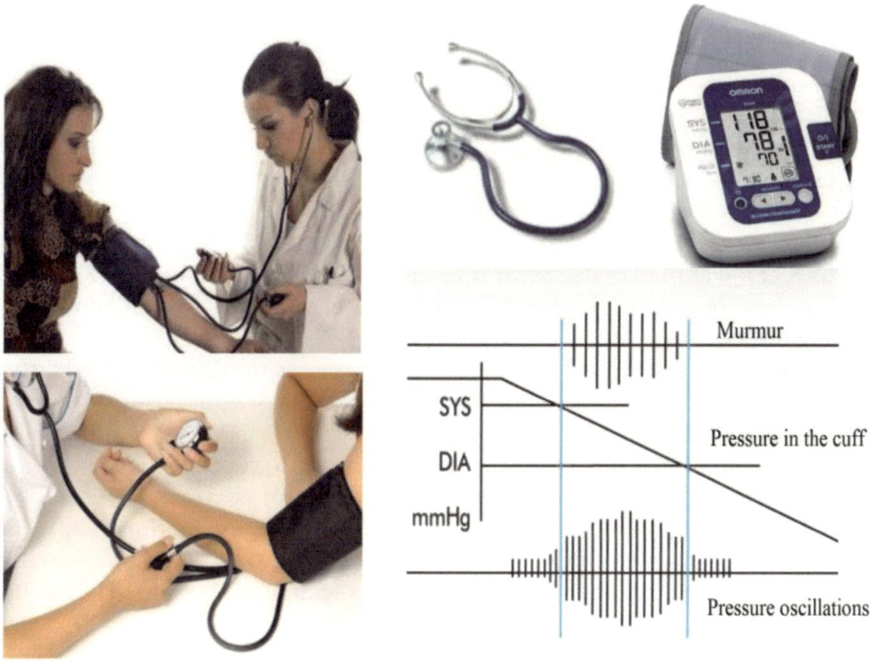

Figure 16.
Auscultation and oscillometric measurement of blood pressure.

same time listens to the murmurs with a stethoscope. In such a way, the doctor determines systolic pressure at the first hearing of murmurs and diastolic pressure at their extinction.

In addition to this auscultation method, there also exists an oscillometric method. Because of the blood pressure pulsation, small periodic pressure changes occur in the inflated cuff. The device has a pressure sensor connected with the tube inflating the cuff, which picks up these pressure pulses. The initial cuff inflation realises a built-in compressor. The pressure pulses in the cuff are similar time-course of the murmurs (**Figure 16**). After the digital processing of the signal of the pressure sensor, the display of the device shows numerical values of the systolic and diastolic pressure and the heart rate. Oscillometric instruments are simple and do not require any special operation. Therefore, they are used for home blood pressure control or continuous pressure monitoring. In the case of a one-time medical examination, doctors prefer the auscultation method because of its better accuracy.

1.9.3 Ultrasonography

1.9.3.1 Basic ultrasonographic imaging

Ultrasonography is a diagnostic method that uses the propagation of ultrasound in substances and its reflection on the impedance interfaces, for example, LABUDA [1], SHUNG [2]. In technical practice, there exists ultrasonic flaw detection (engineering, construction), which allows the examination of cracks or inhomogeneities in a material. Medical ultrasonography (USG) enables imaging of the internal organs of the body with different acoustic impedance. The ultrasonic transducer generates a short ultrasonic pulse on the surface of the body. It proceeds into the depth of the body, reflects from the impedance interfaces of the organ's tissue, and returns to the transducer. It now serves as a detector of the reflected pulses. The detected signal is processed by a receiver and then displayed on the screen of the USG device (**Figure 17**).

The imaging indicated in the figure, in which the magnitude of the reflected signal is displayed by the height of the pulse is called the A-mode (amplitude). Each pulse displays the impedance interface. The time delay t corresponds to the depth $d = c\ t/2$ of the interface under the surface, where c is the speed of ultrasound inside the body.

Structured piezoelectric transducers are the main part of the probes with shapes adapted to specific applications. Several examples of USG probes are in **Figure 18**. The USG probes consist of an array of many small transducers, which allows forming the ultrasound beam.

In the case of 2D imaging, the B-mode (brightness) is used. In this mode, the signal modulates the brightness of the track. An example of comparing A-mode and B-mode is in **Figure 19**.

If a series of parallel or diverging ultrasonic beams are successively sent into the object under investigation, brightness modulated lines are obtained for each of them. By displaying these lines on the monitor, a 2D brightness modulated profile of the internal structure of the object occurs, **Figure 20**. **Figure 20(a)** shows an image of a vessel provided by a series of parallel beams (rectangular image). **Figure 20(b)**

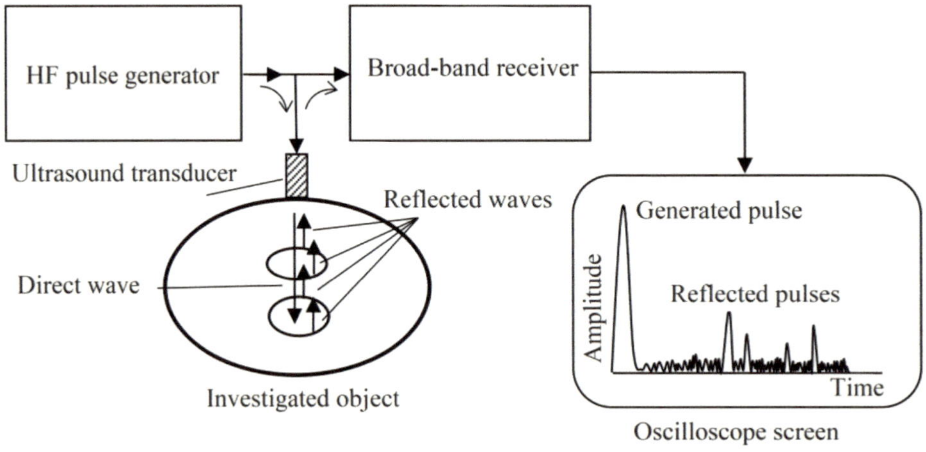

Figure 17.
Displaying of reflected ultrasonic signals in the A-mode.

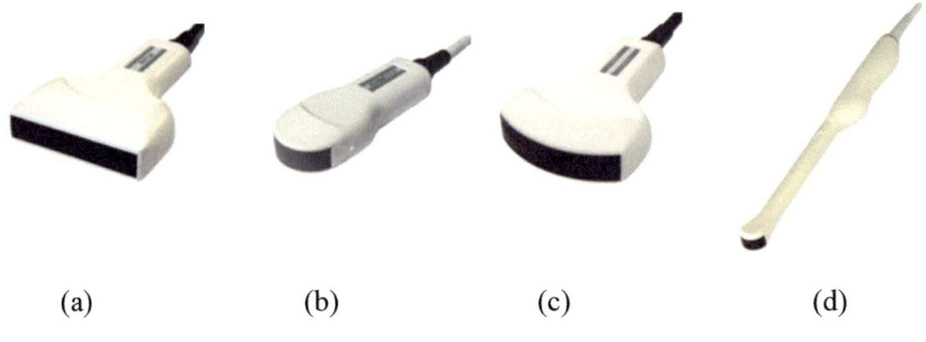

Figure 18.
Several types of USG probes - linear (a), convex (b) and (c), endoscopic (d).

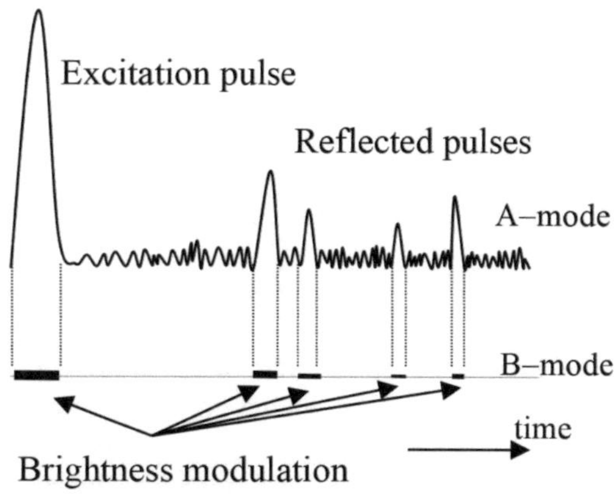

Figure 19.
Comparison of A-mode and B-mode of imaging.

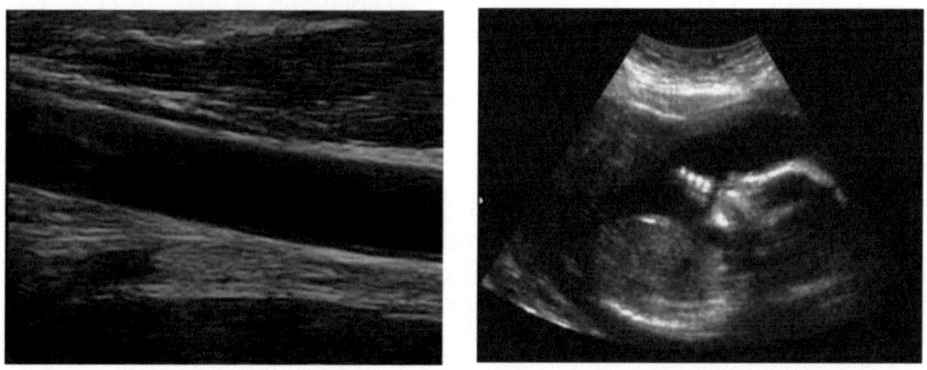

Figure 20.
Ultrasonographic 2D-imaging: (a) rectangular imaging of a vessel with a linear probe, (b) sectoral imaging of a foetus in the mother's body by a convex probe. (royalty free stock photos: https://www.123rf.com).

shows a foetus in the body of a mother by a series of diverging beams, arranged in a certain angular sector.

As ultrasonography utilises the principle of ultrasound reflection, it is not suitable for imaging structural parts with an extreme value of the acoustic impedance, gas-filled cavities with a very low impedance, or solid tissues (bones) with a very high impedance. Ultrasound is practically completely reflected from the surface of such objects, and therefore, it is not possible to obtain information about the structures behind these surfaces. The method is suitable for imaging soft tissues, for example, imaging of the heart, kidney, liver, digestive tract, etc. Since ultrasonography has no adverse effects on the human body, it is even used to examine the foetus in the mother's body, **Figure 20(b)**.

1.9.3.2 Doppler sonography

The Doppler effect is used in acoustic diagnostics to track moving objects, for example, heart, blood flow, etc. When ultrasound reflects from the object that moves in the direction of the ultrasound beam, the frequency of the reflected ultrasound is changed due to the Doppler effect. Doppler sonography device has an electrical circuit for separating signals with the shifted frequency (frequency discriminator), which have been generated by reflection from moving parts of organs, for example, from the beating heart, or from flowing blood. These signals are digitally colour-coded and displayed in a sonogram. Doppler detection also allows suppressing reflections with the original frequency from stationary parts, thus improving the contrast of the image of moving organs. Since the processing of the frequency-shifted signal is time and memory-consuming due to every pixel of the image colour-coding, the Doppler mode is not used for the whole image. The doctor chooses Doppler mode only for a selected demanded part of the image, see **Figure 21**.

The left image is a picture of blood flow through *stenosis* (narrowing of a blood vessel) from the left side rightwards. The ultrasound image is approximately parallel to the vessel, that is, laminar blood flow before stenosis (left side) is red-coloured (see coding on the left side of the image). Behind the stenosis (right side), the blood flow is complex—turbulent, while some blood flowing towards the transducer is yellow-coloured, and blood flowing from the transducer is blue-coloured.

The right image is a picture of the blood flow through the ventricle. Current technical means, especially fast computers, allow obtaining an image in a few tenths of a second so that it is possible to observe the motion of the object online. An example of an online Doppler image of the ventricle in motion can be seen at the page http://cs.wikipedia.org/wiki/Soubor:Doppler_mitral_valve.gif.

1.9.4 Ultrasonic measurement of blood flow in vessels

The Doppler effect allows measuring blood flow in vessels. A principle of the device is in **Figure 22**. It uses a continuous harmonic ultrasonic wave with a frequency of 4–8 MHz, which generates a transmitting transducer T of the probe. Erythrocytes in the blood (the largest blood particles) disperse the ultrasonic wave, and the Doppler-shifted wave returning to the probe detects the receiving transducer R.

The device evaluates the Doppler shift of frequency and displays it in units of blood flow velocity. If we know the cross-section of the vessel, for example, from ultrasonographic measurement, one can determine the volume flow of blood in the vessel. The specific shape of the course of the blood velocity versus time, (**Figure 22** right), the leading and trailing edges of the pulses, various maxima, and minima provide information about the state of the vascular system.

The method is relatively simple and therefore is suitable for indicative angiological investigation. The disadvantage of the method is that the probe reads a response from all vessels, and it is problematic to evaluate only the single one. On the other hand, it is advantageous for an examination of vessels with high blood velocity and of subsurface vessels, for example, in dermatology and phlebology.

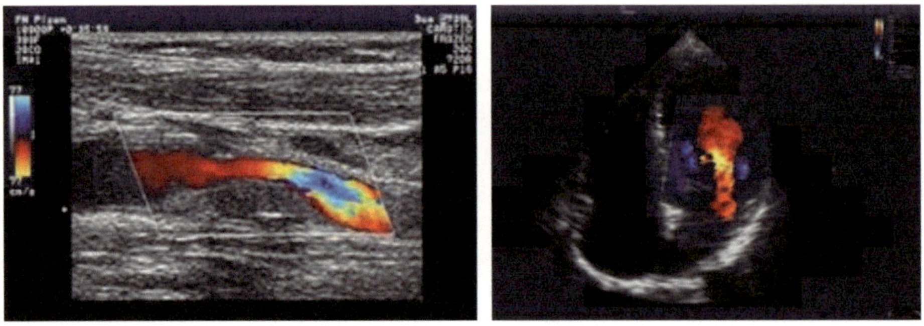

Figure 21.
Doppler ultrasonography images.

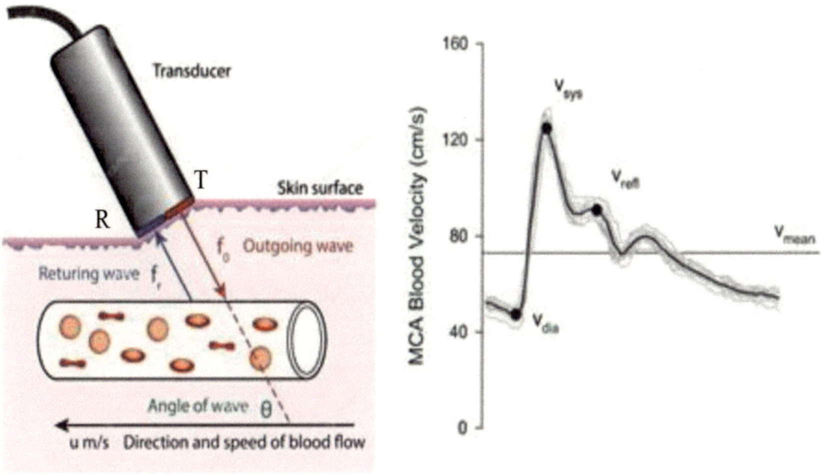

Figure 22.
Blood flow rate probe.

Author details

Ivo Čáp*, Klára Čápová, Milan Smetana and Štefan Borik
Faculty of Electrical Engineering and Information Technology, University of Žilina, Slovakia

*Address all correspondence to: ivo.cap@fel.uniza.sk

References

[1] Labuda M, Vaverka F, Borik S. Ultrasound based distance measurement and assessment of obstacles in the area– a concept for educational purposes. In: 2020 ELEKTRO. IEEE; Žilina: 2020. pp. 1-4

[2] Shung KK. Diagnostic Ultrasound – Imaging and Blood Flow Measurement. Boca Raton: CRC Press; 2006. ISBN: 978-0-8247-4096-2

Chapter 5

Electromagnetic Waves

Ivo Čáp, Klára Čápová, Milan Smetana and Štefan Borik

1. Introduction

There exist various forms of energy in the universe, for example, the kinetic and potential energy of bodies, the internal energy of substances, associated with bonding and microscopic motion of atoms and molecules, nuclear energy associated with atomic nuclei composition, the energy of the gravitational and electromagnetic field. The universal law of energy conservation expresses that energy cannot arise or disappear, and it can only change from one form to another. An important part of the energy of the universe is electromagnetic energy that we perceive through various electrical, magnetic, and electromagnetic phenomena. They are widely used in biomedicine both in diagnostics, e.g., thermography, microscopy, MRI, endoscopy, fluoroscopy, computed tomography, PET, SPECT, and in therapy, e.g., diathermy, microwave hyperthermia, phototherapy, laser scalpel, exposition to ionizing radiation. We present an overview of basic knowledge, which provides a deeper understanding of biomedical applications of electromagnetic waves and the possibilities of their practical use, see also Rajeev [1, 2], Someda [3].

Classical electrodynamics is based on the definition of the basic field quantities, which are the intensity of electric field $\boldsymbol{E}$ and induction of the magnetic field $\boldsymbol{B}$, defined by the force $\boldsymbol{F}$ of the electromagnetic (EM) field on a particle with a charge Q moving at velocity $\boldsymbol{v}$ by the Lorentz relation

$$\boldsymbol{F} = Q\boldsymbol{E} \; + \; Q \; \boldsymbol{v} \times \boldsymbol{B}. \tag{1}$$

In addition to the electric charge, the particles also have a magnetic dipole moment $\boldsymbol{m}$, which describes another type of interaction of a particle, of a magnetic dipole, with a magnetic field with the induction $\boldsymbol{B}$ by.

$$\boldsymbol{M} = \mathbf{m} \times \boldsymbol{B}, \quad \boldsymbol{F} = \mathbf{m} \; \text{grad} \; \boldsymbol{B}, \quad E_\text{p} = -\mathbf{m} \cdot \boldsymbol{B} + E_{\text{p}0}, \tag{2}$$

where $\boldsymbol{M}$ is the moment (torque) of the force $\boldsymbol{F}$ exerting on the dipole, and E_p is the potential energy of the magnetic dipole in the magnetic field.

In addition to the primary quantities $\boldsymbol{E}$, $\boldsymbol{B}$, other ones, electric induction $\boldsymbol{D}$, and magnetic intensity $\boldsymbol{H}$, are defined. They take the properties of the medium into account, in which we follow the EM field.

The classical description of the EM field is based on Maxwell's equations

$$\textbf{curl}\,\mathbf{H} = \mathbf{J} + \frac{\partial \mathbf{D}}{\partial t}, \tag{3}$$

$$\textbf{curl}\,\mathbf{E} = -\frac{\partial \mathbf{B}}{\partial t}, \tag{4}$$

$$\text{div}\,\mathbf{B} = 0, \tag{5}$$

$$\text{div}\,\mathbf{D} = \rho, \tag{6}$$

IntechOpen

where $\boldsymbol{J}$ is the current density of free charge carriers and ρ is the free charge density.

The quantities $\boldsymbol{D}$ and $\boldsymbol{E}$, and quantities $\boldsymbol{H}$ and $\boldsymbol{B}$ are mutually connected by the material relations, which reflect the properties of the medium as homogeneity-inhomogeneity, linearity-nonlinearity, isotropy-anisotropy, etc.

In the case of a linear, homogeneous, and isotropic medium are valid simple relations between the field quantities.

$$\boldsymbol{B} = \mu\,\boldsymbol{H}, \boldsymbol{D} = \varepsilon\,\boldsymbol{E}, \tag{7}$$

where constant coefficients μ, ε are permeability and permittivity of the medium.
The current density has two components.

$$\boldsymbol{J} = \boldsymbol{J}_0 + \gamma\,\boldsymbol{E}, \tag{8}$$

where $\boldsymbol{J}_0$ is the current density of the forced source current, the component $\gamma\boldsymbol{E}$ is the current density of the passive current induced by the electric field in the conductive medium, and γ is the conductivity of the medium.

From the Maxwell Eqs. (3) and (4), using relations (7) and (8), we can express separately the equation for electric intensity $\boldsymbol{E}$ and magnetic induction $\boldsymbol{B}$. In the first Maxwell equation we differentiate according to time, on the second one we apply operator **curl,** and we consider the relation $\partial/\partial t$ **curl** $\boldsymbol{B}$ = **curl** $\partial\boldsymbol{B}/\partial t$

$$\frac{\partial}{\partial t}\ \mathbf{curl}\ \mathbf{B} = \mu\ \frac{\partial \mathbf{J}_0}{\partial t} + \mu\gamma\ \frac{\partial \mathbf{E}}{\partial t} + \mu\varepsilon\ \frac{\partial^2 \mathbf{E}}{\partial t^{\ 2}}, \tag{9}$$

$$\mathbf{curl}\ \mathbf{curl}\ \mathbf{E} = -\mathbf{curl}\ \frac{\partial \mathbf{B}}{\partial t} = \mathbf{grad}\ \mathrm{div}\ \mathbf{E} - \Delta\mathbf{E} \tag{10}$$

We get the equation

$$\Delta\,\mathbf{E} - \mu\gamma\ \frac{\partial \mathbf{E}}{\partial t} - \mu\varepsilon\ \frac{\partial^2 \mathbf{E}}{\partial t^{\ 2}} = \mu\ \frac{\partial \mathbf{J}_0}{\partial t} + \mathbf{grad}\ \frac{\rho}{\varepsilon}. \tag{11}$$

In the same way, we get the equation for magnetic induction

$$\Delta\mathbf{B} - \mu\gamma\ \frac{\partial \mathbf{B}}{\partial t} - \mu\varepsilon\ \frac{\partial^2 \mathbf{B}}{\partial t^{\ 2}} = -\mu\ \mathbf{curl}\mathbf{J}_0. \tag{12}$$

The left sides of the equations are typical for the wave equation (compare with the mechanical one). They are wave equations of a damped wave. The right sides of the equations represent the source functions of the wave. The source of the EM field is the gradient of charge density and the charge movement described by the curl of the current density. Nonhomogeneous distribution of charge is the source of the electrostatic field component, while the charge motion is the source of the magnetic component of the electromagnetic field. From the equations (11) and (12) follows that the EM field propagates in space as a wave and the electric component, given by the vector $\boldsymbol{E}$, and magnetic component given by the vector $\boldsymbol{B}$, have the common space-time dependence and represent only one physical object—the electromagnetic wave. In the space out of the source, the right sides of the wave equations are equal to zero, from which follows that EM wave can propagate in the space independently without the presence of other sources.

1.1 Plane electromagnetic wave

The basic characteristics of EM wave best explain the simplest example of the plane wave, in which the quantities depend only on one space variable z-coordinate in the direction of the wave propagation. The plane wave quantities $\boldsymbol{E}$ and $\boldsymbol{B}$ are not dependent on space coordinates x and y in the directions perpendicular to the wave propagation direction.

Let us consider the wave which propagates in linear homogeneous and isotropic medium out of sources (where ε, μ, g are constants, $\rho = 0, \boldsymbol{J}_0 = 0$). Under these assumptions, the Maxwell equations have the form

$$-\frac{\partial B_x}{\partial z}\ \mathbf{y}^0 + \frac{\partial B_y}{\partial z}\ \mathbf{x}^0 = \mu\gamma\ \left(E_x\mathbf{x}^0 + E_y\mathbf{y}^0 + E_z\mathbf{z}^0\right) + \mu\varepsilon\ \frac{\partial}{\partial t}\left(E_x x^0 + E_y\mathbf{y}^0 + E_z\mathbf{z}^0\right)$$

$$-\frac{\partial E_x}{\partial z}\ \mathbf{y}^0 + \frac{\partial E_y}{\partial z}\ \mathbf{x}^0 = -\mu\ \frac{\partial}{\partial t}\left(B_x x^0 + B_y\mathbf{y}^0 + B_z\mathbf{z}^0\right),$$

$$\frac{\partial E_z}{\partial z} = 0 \text{ and } \frac{\partial B_z}{\partial z} = 0,$$

where $\boldsymbol{x}^0, \boldsymbol{y}^0, \boldsymbol{z}^\mathbf{0}$ are unit vectors in the directions x, y, z of a rectangular coordinate system.

Comparing the vector components of both sides of the equations we get.

$$\frac{\partial B_y}{\partial z} = \mu\varepsilon\ \frac{\partial E_x}{\partial t},\ -\frac{\partial B_x}{\partial z} = \mu\varepsilon\ \frac{\partial E_y}{\partial t}, \tag{13}$$

$$\frac{\partial E_y}{\partial z} = -\mu\ \frac{\partial B_x}{\partial t},\ -\frac{\partial E_x}{\partial z} = -\mu\ \frac{\partial B_y}{\partial t}, \tag{14}$$

$$0 = \mu\varepsilon\ \frac{\partial E_z}{\partial t}, \frac{\partial E_z}{\partial z} = 0, 0 = -\mu\ \frac{\partial B_z}{\partial t}, \frac{\partial B_z}{\partial z} = 0. \tag{15}$$

From Eq. (15) follow that the time and space-dependent longitudinal components of electric intensity and magnetic induction are zero. Non-zero wave components are only transversal ones.

Let us apply the axes x, y, z in the way, that axis x has the direction of the vector of electric intensity, which means $\boldsymbol{E} = E_z\,\boldsymbol{x}^0$, and $E_y = 0$. It results from the Eqs. (13) and (14) that wave component $B_z = 0$. Magnetic induction is then $\boldsymbol{B} = B_y\,\boldsymbol{y}^0$.

The electromagnetic wave has transversal polarization, vectors $\boldsymbol{E}, \boldsymbol{B}$ are mutually perpendicular and perpendicular to the direction of wave propagation.

Eqs. (11) and (12) have the form

$$\frac{\partial^2 E_x}{\partial z^{\ 2}} - \ \mu\gamma\ \frac{\partial E_x}{\partial t} - \mu\varepsilon\ \frac{\partial^2 E_x}{\partial t^{\ 2}} = 0, \qquad E_y = E_z = 0, \tag{16}$$

$$\frac{\partial^2 B_y}{\partial z^{\ 2}} - \ \mu\gamma\ \frac{\partial B_y}{\partial t} - \mu\varepsilon\ \frac{\partial^2 B_y}{\partial t^{\ 2}} = 0, \qquad B_x = B_z = 0. \tag{17}$$

1.1.1 Plane EM wave in a lossless medium

In the medium with the non-zero conductance, $\gamma \neq 0$, arises electric current with the current density $\boldsymbol{J}$. The current in the material relates to the transformation of EM wave energy into heat. This energy loss causes EM wave attenuation.

If the medium conductance is zero (vacuum or the ideal dielectrics), $\gamma = 0$, the plane wave equations have the form

$$\frac{\partial^2 \mathbf{E}}{\partial z^{\ 2}} - \mu\varepsilon\ \frac{\partial^2 \mathbf{E}}{\partial t^{\ 2}} = 0, \tag{18}$$

$$\frac{\partial^2 \mathbf{B}}{\partial z^{\ 2}} - \mu\varepsilon \ \frac{\partial^2 \mathbf{B}}{\partial t^{\ 2}} = 0. \tag{19}$$

These are wave equations of a non-damped EM wave that propagates in the direction of the z- axis with a speed

$$c = \sqrt{\frac{1}{\mu\varepsilon}} = \sqrt{\frac{1}{\mu_0\,\varepsilon_0}} \ \frac{1}{\sqrt{\mu_r\,\varepsilon_r}} = \frac{c_0}{n}, \tag{20}$$

where c_0 is the speed of EM wave in a vacuum and $n = \sqrt{\mu_r\,\varepsilon_r}$ is the absolute refraction index of the medium in which the wave propagates. If the medium is homogeneous one, and the refraction index is independent on frequency, i.e., n = const., the generated EM wave propagates in space with the speed c without any distortion.

Example 1. Propagation of EM wave in a dielectric medium.

As an example, we introduce the speed of EM wave in vacuum ($\varepsilon_0 = 8.85 \times 10^{-12}$ F m^{-1}, $\mu_0 = 4\pi \times 10^{-7}$ H m^{-1}), $c_0 = 3.00 \times 10^8$ m s^{-1}).

At the frequency of 100 Hz is the relative permittivity of water $\varepsilon_{\,r1} = 81$ and $\mu_{\,r} = 1$, i.e., the refraction index $n_1 \sim 9.0$, and the speed of the EM wave $c_1 = 3.3 \times 10^7$ m s^{-1}.

The relative permittivity of water depends on frequency. In the optical range of frequencies, the relative permittivity $\varepsilon_{r2} = 1.77$, refraction index $n \approx 1.33$, and the speed of light $c_2 = 2.25 \times 10^8$ m s^{-1}.

Glass refraction index n = 1.5–1.9 according to the sort of glass, i.e., the speed of light $c \approx (1.58–2.00) \times 10^8$ m s^{-1}.

Air refraction index at the standard conditions $n = 1.00059$, i.e., the speed of EM wave in the air is $c = 2.99283 \times 10^8$ m s^{-1}. For most of the applications is used $c \approx c_0$. When considering inhomogeneity of the air or a wave dispersion, it is necessary to take the speed of light in the air with an accuracy of 5 decimal numbers.

1.1.2 Harmonic plane electromagnetic wave

1.1.2.1 Wave function of harmonic EM wave

If the exciting current of the EM wave has the harmonic time dependence with the angular frequency ω, then in a linear medium, all quantities of EM field also have the harmonic time dependence with the same angular frequency ω. Let us consider the EM wave in the loss medium.

The complex harmonic functions we express by relations.

$$\mathbf{E}(z,t) = \mathbf{E}(z)\ \mathrm{e}^{\mathrm{j}\omega\, t}, \mathbf{H}(z,t) = \mathbf{H}(z)\ \mathrm{e}^{\mathrm{j}\omega\, t}, \tag{21}$$

where $\mathbf{E}(z)$, $\mathbf{H}(z)$ are phasors of the EM wave.

The complex quantities we introduce into wave equations (11) and (12), we realize time derivatives and reduce time function.

For the wave out of the source, we get equations for the phasors of the field quantities

$$\frac{\mathrm{d}^2\mathbf{E}(z)}{\mathrm{d}z^2} - \left(\mathrm{j}\omega\mu\gamma - \omega^2\mu\,\varepsilon\right)\ \mathbf{E}(z) = 0, \tag{22}$$

$$\frac{\mathrm{d}^2\mathbf{H}(z)}{\mathrm{d}z^2} - \left(\mathrm{j}\omega\mu\gamma - \omega^2\mu\,\varepsilon\right)\ \mathbf{H}(z) = 0. \tag{23}$$

Their solutions are the following functions.

$\mathbf{E}(z) = \mathbf{E}_\mathrm{m}\ \mathrm{e}^{\pm \mathbf{k} z}$, $\mathbf{H}(z) = \mathbf{H}_\mathrm{m}\ \mathrm{e}^{\pm \mathbf{k} z}$, where

$$\mathbf{k} = \sqrt{\mathrm{j}\,\omega\mu\,(\gamma + \mathrm{j}\,\omega\varepsilon)} = \beta + \mathrm{j}\,\alpha \tag{24}$$

is complex propagation constant of the EM wave.

The complex wave functions are

$$\mathbf{E}(z,t) = \mathbf{E}_\mathrm{m}^{+}\ \mathrm{e}^{-\beta z}\ \mathrm{e}^{\mathrm{j}\,(\omega\, t - \alpha z)} + \mathbf{E}_\mathrm{m}^{-}\ \mathrm{e}^{\beta z}\ \mathrm{e}^{\mathrm{j}\,(\omega\, t + \alpha z)} \tag{25}$$

$$\mathbf{H}(z,t) = \mathbf{H}_\mathrm{m}^{+}\ \mathrm{e}^{-\beta z}\ \mathrm{e}^{\mathrm{j}\,(\omega\, t - \alpha z)} + \mathbf{H}_\mathrm{m}^{-}\ \mathrm{e}^{\beta z}\ \mathrm{e}^{\mathrm{j}\,(\omega\, t + \alpha z)}. \tag{26}$$

The relations consist of a superposition of direct and reflected waves. The phase argument $\omega\, t - a\, z$ represents the direct wave propagating in the z-direction, and argument $\omega\, t + a\, z$ is the reflected wave in the opposite direction. Both waves exponentially damp in their propagation directions with the attenuation factor β.

The real and imaginary parts of the coefficient **k** we obtain by decomposition of the definition relation (24)

$$\mathbf{k}^2 = \mathrm{j}\,\omega\mu\,(\gamma + \mathrm{j}\,\omega\varepsilon) = \beta^2 - \alpha^2 + \mathrm{j}\,2\alpha\beta. \tag{27}$$

By comparing real parts and imaginary parts on the left and right side we get two equations for α and β, from which we get

$$\beta = \sqrt{\frac{\omega^2\mu\,\varepsilon}{2}}\ \sqrt{-1 + \sqrt{1 + \left(\frac{\gamma}{\omega\,\varepsilon}\right)^2}}, \tag{28}$$

$$\alpha = \sqrt{\frac{\omega^2\mu\,\varepsilon}{2}}\ \sqrt{\ 1 + \sqrt{1 + \left(\frac{\gamma}{\omega\,\varepsilon}\right)^2}}. \tag{29}$$

The attenuation coefficient β determines the effective wave propagation length $\delta = 1/\beta$, at which the amplitude of the wave decreases due to the attenuation in the ratio $\mathrm{e}^{-1} \approx 37\%$.

The coefficient α determines the wavenumber,

$$\textit{the wavelength } \lambda = \frac{2\pi}{\alpha}, \text{and the } \textit{phase velocity of the wave } c = \frac{\omega}{\alpha}. \tag{30}$$

EM waves can propagate in free space, e.g., light from a light source, or in wires, e.g., two-wire line, coaxial line, waveguide, optical fiber, etc. In the case of EM wave propagation in confined structures, the propagation parameters (phase velocity and attenuation) also depend on the geometrical arrangement of the line.

1.1.2.2 EM wave propagation in a low-loss medium

In the case of a low-loss medium, for which $\gamma \ll \omega\,\varepsilon$ at low conductivity γ of the medium, and/or high-frequency ω, the propagation constants α and β are given by approximate relations

$$\beta \approx \frac{\gamma}{2}\ \sqrt{\frac{\mu}{\varepsilon}}, \qquad \alpha = \omega\sqrt{\mu\,\varepsilon}\ , \tag{31}$$

from which we get the phase velocity c of the wave and the effective propagation length δ.

$$c = \frac{1}{\sqrt{\mu\,\varepsilon}} = \frac{1}{\sqrt{\mu_0\,\varepsilon_0}}\,\frac{1}{\sqrt{\mu_r\,\varepsilon_r}} = \frac{c_0}{n}, \text{and } \delta \approx \frac{2}{\gamma}\,\sqrt{\frac{\varepsilon}{\mu}}. \tag{32}$$

If the material parameters of the medium are constant, then both quantities are constant and independent of the frequency. However, when moving from one frequency domain to another, e.g., from the radio waves to the optical region, the parameters may change significantly, resulting in a change in phase velocity and effective wave propagation length.

1.1.2.3 EM wave propagation in a conductive medium

In the case of a conductive medium where $\gamma \gg \omega\,\varepsilon$, the propagation coefficients are given by approximate relations.

$$\beta \approx \sqrt{\frac{\omega\,\mu\,\gamma}{2}} \text{ and } \alpha \approx \sqrt{\frac{\omega\,\mu\,\gamma}{2}}\ . \tag{33}$$

Effective wave propagation length $\delta \approx \sqrt{\frac{2}{\omega\,\mu\,\gamma}}$ decreases with increasing frequency.

The phase velocity of a wave $c = \frac{\omega}{\alpha} = \sqrt{\frac{2\omega}{\mu\gamma}}$ depends on the frequency.

The wavelength $\lambda = \frac{2\pi}{\alpha} = 2\pi\ \delta$, i.e., the length δ is about 1/6 of λ.

Example 2. EM wave in a conductor.

Consider an EM wave with a frequency of 10 MHz propagating in the copper with γ = 56 MS m^{-1}, and μ_r = 1.00. The wave propagates in the medium as damped one with parameters: $\delta \approx$ 21.3 μm, $c \approx$ 1340 m s^{-1}, λ = 134 μm.

As a result, we can see that the EM wave incident on the surface of the metal penetrates only a very thin surface layer. This effect calls the *skin effect*.

The penetrating EM wave causes an eddy current in the surface layer of the conductor. Due to the current flow, the energy of the EM wave changes into heat in the medium. This loss of energy causes wave attenuation. On passing the depth δ, the amount of 86% of the EM wave power penetrating the conductor is consumed. Changing the frequency allows controlling the penetration depth δ. The absorption of wave energy is utilized for heating conducting bodies. For example, a microwave oven uses an EM field with a frequency of 2.45 GHz. Assuming a meat conductivity of approximately 0.1 S m^{-1}, we obtain $\delta \approx$ 3 cm. So, the heat is releases in a thick surface layer of the meat, and the whole volume warms. In the case of a grill that uses infrared radiation with a wavelength of about 10 μm (f = 30 THz), we have $\delta \approx$ 0.3 mm. In this case, the wave energy converts to heat in a very thin surface layer, and such a crispy crust arises. The rest of the meat volume is then warmed by the heat conduction from the surface to the inside. In medicine, the heating of tissues is used for therapeutic purposes.

Hyperthermia (tissue warming) aims to destroy the tumors, which are sensitive to overheating. By selecting a suitable frequency, one can adjust the action to the required depth below the surface of the body.

Thermotherapy utilizes stimulation of some physiological processes and, in such a way, speeds up the treatment (e.g., diathermy using EM waves up to tens of MHz, hyperthermia using microwave radiation, phototherapy using optical radiation, etc.).

A thin layer of skin protects the subcutaneous organs from the effects of light and UV radiation. A thin layer of eyelids protects the eye from the direct influence of sunlight (looking into the sun with the eyelids closed). Protecting the body against overheating by the direct impact of intensive radiation realizes sweating due to the conversion of the absorbed energy into the latent heat of evaporation.

The electrical conductivity of the tissue varies with the frequency. At frequencies above the infrared band, the conductivity significantly drops. Despite the increasing frequency, the effective depth of the wave penetration increases. While ultraviolet radiation has an effective penetration depth of less than 1 mm, that of X-rays is of about tens centimeters, which allows imaging of body structures by transmission radiology (X-ray, CT-Computed Tomography), utilizing different attenuation of radiation in different tissues.

1.1.2.4 Dielectric parameters of substances

In biomedical applications, we are interested in the propagation of EM waves in non-magnetic media with relative permeability $\mu_r = 1$. Substances thus describe the relative permittivity ε_r and the conductivity γ. We often consider tissues or the surrounding media as lossy dielectrics.

For the harmonic wave, the first Maxwell equation has a form

$$\mathbf{curl\,H} = \gamma\mathbf{E} + \mathrm{j}\omega\varepsilon\mathbf{E} = \mathrm{j}\omega\varepsilon_0\left(\varepsilon_r - \mathrm{j}\frac{\gamma}{\omega\varepsilon_0}\right) = \mathrm{j}\omega\;\varepsilon_0\boldsymbol{\varepsilon}_r, \tag{34}$$

where $\boldsymbol{\varepsilon}_r = \varepsilon_r' - \mathrm{j}\varepsilon_r''$ is a complex relative permittivity. The real part ε_r' determines the displacement current in the substance, the imaginary part ε_r'' is called the loss factor, and it is related to the attenuation of the wave by the conversion of the EM field energy into heat. Quantities ε_r', ε_r'', and γ are complicated functions of the frequency of the harmonic wave.

The permittivity of the substances is influenced by internal relaxation processes, especially in liquid substances, that characterizes the relationship

$$\boldsymbol{\varepsilon}_r = \varepsilon_\infty + \frac{\varepsilon_s - \varepsilon_\infty}{1 + \mathrm{j}\omega\tau},$$

where ε_s is the static value, ε_∞ the high-frequency (optical) value, and τ is the characteristic relaxation time. The real part corresponds to ε_r', and the imaginary one is a part of the loss factor ε_r'' together with conductivity γ.

An example of the frequency dependence of ε_r' and ε_r'' for water and ice is shown in **Figure 1**. The value drops from the initial value ε_s to the optical level ε_∞ after the relaxation process. E.g., for water, at low frequencies $\varepsilon_r' \approx 81$, but in the optical band $\varepsilon_r' \approx 1.77$. In the interval around the relaxation frequency, the value of the loss factor ε_r'' significantly increases (dashed line in the figure). The relaxation frequency of pure water is approximately 10 GHz. For water bound in tissues, the frequency of the maximum loss factor is lower. Therefore, EM wave with a frequency of 2.45 GHz uses the microwave oven for the most efficient heating of food.

In **Table 1**, there are some typical values of the conductivity of selected tissues for different frequencies. We see that the conductivity at low frequencies is of the order of 0.01–1.00 S m^{-1} (except for dry skin) and increases significantly with the frequency above 1 GHz.

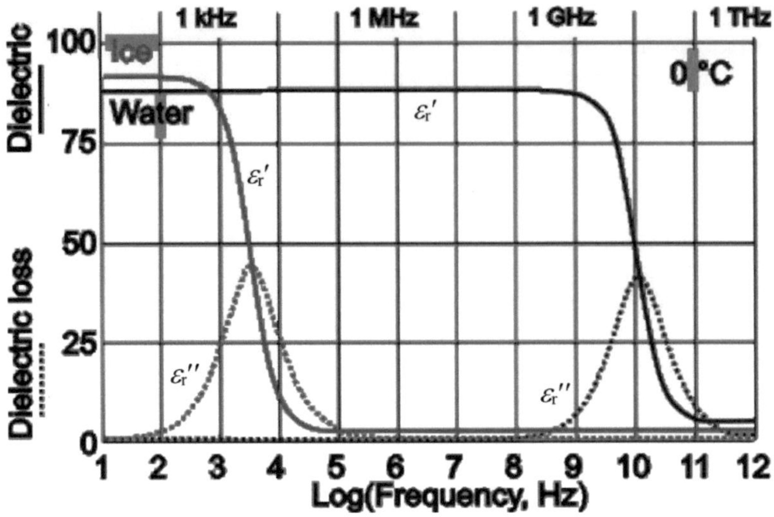

Figure 1.
Frequency dependence of components of complex relative permittivity (source: http://www1.lsbu.ac.uk/water/microwave_water.html).

	Tissue conductivity at different frequencies γ/(S/m)				
	100 Hz	100 kHz	10 MHz	1 GHz	100 GHz
Blood	0.700	0.70	1.10	1.58	63.4
Brain	0.109	0.154	0.378	1.31	48.2
Nerve	0.0280	0.0808	0.223	0.600	30.9
Liver	0.0381	0.0846	0.317	0.897	42.9
Lungs inhaled	0.0730	0.107	0.225	0.474	21.4
Kidney	0.102	0.171	0.508	1.45	57.1
Muscles	0.267	0.362	0.617	0.978	62.5
Tendons	0.305	0,389	0.408	0.760	34.9
Fat	0.0406	0.0434	0.0526	0,116	10.6
Bone cortical	0.0201	0.0208	0.0428	12.4	8.66
Dry skin	2.00×10^{-4}	4.51×10^{-4}	0.197	0.900	39.4
Water	2.30×10^{-15}	2.30×10^{-9}	2.30×10^{-5}	0.229	84.4

Table 1.
Tissue conductivity (https://www.itis.ethz.ch/virtual-population/tissue-properties/database/dielectric-properties/).

Tissues with a high content of water are not typical dielectrics. As you see in **Table 2**, the low-frequency relative permittivity is very high, of the order up to10^6. After the first relaxation around 1 MHz, it decreases to the values of the order of 10^1 to 10^2 and then above 10 GHz to values of the order of units. High values at low frequencies cause organic components (macromolecules) in the tissue, which contribute only a little to the alternating polarization at high frequencies.

Knowledge of these values is important for various applications, e.g., diathermy at frequencies of tens of MHz or hyperthermia at frequencies above 1 GHz.

	Relative permittivity at different frequencies $\varepsilon_r'/(-)$				
	100 Hz	**100 kHz**	**10 MHz**	**1 GHz**	**100 GHz**
Blood	5.26×10^3	5.12×10^3	280	61.1	8.30
Brain	3.91×10^6	3.52×10^3	465	48.9	7.38
Nerve	4.66×10^5	5.13×10^3	155	32.3	6.18
Liver	6.78×10^5	7.50×10^3	223	46.4	6.87
Lungs inhaled	1.77×10^6	2.58×10^3	124	21.8	4.00
Kidney	3.52×10^6	7.65×10^3	371	57.9	8.04
Muscles	9.33×10^6	8.09×10^3	171	54.8	8.63
Tendons	1.19×10^7	472	103	45.6	5.98
Fat	1.52×10^5	101	29.6	11.3	3.67
Bone cortical	5.85×10^3	228	36.8	0.156	3.30
Dry skin	1.14×10^3	1.12×10^3	362	40.9	5.6
Water	84.6	84.6	84.6	84.4	8.48

Table 2.
Relative permittivity of tissues.

Example 3. At the frequency of 100 MHz, the muscle parameters are γ = 0.708 S m^{-1}, ε_r = 66, and μ_r = 1.00. The value $\omega\,\varepsilon$ = 0.367 S m^{-1}, which is comparable with the value of γ. For the calculation, we use formulas (28) and (29). After substitution, we have $\beta \approx 3.93$ m^{-1}, $\alpha \approx 21.4$ m^{-1}. From here we get an effective EM wave propagation length of $\delta \approx 25$ cm, a phase velocity of 2.94×10^7 m s^{-1}, and a wavelength of $\lambda \approx 29$ cm.

Thus, most of the energy of EM radiation is absorbed in the tissue in a layer with a depth of approximately $\delta/2 \approx 12.5$ cm.

1.1.2.5 Wave impedance

A quantity, important especially in the transition of waves from one medium to another, is the wave impedance **Z** of the medium, which is the ratio of the phasors of the electric intensity **E** and the magnetic intensity **H**.

From Maxwell's equations for the planar EM wave, which propagates in the direction of the axis z, see equations (14), we obtain the relation for the wave impedance of a direct harmonic wave

$$-\mathbf{k}\ \mathbf{E}^+(z,t) = -\mathrm{j}\,\omega\mu\ \mathbf{H}^+(z,t) \tag{35}$$

from where

$$\mathbf{Z} = \frac{\mathbf{E}_\mathrm{m}^+}{\mathbf{H}_\mathrm{m}^+} = \frac{\omega\mu}{\mathbf{k}} = \sqrt{\frac{\mathrm{j}\,\omega\mu}{\gamma + \mathrm{j}\,\omega\varepsilon}}. \tag{36}$$

Z is the *complex wave impedance* of the medium.

For the back wave, we get similarly

$$\mathbf{Z} = -\frac{\mathbf{E}_\mathrm{m}^-}{\mathbf{H}_\mathrm{m}^-}. \tag{37}$$

The complex wave impedance is a complex number.

$$\mathbf{Z} = Z\ \mathrm{e}^{\mathrm{j}\varphi}, \text{where } Z = \frac{E_\mathrm{m}}{H_\mathrm{m}} = \sqrt{\frac{\omega\mu}{\sqrt{\gamma^2 + (\omega\varepsilon)^2}}}, \text{ and } \varphi = \frac{\pi}{4} - \frac{1}{2}\ \arctan\frac{\omega\varepsilon}{\gamma}. \quad (38)$$

The absolute value Z of the complex impedance indicates the ratio of the amplitudes of the electric field intensity and the magnetic field intensity. The argument φ of the complex impedance represents the phase shift of the electric field intensity wave function relative to the magnetic field intensity.

For low loss medium $\gamma \ll \omega\,\varepsilon$ (dielectrics).

$$Z \approx \sqrt{\frac{\mu}{\varepsilon}}, \text{ and} \qquad \varphi \approx 0. \quad (39)$$

For high-conductivity medium $\gamma \gg \omega\,\varepsilon$ (conductor).

$$Z \approx \sqrt{\frac{\omega\mu}{\gamma}}, \text{ and } \varphi \approx \pi/4 \text{ rad} = 45°. \quad (40)$$

Example 4. Wave impedance of selected materials.

Vacuum wave impedance $Z_0 = \sqrt{\mu_0/\varepsilon_0} \approx 377\ \Omega$ is practically the wave impedance of air. The dielectric wave impedance ($\gamma \approx 0$ and $\mu_\mathrm{r} = 1$) is a real quantity, e.g., distilled, and deionized water is a non-conductor with a permittivity $\varepsilon_\mathrm{r} = 81$ in the radiofrequency range. The wave impedance is $Z = Z_0/\sqrt{\varepsilon_r} \approx 42\ \Omega$. For glass with a relative permittivity $\varepsilon_\mathrm{r} \approx 7.6$ for the order of magnitudes, $Z \approx 137\ \Omega$), but with a refractive index $n = 1.7$ for light, $Z = 222\ \Omega$. The wave impedance of copper ($\gamma = 56$ MS m^{-1}, $\mu_\mathrm{r} = 1$), for which $\omega\varepsilon < < \gamma$ holds, has an absolute value $Z \approx 1.2$ mΩ for the frequency $f = 10$ MHz, while the real value $R \approx 0.84$ mΩ is the same size as the imaginary part. The conductor surface is inductive for EM wave.

The wave impedance of vacuum $Z_0 = \sqrt{\mu_0/\varepsilon_0} \approx 377\ \Omega$ is practically the wave impedance of the air. The wave impedance of a dielectric substance ($\gamma \approx 0$ and $\mu_\mathrm{r} = 1$) is a real quantity. E.g., distilled, and deionized water is a non-conductor with a permittivity of $\varepsilon_\mathrm{r} = 81$ in the radio-frequency range. The wave impedance is $Z = Z_0/\sqrt{\varepsilon_r} \approx 42\ \Omega$. For the glass with a relative permittivity $\varepsilon_\mathrm{r} \approx 7.6$ and the radio-frequency range is $Z \approx 137\ \Omega$, but with a refractive index $n = 1.7$ for light is $Z = 222\ \Omega$. The wave impedance of copper ($\gamma = 56$ MS·m^{-1}, $\mu_\mathrm{r} = 1$), for which $\omega\,\varepsilon \ll \gamma$ absolute value $Z \approx 1.2$ mΩ for the frequency $f = 10$ MHz, while the real value $R \approx 0.84$ mΩ is of the same size as the imaginary part. The conductor surface is inductive for the EM wave.

1.2 Power transmitted by electromagnetic waves

Electromagnetic waves also transmit power, which causes, e.g., heating the surface of the body, or a mechanical effect on the body on which the wave incidents. It utilizes hyperthermia, laser scalpel, laser lithotripsy, photoacoustic tomography, and the like. Also, visual perception is proportional to the power of light.

If an electric current flow through the medium, work takes place. The electric power density p is the scalar product $p = \boldsymbol{J} \times \boldsymbol{E}$ of the current density and electric field intensity. If we express the current density by Eq. (3), we get

$$p = \mathbf{E} \cdot \left(\mathbf{curl}\,\mathbf{H} - \frac{\partial \mathbf{D}}{\partial t}\right) = -\mathrm{div}\,(\mathbf{E} \times \mathbf{H}) + \mathbf{H} \cdot \mathbf{curl}\,\mathbf{E} - \mathbf{E} \cdot \frac{\partial \mathbf{D}}{\partial t}. \quad (41)$$

Using equation (4) we have

$$\mathbf{E} \cdot \mathbf{J} = -\text{div}\,(\mathbf{E} \times \mathbf{H}) - \mathbf{H} \cdot \frac{\partial \mathbf{B}}{\partial t} - \mathbf{E} \cdot \frac{\partial \mathbf{D}}{\partial t}. \tag{42}$$

If ε and μ do not depend on time, there is

$$\mathbf{H} \cdot \frac{\partial \mathbf{B}}{\partial t} + \mathbf{E} \cdot \frac{\partial \mathbf{D}}{\partial t} = \frac{\partial}{\partial t}\left(\frac{1}{2}\mathbf{H} \cdot \mathbf{B} + \frac{1}{2}\mathbf{E} \cdot \mathbf{D}\right). \tag{43}$$

We can write the power equation in the form

$$-\frac{\partial}{\partial t}\left(\frac{1}{2}\mathbf{H} \cdot \mathbf{B} + \frac{1}{2}\mathbf{E} \cdot \mathbf{D}\right) = \mathbf{E} \cdot \mathbf{J}_0 + \gamma E^2 + \text{div}\,(\mathbf{E} \times \mathbf{H}). \tag{44}$$

The term

$$e_{\text{EM}} = \frac{1}{2}\mathbf{H} \cdot \mathbf{B} + \frac{1}{2}\mathbf{E} \cdot \mathbf{D} \tag{45}$$

represents the energy density of the electromagnetic field.

Eq. (44) describes the energy balance in the volume element of the medium. The left side represents a negative time change (loss) in energy density. The right side reviews the causes of this change. The first term $\boldsymbol{E} \times \boldsymbol{J}_0$ is the power density of the source current $\boldsymbol{J}_0$ and the second γE^2 the power dissipation density caused by the medium conductivity. Joule losses cause medium heating and EM wave attenuation. The last term in (44) is a decrease in the energy density of the element due to the irradiation of electromagnetic waves to the surroundings.

If we integrate the equation (44) in volume V of the body, we get

$$-\frac{\mathrm{d}}{\mathrm{d}t}\iiint_V e_{\text{EM}}\,\mathrm{d}V = -P_{\text{source}} + P_{\text{loss}} + \oiint_S (\mathbf{E} \times \mathbf{H}) \cdot \mathbf{dS}, \tag{46}$$

where S is the surface that enclose the volume V.

The quantity

$$\mathbf{\Pi} = \mathbf{E} \times \mathbf{H} \tag{47}$$

is called the Poynting vector and represents the areal power density of EM radiation. The radiation power passing through the surface S (radiation power) is

$$P_{\text{rad}} = \iint_S \mathbf{\Pi} \cdot \mathbf{dS}. \tag{48}$$

Mean value of the Poynting vector

$$I = \langle |\mathbf{E} \times \mathbf{H}| \rangle \tag{49}$$

represents the *intensity of radiation*. It is expressed in W m^{-2} units.

In the case of harmonic waves, the intensity of radiation

$$I = E_{\text{m}} H_{\text{m}} \cos\varphi \,\left\langle \cos^2 \omega t \right\rangle = \frac{1}{2} E_{\text{m}} H_{\text{m}} \cos\varphi = EH \cos\varphi, \tag{50}$$

where φ is the phase shift between the phasors **E** and **H** and E, H are the RMS values.

1.3 Transmission of EM waves between two media

When the wave propagates through different spatial structures, various phenomena such as reflection, scattering, interference, diffraction, and the like occur. These phenomena can be both desirable and undesirable. The reflection utilizes, e.g., mirror. The mirror effect also uses EM shielding. On the other hand, due to the reflection of light from the lens surface, the intensity of the radiation entering the glass and passing the lens decreases, and it is, therefore, proper to eliminate the reflection. Waveguides and optical fibers utilize a total reflection of the radiation on the walls. The following paragraphs are devoted to explaining some basic principles and contexts of the mentioned effects.

1.3.1 Reflection and refraction of electromagnetic waves

If the wave incident on the interface of two homogeneous media, there is always a partial reflection from the interface, and a partial crossing of the wave the interface. The phenomena obey the fundamental laws of reflection and refraction, see **Figure 2**.

All three rays, and the normal line (dashed) at the point of impact of the beam to the interface, lie in one plane. If the wave is incident at angle α concerning the normal line to the interface, the angles of reflection α' and refraction β are as follows.

$$\alpha' = \alpha \text{ and } \sin\beta = \frac{c_2}{c_1} \sin\alpha, \text{resp. } \sin\beta = \frac{n_1}{n_2} \sin\alpha. \tag{51}$$

where c_1 and c_2 are the speeds of wave in the individual media, and n_1, n_2 the refractive indices of both media.

1.3.2 Transition of EM waves energy between two media

When assessing the intensity of the wave reflected from the interface and passing through the interface, we will start from the simplifying assumption of the

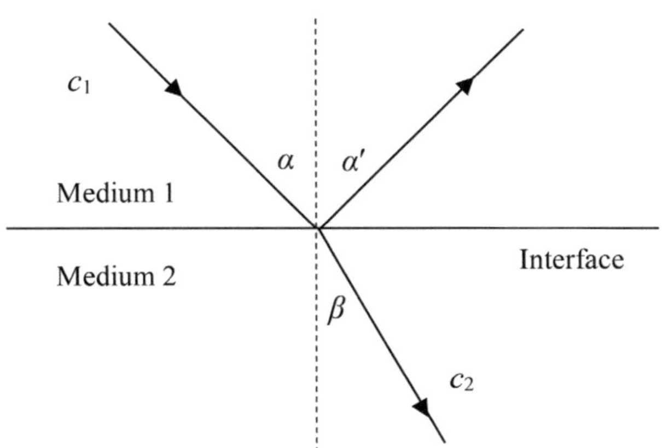

Figure 2.
Reflection and refraction of waves at the interface of two media.

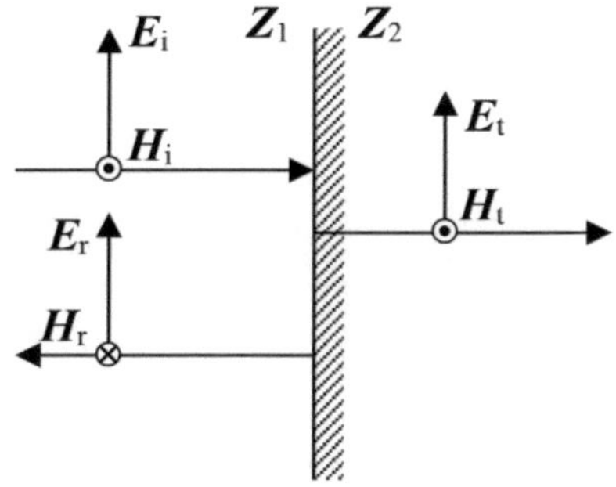

Figure 3.
EM wave transition Prechod EM vlny rozhraním.

perpendicular impact of the harmonic EM wave on the plane interface of two homogeneous environments.

The situation illustrates in **Figure 3**. Indices refer to "i"—incident wave, "t"—transmitted wave, and "r"—reflected wave. The solution of the field at the interface results from the boundary conditions for the EM field. The tangent components of electric and magnetic field intensity are maintained at the interface, i.e.,

$$\mathbf{E}_i + \mathbf{E}_r = \mathbf{E}_t, \tag{52}$$

$$\mathbf{H}_i + \mathbf{H}_r = \mathbf{H}_t, \tag{53}$$

where we have $\mathbf{E}_i = \mathbf{Z}_1\, \mathbf{H}_i$, $\mathbf{E}_t = \mathbf{Z}_2\, \mathbf{H}_t$, and $\mathbf{E}_r = -\mathbf{Z}_1\, \mathbf{H}_r$.

After replacing and adjusting the system of equations, we get relationships.

$$\mathbf{E}_r = \frac{\mathbf{Z}_2 - \mathbf{Z}_1}{\mathbf{Z}_2 + \mathbf{Z}_1}\, \mathbf{E}_i, \mathbf{E}_t = \frac{2\mathbf{Z}_2}{\mathbf{Z}_2 + \mathbf{Z}_1}\, \mathbf{E}_i, \tag{54}$$

$$\mathbf{H}_r = -\frac{\mathbf{Z}_2 - \mathbf{Z}_1}{\mathbf{Z}_2 + \mathbf{Z}_1}\, \mathbf{H}_i, \mathbf{H}_t = \frac{2\mathbf{Z}_1}{\mathbf{Z}_2 + \mathbf{Z}_1}\, \mathbf{H}_i. \tag{55}$$

$$I_r = \left|\frac{\mathbf{Z}_2 - \mathbf{Z}_1}{\mathbf{Z}_2 + \mathbf{Z}_1}\right|^2 I_i, I_t = \frac{4\,\mathrm{Re}\left\{\mathbf{Z}_2 \mathbf{Z}_1^*\right\}}{\left|\mathbf{Z}_2 + \mathbf{Z}_1\right|^2}\, I_i. \tag{56}$$

As a result, we can see that the EM wave impact on any interface of media with different impedances, leads to the reflection of the wave and thus to the loss of intensity of the penetrating wave.

In the case of non-magnetic dielectric substances $\mu_r = 1$ and $Z = \frac{Z_0}{\sqrt{\varepsilon_r}} = \frac{Z_0}{n}$, where $Z_0 = \sqrt{\frac{\mu_0}{\varepsilon_0}}$ is the wave impedance of vacuum and $n = \sqrt{\varepsilon_r}$ the refractive index.

The intensity of the reflected and transmitted waves are expressed by means of the refractive indices.

$$I_r = \left(\frac{n_1 - n_2}{n_1 + n_2}\right)^2 I_i, \qquad I_t = \frac{4 n_1 n_2}{(n_2 + n_1)^2}\, I_i. \tag{57}$$

Note: Since we have not considered losses, $I_r + I_t = I_i$ is valid, which can be proved by the simple addition of relations (57).

Example 5. Reflection of light from the glass.

When light falls on the optical lens of glasses, telescopes, cameras, etc., some of the light power reflects from the lens surface. Consider the refractive index of glass $n_2 = 1.7$. Then we get the intensity of reflected and transmitted light for $n_1 = 1$ (air), $I_r \approx 0.067\, I_i$, and $I_t \approx 0.933\, I_i$. As we see, 6.7% of the incident power reflects from the surface. This intensity is usually enough to see our mirror image in a glass window, especially if the dark background is behind it. An anti-reflective layer (which discusses the next paragraph) is applied to the surface of the glass optical elements to prevent the intensity loss by the reflection.

Example 6. Reflection of EM wave from the conductor surface.

If an EM wave with a frequency of 10 MHz falls from the air onto the aluminum surface (γ = 37 MS m^{-1}, μ_r = 1.0), due to inequality $Z_1 \gg Z_2$, the reflection factor is $I_r/I_i \approx 1$. Transition factor

$$\frac{I_t}{I_i} = \frac{4\,\mathrm{Re}\left\{\mathbf{Z}_2\mathbf{Z}_1^*\right\}}{|\mathbf{Z}_2 + \mathbf{Z}_1|^2} \approx \frac{4\,\mathrm{Re}\,\mathbf{Z}_2}{Z_1} = \frac{4}{Z_0}\sqrt{\frac{\omega\mu_0}{2\gamma}} = 4\sqrt{\frac{\omega\varepsilon_0}{2\gamma}} \approx 1,1 \times 10^{-5}.$$

As a result, we can see that the conductive layer on the body surface almost perfectly shields the internal volume from the external EM field in the radio frequency region. Despite such a small amount of power penetrating the body, we can achieve the demanded surface heating.

For tissue with significantly lower conductivity, the power transfer factor is up to three orders greater (up to 10%). The tissue at higher frequencies is no more a good conductor. The condition $\gamma \gg \omega\,\varepsilon$ at higher frequencies is not valid, and the tissue behaves more like a lossy dielectric.

1.3.3 Transition of EM waves through a dielectric layer

To achieve a higher reflection factor (e.g., reflective UV filters on glasses or cameras), or to reduce the reflectivity (e.g., anti-reflective layers on glasses or lenses), the thin layers are applied to the glass surface.

Consider a set of three media, in which layer 2 is between media 1 and 3, **Figure 4**. There are two interfaces in the system. We are interested in the transition of EM waves through this structure and reflection from the first interface.

Again, we consider a simple case of the perpendicular impact of the harmonic wave with the $\boldsymbol{E}_0$, $\boldsymbol{H}_0$ electric, and magnetic field intensities. Reflected wave r1 propagates back from the first interface. Inside the layer, the resulting wave consists of the direct wave t1 and the reflected one r2. From the second interface, the wave t2 propagates into the third medium.

Boundary conditions apply to the phasors of the EM field quantities at the interfaces.

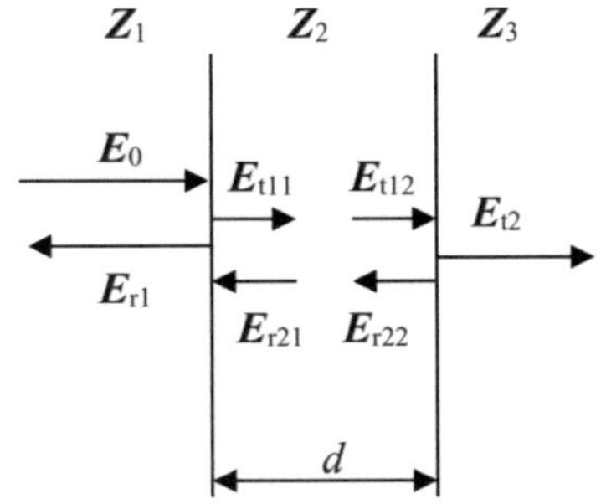

Figure 4.
Transition of an EM through a thin layer.

$$\begin{aligned} \mathbf{E}_0 + \mathbf{E}_{r1} = \mathbf{E}_{t11}, \quad \mathbf{H}_0 + \mathbf{H}_{r1} = \mathbf{H}_{t11}, \\ \mathbf{E}_{t12} + \mathbf{E}_{r22} = \mathbf{E}_{t2}, \quad \mathbf{H}_{t12} + \mathbf{H}_{r22} = \mathbf{H}_{t2}, \end{aligned} \tag{58}$$

with relationships

$$\mathbf{E}_0 = \mathbf{Z}_1 \mathbf{H}_0, \quad \mathbf{E}_{r1} = -\mathbf{Z}_1 \mathbf{H}_{r1}, \; \mathbf{E}_{t1} = \mathbf{Z}_2 \mathbf{H}_{t1}, \quad \mathbf{E}_{r2} = -\mathbf{Z}_2 \mathbf{H}_{r2}, \quad \mathbf{E}_{t2} = \mathbf{Z}_3 \mathbf{H}_{t3}, \tag{59}$$

and further

$$\mathbf{E}_{t12} = \mathbf{E}_{t11}\ \mathrm{e}^{-\mathrm{j}\mathbf{k}d}, \qquad \mathbf{E}_{r21} = \mathbf{E}_{r22}\ \mathrm{e}^{\mathrm{j}\mathbf{k}d}, \tag{60}$$

where d is the thickness of the middle layer and $\mathbf{k}$ is the coefficient of wave propagation in it.

From these equations and relations, we get after adjustment the complex factors $\mathbf{r}$ of reflection from the middle layer and $\mathbf{t}$ of the transition through the layer.

$$\mathbf{r} = \frac{\mathbf{E}_{r1}}{\mathbf{E}_0} = \frac{(\mathbf{Z}_2 - \mathbf{Z}_1)(\mathbf{Z}_2 + \mathbf{Z}_3) + (\mathbf{Z}_2 + \mathbf{Z}_1)(\mathbf{Z}_3 - \mathbf{Z}_2)\mathrm{e}^{-\mathrm{j}2\mathbf{k}d}}{(\mathbf{Z}_2 + \mathbf{Z}_1)(\mathbf{Z}_2 + \mathbf{Z}_3) + (\mathbf{Z}_2 - \mathbf{Z}_1)(\mathbf{Z}_3 - \mathbf{Z}_2)\,\mathrm{e}^{-\mathrm{j}2\mathbf{k}d}}, \tag{61}$$

$$\mathbf{t} = \frac{\mathbf{E}_{t2}}{\mathbf{E}_0} = \frac{4\mathbf{Z}_3\,\mathbf{Z}_2\,\mathrm{e}^{-\mathrm{j}\mathbf{k}d}}{(\mathbf{Z}_2 + \mathbf{Z}_1)(\mathbf{Z}_2 + \mathbf{Z}_3) + (\mathbf{Z}_2 - \mathbf{Z}_1)(\mathbf{Z}_3 - \mathbf{Z}_2)\,\mathrm{e}^{-\mathrm{j}2\mathbf{k}d}}. \tag{62}$$

Compare with the same result for acoustic waves (see Chapter 3).

As we can see from these relations, the coefficients $\mathbf{r}$ and $\mathbf{t}$ depend on the thickness d of the middle layer.

To give an idea of the nature of the phenomenon, let us analyze the case of lossless dielectric and non-magnetic media with real impedance and wavenumber values.

$$Z_i = \frac{Z_0}{\sqrt{\varepsilon_{ri}}} = \frac{Z_0}{n_i}, \text{ for } i = 1, 2, 3, \text{ and } k = \frac{\omega}{c_0}\ \sqrt{\varepsilon_{r2}} = \frac{\omega}{c_0}\ n_2,$$

where Z_0, c_0 are vacuum impedance and EM wave speed in a vacuum.

Taking these relations into account, we adjust equations (61), (62) to form

$$\mathbf{r} = \frac{\mathbf{E}_{r1}}{\mathbf{E}_0} = \frac{(n_1 - n_2)(n_2 + n_3) + (n_1 + n_2)(n_2 - n_3)\mathrm{e}^{-\mathrm{j}2kd}}{(n_1 + n_2)(n_2 + n_3) + (n_1 - n_2)(n_2 - n_3)\,\mathrm{e}^{-\mathrm{j}2kd}}, \tag{63}$$

$$\mathbf{t} = \frac{\mathbf{E}_{t2}}{\mathbf{E}_0} = \frac{4 n_1 n_2\,\mathrm{e}^{-\mathrm{j}kd}}{(n_1 + n_2)(n_3 + n_2) + (n_1 - n_2)(n_2 - n_3)\,\mathrm{e}^{-\mathrm{j}2kd}}. \tag{64}$$

We express the intensity of radiation for individual media $I = E^2/Z$ and determine the rates of reflected and transmitted wave intensities

$$\frac{I_{r1}}{I_0} = \frac{[(n_1 - n_2)(n_2 + n_3) + (n_1 + n_2)(n_2 - n_3)\cos 2kd]^2 + [(n_1 + n_2)(n_2 - n_3)\sin 2kd]^2}{[(n_1 + n_2)(n_2 + n_3) + (n_1 - n_2)(n_2 - n_3)\cos 2kd]^2 + [(n_1 - n_2)(n_2 - n_3)\sin 2kd]^2}, \tag{65}$$

$$\frac{I_{t2}}{I_0} = \frac{16 n_1 n_2^2 n_3}{[(n_1 + n_2)(n_3 + n_2) + (n_1 - n_2)(n_2 - n_3)\cos 2kd]^2 + [(n_1 - n_2)(n_2 - n_3)\sin 2kd]^2}. \tag{66}$$

The graph of the reflection and transmission factors is in **Figure 5** for $n_1 = 1.00$ (air), $n_2 = 1.40$ (layer), and $n_3 = 1.90$ (glass). The graph shows that if $k\,d = \pi/2$ rad,

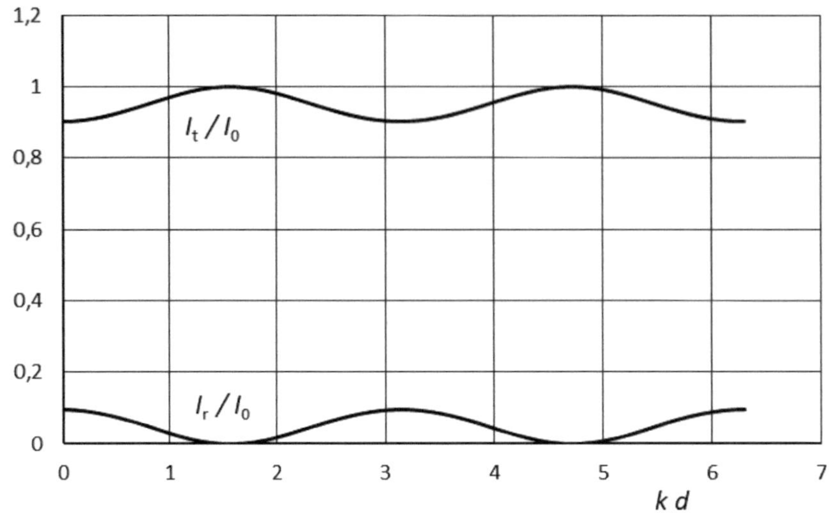

Figure 5.
Graf of reflection and intensity transition factors versus wave thickness k d (n_1 = 1.00, n_2 = 1.40, n_3 = 1.90).

i.e., $d = \lambda/4$, is zero reflection and 100% transition. It represents an anti-reflective layer (e.g., on reading glasses). On the other hand, for the $k\,d = \pi$ rad, the reflection is maximum (reflective layer as a UV filter on sunglasses). Thin layers on the optical elements (*antireflective or reflective*) control the reflection of light from their surfaces. The condition of zero reflection, resp. maximum reflection is fulfilled only for one wavelength, i.e., light color. In practice, antireflective layers are composed of several layers of different materials placed successively on each other.

1.4 Quantum properties of EM waves

At the beginning of the twentieth century, the quantum nature of EM radiation was discovered. According to quantum theory, radiation generates in elementary quanta—*photons* that have properties as the classical particles. Similarly, in the interaction of EM radiation with the structure of the substance, radiation is also absorbed in these quanta. Quantum theory explains the nature of spectra of the bodies' thermal radiation, the external photoelectric effect, the optical properties of substances, the electrical conductivity of semiconductors, and many other phenomena.

Electromagnetic radiation has two forms of manifestation. In some contexts, it behaves like a wave with frequency f and wavelength λ (wave parameters), in other ones, like a flow of particles (photons) with energy E_{ph} and momentum p_{ph} (mechanical parameters). The relations between wave and particle parameters describe de Broglie equations.

$$E_{\mathrm{ph}} = h\,f, \text{and}\, p_{\mathrm{ph}} = \frac{h}{\lambda}, \tag{67}$$

where h is the Planck's constant.

At the Sun's surface temperature T = 5780 K, the Sun most intensively radiates light with a wavelength $\lambda \approx 500$ nm, which corresponds to a photon energy $E_{\mathrm{ph}} \approx 2.1$ eV ($\approx 4.0 \times 10^{-19}$ J) and a yellow-green color. To this color, the human eye is most sensitive.

Spatially confined structures (atoms, molecules, crystals, etc.) have discrete energy levels of stationary states, e.g., electrons in atoms have only specific values of energy. If the system is in a state with energy E_1, it can go into a state with energy $E_2 > E_1$ (excitation) due to the absorption of a photon of the radiation with energy $E_{ph} = E_2 - E_1$. If the system is excited with the energy E_2, it spontaneously returns to a lower state with energy $E_1 < E_2$ (relaxation). The energy difference $\Delta E = E_2 - E_1$ is usually released in the form of a photon. This results in the *emission of a photon* (radiation) with a wavelength

$$\lambda = \frac{h\,c}{E_2 - E_1}. \tag{68}$$

When EM radiation passes through a certain substance, it absorbs the photons with energy corresponding to the transitions between its energy levels. The corresponding wavelengths will miss in the transmitted radiation. It results in *the absorption spectrum* of the substance. On the other hand, if we excite the substance, e.g., by electric discharge, the system relaxes to the lower state and emits photons of corresponding transition energies. Thus, the radiation contains only radiation with certain characteristic wavelengths. In such a way arises the *emission spectrum* of the substance. The emission or absorption spectrum is typical for any substance. This phenomenon is a base of *emission or absorption spectroscopy*. In medicine, *optical spectroscopy* is useful for biochemical analyses and in hematology. Another tool of biomedicine is magnetic resonance spectroscopy.

Each system has its characteristic values of binding energy E_b (energy for separation of some part of the system or the overall disintegration of the system into elementary parts). If a photon with the energy $E_{ph} \geq E_b$ enters the system, it may cause its dissociation (decay). E.g., if an atom or group of atoms belonging to the DNA macromolecule with the binding energy E_b, the EM radiation with the wavelength $\lambda \leq h\,c/E_b$ can break the binding and release some of its parts. Such a damaged DNA molecule may originate a tumor formation. Since the binding energies of molecules reach values of several eV (electron-volts), the corresponding wavelengths of radiation are several hundred nm. It corresponds to the ultraviolet radiation, e.g., for $E_b \sim 4$ eV, the wavelength $\lambda \sim 310$ nm (ultraviolet UVB band). The O_2 molecule has a binding energy of 5.1 eV, so that if the radiation with a wavelength $\lambda < 244$ nm (UVC band) irradiates, the dissociation of the molecules results in arising of one atomic oxygen. The free O atoms then bind to the O_2 molecules and form O_3 molecules (ozone). In such a way, solar ultraviolet UVC radiation absorbs in the upper atmosphere and creates the ozonosphere.

Electrons in atoms and molecules are bound by binding energy, which calls *ionizing energy*. The substance with ionizing energy E_i ionizes when exposed to radiation with a wavelength $\lambda \leq h\,c/E_i$. For the oxygen and nitrogen binding energies $E_i\,(O_2) = 13.6$ eV and $E_i\,(N_2) = 14.5$ eV, air ionization occurs, if EM wavelengths $\lambda < 90$ nm. Due to the far UV and X radiation from the sun, the highest atmospheric layer ionizes, creating an ionosphere.

In such a way atmosphere protects the surface of the Earth against the dangerous short-wavelengths radiation from the Sun.

From the above examples, we see that the interface between ionizing and non-ionizing EM radiation is approximately the wavelength of about 100 nm and the corresponding photon energy about 12 eV.

The photon energies of the EM radiation in the different bands of EM radiation are given in the last column in **Table 3**.

Band	Wavelength λ (approx.)	Frequency f (approx.)	Photon energy E_{ph} (approx.)
Very long waves	>1 km	<300 kHz	<1 neV
Radio waves (RF)	1 km–1 m	300 kHz–300 MHz	1 neV–1 μeV
Microwaves (MW)	1 m–1 mm	300 MHz–300 GHz	1 μeV–1 meV
Infrared radiation (IR)	1 mm–700 nm	300 GHz–430 THz	1 meV–1.8 eV
Visible light (VL)	700–400 nm	430–750 THz	1.8–3.1 eV
Ultraviolet radiation (UV)	400–100 nm	750 THz–3 PHz	3.1–12 eV
Edge of ionizing radiation	100 nm	3 PHz = $3 \cdot 10^{15}$ Hz	12 eV
Extreme ultraviolet radiation (EUV)	100–10 nm	$3 \cdot 10^{15}$–$3 \cdot 10^{16}$ Hz	12–100 eV
Roentgen radiation (X)	10 nm–1 pm	$3 \cdot 10^{16}$–$3 \cdot 10^{20}$ Hz	100 eV–1 MeV
Gamma radiation (γ)	1 pm–1 fm	$3 \cdot 10^{20}$–$3 \cdot 10^{23}$ Hz	1 MeV–10 GeV
High-energy gamma rays	<1 fm	>$3 \cdot 10^{23}$ Hz	>10 GeV

Table 3.
Characteristic bands of electromagnetic waves. The boundaries of the bands are only approximate, the wavelength is calculated for the vacuum, where $\lambda = c_o/f$*, photon energy* $E_{ph} = h\,f$*.*

1.5 Spectrum of EM waves

Although the nature of EM waves is the same for all frequencies, the characteristics, effects of EM waves, and practical applications vary across different frequency bands. **Table 3** shows the classic distribution.

Very long waves up to a wavelength equal to the length of the Earth's perimeter occur in nature, caused by, e.g., atmospheric discharges (lightning), affecting living organisms as a part of the environment. We can mention, e.g., Schumann resonances, which correspond to a wavelength $\lambda = 2\,\pi\,R_z \approx 40{,}000$ km, and a frequency of 7.5 Hz, which falls within the range of the human brain waves frequency. It is known that this EM field mainly affects the mental side of the man and affects his immune system. This is used in some forms of therapy at very low-frequency waves, which produce some animals (e.g., dogs—*Canis therapy*, horses—*hippotherapy*, cats—*feline therapy*, *dolphin therapy*, etc.)

Radio-frequency waves (*RF*) are used mainly in the transmission of radio and television signals, radiolocation, electromagnetic flaw detection, surface heating of conductive materials, etc. In medicine, RF waves also use magnetic resonance imaging and diathermy. Research is underway to investigate the effects of the radiofrequency EM field on biological systems with a prognosis of cancer treatment.

Microwaves (*MW*) are used in transmitting signals on the direct visibility, or in waveguides, satellite communication, mobile communication, radiolocation, microwave heating, in medicine, especially in hyperthermia and tumor treatment.

Infrared radiation (*IR*) is typical for radiant heat transfer. It is used for signal transmission by optical fibers, measuring the surface temperature of bodies, in medicine, especially for diagnostics by the method of thermography. IR laser radiation uses laser scalpels and lithotripsy, or IR spectroscopy (oximetry, photoplethysmography, e.g., Borik and Cap [4], measurement of blood flow), etc.

Visible light (*VL*) is the dominant information channel of a human being and is used in various optical devices such as binoculars, microscopes, magnifying glasses, glasses, lighting tools, etc. In medicine, light use, also, optical imaging and lighting in surgery, phototherapy, endoscopy, and the like. Different light attenuation or light dispersion in substances at different wavelengths uses optical spectroscopy of biological materials, photoplethysmography Borik et al. [5], Borik and Cap [4, 6], Blazek et al. [7], ophthalmic surgery using optical lasers, etc.

Ultraviolet radiation (*UV*) reaches the limit of ionizing radiation (wavelength of approximately 100 nm). According to the wavelength, the UV band is divided into three parts: UVA (400–320) nm, UVB (320–280) nm, and UVC (280–100) nm. UVA radiation has greater penetration depth than light. It uses, e.g., dermatology. The UVA component of the Sun's radiation disperses in the atmosphere and reaches the Earth's surface (like light). UVB takes place in the production of vitamin D. Its greater exposure leads to erythema (skin inflammation) and pigmentation during tanning. The ozone layer reduces the UVB component of the sun. Its intensity significantly increases with altitude, and therefore tanning is dangerous at the high mountains. UVC has a profound effect on chemical bonds. It can cause skin cancer and has a significant disinfectant effect due to destroying microorganisms. The UVC component of the sun's radiation is attenuated by the atmosphere so that it practically does not reach the earth's surface. UVC and UVB contribute to the formation of the ozone layer of the Earth's atmosphere, which protects the biosphere at the earth's surface from the effects of UVC, EUV, and the X-rays from the Sun. UV radiation harms human vision and leads to damage of the retina at a greater intensity. Because the retina of the eye is not sensitive to UV radiation, it does not have a reflexive protective narrowing of the pupil. The retina is thus exposed to high radiation intensity, and therefore quality sunglasses contain a UV filter.

The edge of ionizing radiation is derived from photon energy, at which the ionization of air molecules begins to take place. The edge is for reference only. Ionization processes and disruption of chemical bonds can also occur in the energy field below this threshold.

Extreme Ultraviolet radiation (*EUV*) or far ultraviolet radiation causes ionizing effects and modification of chemical bonds. On the Earth, it originates only from artificial sources. The EUV and X components of solar radiation are trapped in the upper atmosphere (ionosphere) and do not reach the earth's surface.

X-rays are ionizing radiation, which has a high penetration depth. It penetrates through the entire volume of the human body. In technical practice, it uses mainly body electromagnetic testing. In medicine, it is used mainly in radiology from classical X-rays devices to modern CT imaging, **Figure 6**, Röntgen [8]. Due to the destructive effect of X-rays on biological tissue, it uses radiotherapy of tumors and various bone growths. Due to damage to biological structures, the human organism can be safely exposed only to limited doses of radiation determined by hygiene standards.

Gamma radiation is a very penetrating ionizing radiation that is generated by nuclei of atoms (nuclear radiation). It uses *nuclear medicine*. Weak radiation doses utilize diagnostic devices such as gamma camera, PET (Positron Emission Tomography), and SPECT (Single Photon Emission Tomography); often used radioactive radiators are preparations: cobalt ^{60}Co, cesium ^{133}Cs, iridium ^{192}Ir, and others. Modern nuclear therapy facilities include *Leksell's gamma knife* or, less common *cyber-knife*.

High-energy gamma radiation is EM radiation with a wavelength of less than 10^{-15} m. This radiation with photon energy above 10 GeV arises in huge particle accelerators that serve scientific purposes. Before, this radiation was called *cosmic radiation*, because of its origin in cosmic space.

Maxwell's EM field theory is useful for the classical description of EM radiation, which emphasizes its wave character. EM waves characterize wave-quantities as the

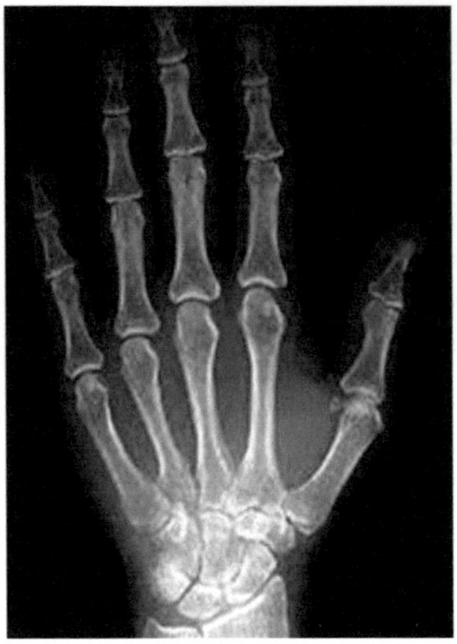
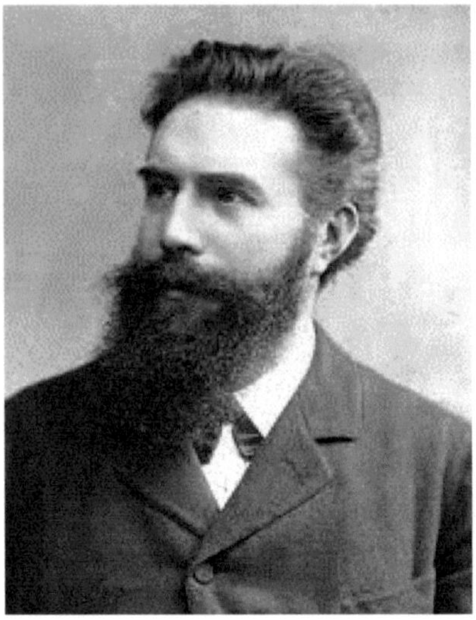

Figure 6.
X-rays image of the hand, Wilhelm Conrad roentgen (1845–1923).

angular frequency ω and wave vector $\boldsymbol{k}$, as described in the previous sections. The components of the wave vector β and α or phase velocity c describe the propagation of EM waves in the medium. The damping coefficient β and the phase shift coefficient α depend on the frequency of the EM wave through the frequency dependence of the quantities μ, ε, and γ.

An example is a seawater, which has a high conductivity $\gamma \sim 1$ S/m. At radiofrequency $f = 10$ MHz, the permittivity of water is $\varepsilon_r \approx 81$. The relation $\omega \varepsilon \approx 4.4 \times 10^{-2}$ S/m $\ll \gamma$ is valid. It is, therefore, a well-conducting medium for which the penetrating depth $\delta \approx 16$ cm. For the visible light, $\delta \sim 10$ m (and transparency up to 200 m) is given for clean seawater. It is known that radio communication is not possible with submarines, while optical visibility is very good in pure seawater. Another example is a soft tissue that is opaque for the visible light but permeable for X-rays. In some cases, quantum processes influence the frequency dependence of the attenuation coefficient β. E.g., the Ge semiconductor monocrystal is transparent (like glass) for wavelengths $\lambda > 1.7$ μm, while for shorter wavelengths $\lambda < 1.7$ μm the Ge monocrystal is opaque (looks like shiny metal). It uses infrared optics in thermographic cameras.

The relatively low attenuation of X-rays in substances is used in medical diagnostics. X-rays have been used in medicine practically since the discovery of X-rays in 1895.

Imaging the internal structure of the body uses different attenuation of X-rays in different tissues, **Figure 6**. The original direct method—*skiascopy (gr. skias—shadow)*, uses the detection of radiation penetrating the body on the screen of the device. The more complex CT (Computed Tomography) method uses the detection of passing X-rays by a series of detectors and computer signal processing. As this is ionizing radiation, human exposition must be kept to a minimum under hygiene standards.

1.6 Sources of electromagnetic radiation

EM radiation sources have a very diverse character, which depends on the wavelength of the generated radiation. The diversity of resources also depends on the purpose of their use. We divide the sources into three groups according to the dominance of the manifestation of the generated radiation:

- sources of coherent waves.
- sources of energy radiation.
- photon radiation sources (dominated by quantum behavior).

The same EM radiation can occur in all three groups according to its further use, e.g., in the case of light, its wave properties can be used in the event of interference; a focused light beam can induce a thermal (energetic) effect, e.g., laser scalpel, or light can be used in typically quantum phenomena such as photoemission of electrons from a metal surface or optical spectroscopy.

1.6.1 Coherent and incoherent resources

If EM radiation behaves like waves, the wave sources are *coherent (coherent = interrelated)* or *incoherent*. Two waves are coherent if they have the same frequency and have a constant phase difference at any point in the space. The coherent source generates a wave with a constant initial phase so that the wave function is unambiguously defined. A coherent source is, e.g., a radio wave antenna supplied by a harmonic voltage source. The optical coherent source is, e.g., LASER, which achieves coherence using a wave resonator. The waves (sources) in which the phase relationship is not defined, are *incoherent*. Many microscopic sources, not mutually coordinated, generate such radiation, e.g., the individual atoms in the filament lamps generate light with a minimally coordinated phase. Incoherent sources are heat sources, noise sources, light bulbs, discharge lamps, LEDs, sources of X-rays, gamma radiation, etc.

Note: A coherent source can be created from an incoherent optical source using a resonator—e.g., incoherent LED source + resonator → coherent semiconductor LASER.

Incoherent sources emit EM radiation usually in elementary "wavelets". A wavelet itself is coherent, but the different wavelets are incoherent. Each radiation has several periods, in space several wavelengths, of coherence. The *coherence length* is the propagation distance in which the radiation is coherent. Coherence is important in the interference processes. If the phase relationships are random, no interference occurs. In the case of interference, diffraction, or holography, phase relationships are decisive. For such cases, we assess the necessary coherence of radiation by comparing the coherence length with characteristic dimensions of the structure on which interference or diffraction arises.

Waves of radiofrequency sources have the coherence length up to thousands of kilometers, of the LASER hundreds of meters. On the other hand, thermal radiation, e.g., a bulb light, radiation of electric discharge, or radiation of LEDs reaches the coherence length of less than a tenth of a millimeter. X-rays of most sources have a coherence length of the magnitude order comparable to the interatomic distances in substances, gamma rays of the magnitude order comparable to the dimensions of the atomic nucleus.

The particles, e.g., electrons, neutrons, protons, ions, also behave like a wave. In such a case, the coherence is understood differently, and quantum mechanics gives the answers. The wave behavior is also observed when a single particle interacts with a fabric structure if the wavelength of the de Broglie wave is comparable to or greater than the characteristic dimensions of the structure with which the particles interact. This fact is used, e.g., in the electron microscope.

1.6.2 Sources of radiofrequency and microwave EM waves

Conductors with non-stationary electric current generate EM waves. Their sources—*antennas* are essentially oscillating electric or magnetic dipoles. An

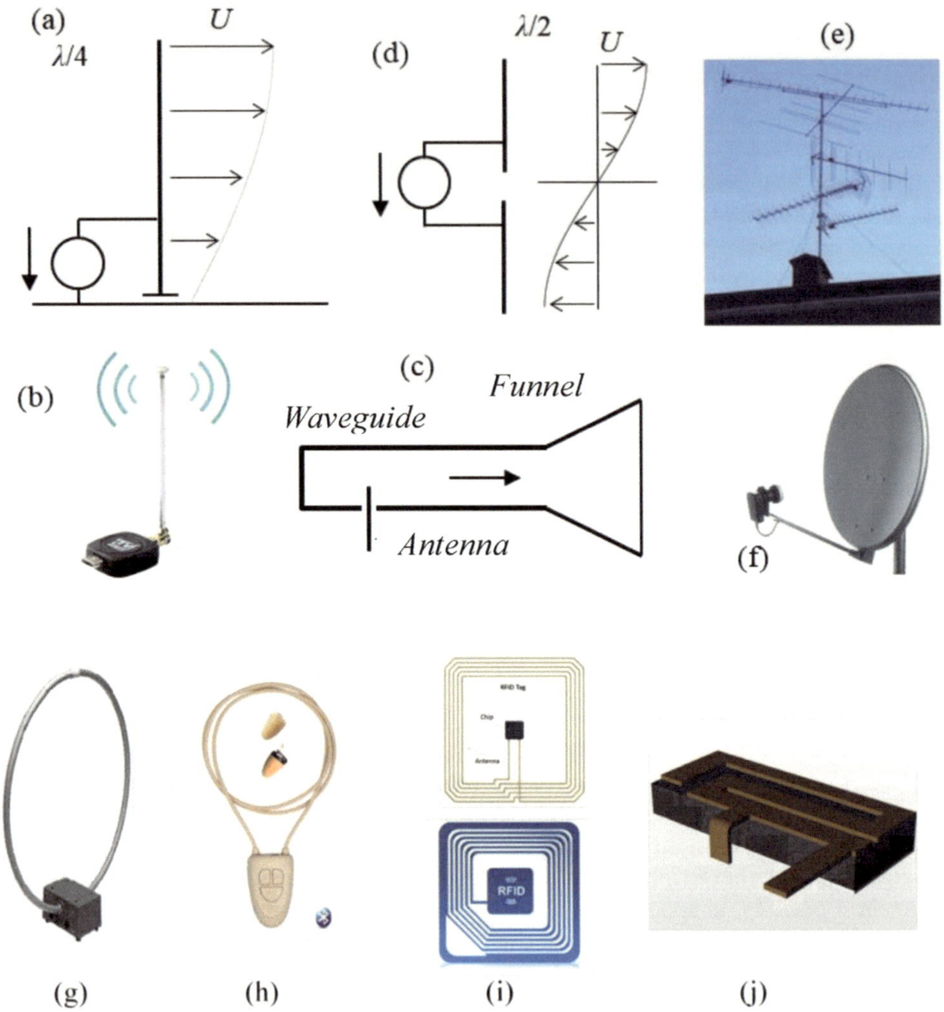

Figure 7.
EM waves antennas.

example of electric dipole antennas for radio and microwave radiation is in **Figure 7**. Figure (a) shows a quarter-wave antenna with the indicated voltage wave distribution. One of its ends is grounded (level of zero potential). Radio transmission on long, medium, and short waves, or short-distance transmission systems (e.g., WIFI—figure (b)), use such antennas. In figure (c) is the dipole antenna for the generation of EM waves in a waveguide. In figure (d) is a half-wave antenna (dipole) with an indicated voltage distribution. Half-wavelength antennas of this type of use wave transmission in VHF and UHF bands (radio, TV, telecommunications), see figure (e). The directivity and thus the gain of the antennas adjust various elements.

The so-called Yagi antenna is in figure (e). Its directionality is adjusted by other elements, in front of and behind the radiating dipole. The directionality of EM wave emission from the waveguide, figure (c), is achieved by a funnel-shaped extension of the waveguide.

The parabolic mirror, figure (f), also serves to form a very narrow radiating characteristic. In this case, the little dipole radiator is placed in the focal plane of the parabolic dish. Satellite communication antennas narrowly directed telecommunication connections, systems of microwave data transmission, etc., use this type of antenna. Some antennas also use a current excitation. They have the shape of loops or coils. The typical loop antenna is in figure (g). The bluetooth connection uses the loop antenna in figure (h). RFID (Radio Frequency Identification) technology uses an antenna in figure (i). It appears, e.g., as security elements of goods, or a smart card identification element. Special planar antennas PIFA (Planar Inverted F-Antennas) with small dimensions, figure (j), is proper for mobile devices, e.g., mobile phones.

1.6.3 Sources of incoherent optical radiation

Incoherent optical sources, which include sources of visible light, infrared, ultraviolet, and X-rays, are divided into temperature sources and quantum sources with spontaneous relaxation.

The principle of the action of these sources relates to photon emission, which accompanies spontaneous transitions of electrons from higher energy states to lower ones. These spontaneous transitions are coherent around the relaxing atom only in a small volume with dimensions of the order of units of the wavelength. The coherence length is, therefore, very small. In the optical region, it is of the order of magnitude of units to tens of micrometers.

Note: Interference phenomena, such as grating diffraction or thin-film interference, occur only if the coherence length is greater than the characteristic dimension of the structure (grating constant, layer thickness, etc.). On the thin oil layer on the surface of the flour, we see color effects if the layer is thin. If it is thicker, it has the appearance of a gray mirror. Since the coherence length of the sunlight is several times its wavelength, it is possible to decompose the light into spectral components by an optical grating. However, this coherence length is not enough to create a hologram.

In the case of substances with electron energy bands, there are many possibilities for a relaxation transition, and the emitted radiation has a wide continuous spectrum. In the case of individual atoms (e.g., gas discharge lamps) with discrete energy levels, the spectrum of the emitted radiation is a discrete one, as well.

1.6.3.1 Heat sources, filament lamps, and arc lamps

Thermal radiation is emitted from the surface of the body in a state of thermodynamic equilibrium. If the thermodynamic temperature of the body surface is T, the spectral composition of the radiation emitted from the body surface gets Planck's law

$$I(\lambda) = \frac{\mathrm{d}I_\lambda}{\mathrm{d}\lambda} = \frac{2\pi h c^2}{\lambda^5} \frac{1}{e^{\frac{hc}{\lambda k_B T}} - 1}, \tag{69}$$

where $I(\lambda)$ is the spectral density of the radiation. A characteristic property of temperature sources is their continuous frequency spectrum (*polychromatic sources*).

The graph of the spectral density $I(\lambda)$ vs. the wavelength λ is in **Figure 8**. In the picture on the left, we see the spectrum of the Sun's radiation (6000 K) compared to a filament lamp (3000 K). The picture on the right shows the radiation spectrum of the human body surface (37 ± 2°C), which is used in thermography and in the non-contact measurement of body temperature. As can be seen from the figures, the maximum spectral density of the radiation intensity is approximately 500 nm (yellow-green color) for solar radiation and about 9–10 μm (infrared radiation) for the human body.

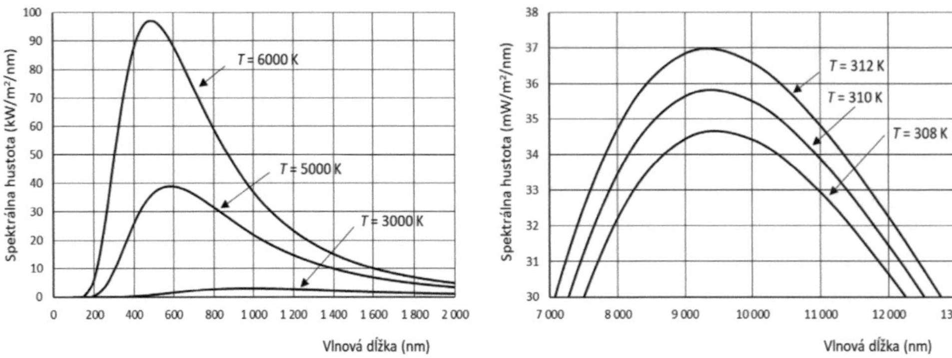

Figure 8.
Spectral density of thermal radiation intensity vs. a wavelength.

High-temperature heat sources are used as heat sources in thermotherapy or as sources for lighting. As can be seen from the graph, the total energy that falls into the optical band (350–700 nm) is only a small part of the total energy expenditure of the source. The light efficiency of these sources is very low, and therefore they are replaced by sources with significantly higher efficiency (discharge lamps, LEDs) for lighting purposes.

From a physiological point of view, the spectrum of heated sources is the most like to the natural light of the Sun. Besides, incandescent sources have high thermal inertia and therefore do not flash when supplied with 50 Hz AC power. The main disadvantage of lighting is low light efficiency. They are preferred as heat sources because most of the radiation spectrum is in the infrared range.

Note: The source temperature results from the analysis of the radiation spectrum. Optical pyrometers use this option to measure very high temperatures. By determining the maximum spectral density in the spectrum of space radiation, the temperature of the Universe was determined to be approximately 3 K. It is one of the pillars of the theory of the origin of the Universe—the Big Bang.

The classical heated sources are incandescent bulbs. The basic modification is a vacuum bulb with a tungsten filament. They have a low light efficiency and a short lifetime due to the evaporation of the tungsten filament, and thus it's thinning. The bulbs filled with inert gas (halogen) improve their efficiency and durability.

Another improvement of light sources represents halogen (krypton, xenon) high-pressure arc lamps, which have a favorable emission spectrum (practically white light), high luminosity, and light efficiency. They use the principle of primary electric arc radiation and subsequent modification of the radiation spectrum using a halogen filling. They are used as sources of intense white light in projectors, sources of white light in optical spectroscopy, and bodies for lighting small or large spaces, e.g., the lighting of the operating area in surgery, dentistry, etc.

1.6.3.2 Thermovision and thermography

Thermovision is a diagnostic imaging method that uses infrared (thermal) radiation from the bodies with non-zero thermodynamic temperature. The average body surface temperature is approximately 310 K (37°C). This corresponds to the spectrum of electromagnetic radiation with a maximum spectral power density at the wavelength of $\lambda_m \approx 9.3$ μm, according to Planck's law. Semiconductor sensors detect the thermal radiation, e.g., InSb is most sensitive to the radiation with a wavelength around $\lambda \sim 5$ μm. At this wavelength, the temperature change of $\Delta T = 1$°C causes the relative power change of 3%. The detector enables detecting the relative change of the power of incident radiation up to 10^{-4}. It allows evaluating the temperature change better than 0.1°C.

A thermographic camera allows the thermal imaging of observed objects. It works on the same principle as a conventional digital camera, but instead of visible light, it is sensitive to infrared radiation. The optical system is transparent only for infrared radiation but is opaque for visible light. CMOS chips are used for the detection of radiation. They are less noisy in the IR region than CCD chips that mainly use conventional cameras. The amplitude of the signal of the individual sensor pixels is color-coded so that a color map of the photographed object displays the monitor of the camera or a connected computer.

In biomedicine, thermovision or thermography is a diagnostic tool allowing to discover diseases that lead to a change of body surface temperature. E.g., inflammatory processes, or not very deep tumors lead to an increase in temperature, reduced blood flow to the limbs due to thrombosis or stenosis results in a decrease in temperature. An example of a thermographic image is in **Figure 9**.

The picture displays a thermographic record of a breast examination, which shows cancer in the right breast (red color indicates an increased temperature). In medical diagnostics, thermography is the most often used for the orientational diagnosis of breast tumors, monitoring the subcutaneous inflammation, or monitoring of the postoperative state. The so-called differential diagnostics, when paired organs, e.g., arms, legs, breasts, are photographed and compared to each other. The different images indicate the changed function of one of them.

1.6.3.3 Low pressure lamps

Another source of incoherent optical radiation is a low-pressure gas discharge lamp. A quantum source is characterized by a discrete frequency spectrum of radiation. The lamp bulb is filled with a low-pressure gas so that the individual atoms are independent and have a line spectrum of electron energy levels. After

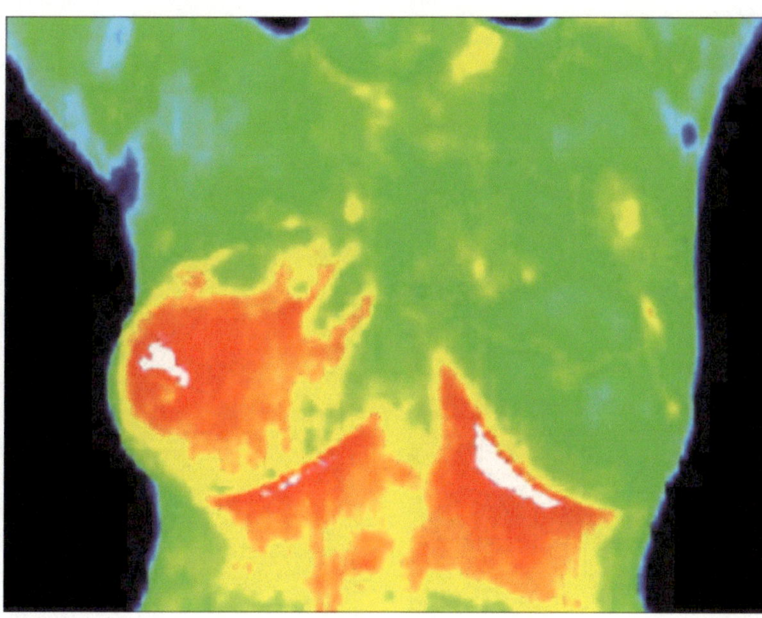

Figure 9.
Example of thermographic record. Source: https://www.researchgate.net/figure/Image-of-digital-infrared-thermal-imaging-Inflammatory-carcinoma-of-right-breast_fig1_260486952.

excitation to a higher energy state, the atom relaxes back to a lower state and emits a photon. The energy of the emitted photon is equal to the difference between the energy of the excitation and the relaxation states. The wavelength of the emitted radiation corresponds to this photon energy, see (68).

The emission spectra of some gases are in **Figure 10**. The upper strip represents a continuous spectrum of a glowing source with a temperature of 6000 K (the Sun). By composing all components of the spectrum, we get white light.

The light intensity of the emission lines, and thus the color of the lamplight, can change as the voltage between the electrodes of the lamp changes. Typical discharge colors are hydrogen—pink to magenta, neon—red to orange, argon—violet to blue, krypton—green to blue-white, xenon—blue to white. Different discharge colors are used for advertising purposes, such as discharge indicators, etc.

Due to the low pressure, and thus the density of the gas, the light intensity of the lamps does not reach too high values. They are, therefore, not suitable for lighting.

Low-pressure discharge lamps also include metal vapor discharge lamps—sodium and mercury. When cold, metals are in a solid or liquid state on the walls of the bulb. The lamps contain a small amount of inert gas (Ne, Ar) so that discharge can arise when switched on the cold lamp. This discharge gradually raises the temperature of the lamp, the metal evaporates and becomes a discharge gas. The light of metallic discharge lamps has a high intensity. These lamps are proper for lighting purposes, e.g., streetlamps. The sodium lamp emits monochromatic light with a wavelength of 589 nm (yellow-orange color). One can encounter sodium lamps in street lighting (yellow lamps).

The mercury vapor discharge contains, in addition to the intense spectral lines: green (546 nm), blue (405 and 436 nm), very intense spectral lines of invisible UV radiation (312 and 365 nm). Mercury lamps, therefore, serve as sources of UV radiation (disinfection of rooms with UV radiation, "mountain sun" in solariums,

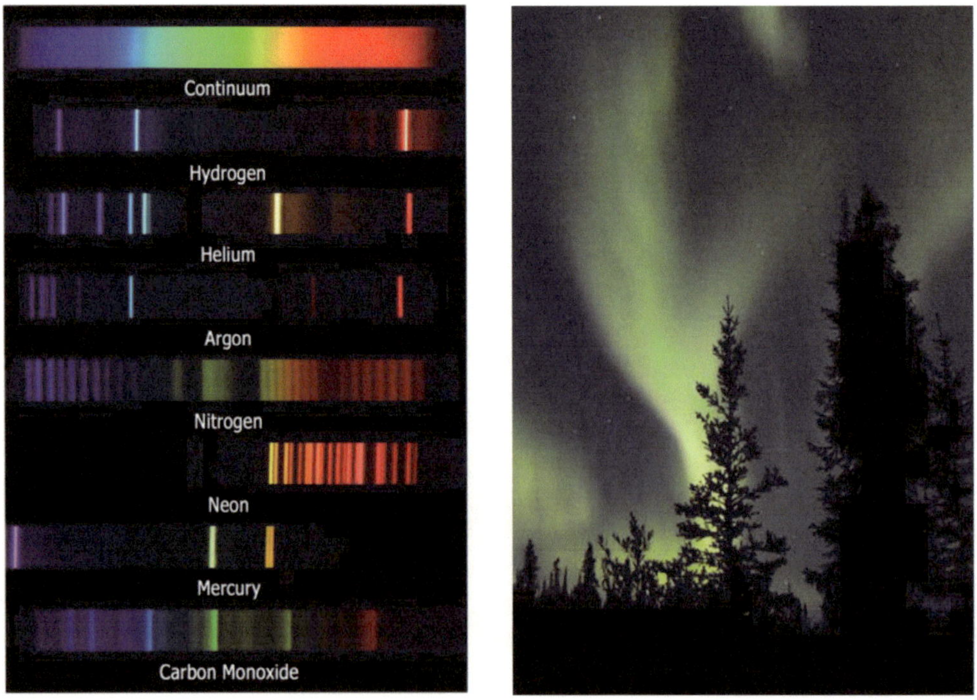

Figure 10.
Emission spectra of some gases and aurora borealis.

for therapeutic purposes in dermatology, etc.). Due to the spectral composition with a predominantly blue color, it is not suitable for lighting purposes.

UV photons excite various substances, which then emit lower energy photons when relaxed. This phenomenon is called *photoluminescence.* This phenomenon is characteristic of substances called *luminophores.* The light emitted from the luminophore has a discrete spectrum typical for the substance. There are known, e.g., banknote security features readable only after UV light illumination.

The mercury lamps are an important example of the use of phosphors. The mercury lamp itself is in a larger bulb, which has a layer of phosphor on the inner surface (most often yttrium-vanadate), which emits red light after irradiation with UV radiation. After combining with the blue and green components of the primary source, it produces white light suitable for illumination. While the mercury lamp bank is of pure silica glass, which transmits UV radiation, the outer bank of the lighting lamp consists of ordinary glass, which does not transmit UV radiation. In this way, the lamp emits only white light without any UV component. It is, therefore, not dangerous for humans.

The lamps of this type can be found in street lighting (white to purple lamps) and lighting in buildings (ordinary fluorescent tubes).

Note: An example of an incoherent quantum source is Aurora Borealis, **Figure 10**. *Air molecules (mostly nitrogen) are excited by high-energy particles of the solar wind, which are concentrated in the pole regions by the Earth's magnetic field. The nitrogen then emits blue-green light typical for Aurora Borealis.*

1.6.3.4 Luminescence

In the previous paragraph, we suggested that atoms of substances can be excited to a higher energy state, with the electrons subsequently relaxed back to lower energy levels, either directly or through several intermediate states. The differences in the energy of the states between which the electrons relax determine the emission lines of radiation. If the relaxation follows immediately after excitation (for a time $< 10^{-8}$ s), we speak about *fluorescence,* if the atoms remain in the excited state longer and the relaxation is delayed (for a time $> 10^{-8}$ s), we speak of *phosphorescence.*

The excitation of atoms can take place in various physical ways, which always have in common the supply of the necessary excitation energy of an atom.

The most common phenomenon is *electroluminescence*. A strong electric field accelerates charged particles (electrons) of the gas. They transfer the received kinetic energy due to impacts to the neutral atoms or molecules of gases—we talk about the so-called *impact excitation*. This phenomenon uses conventional electrically powered lamps. The more exotic cases include the Aurora Borealis or lightning during atmospheric discharges.

Another case is *photoluminescence*, where excitation arises due to EM radiation with sufficiently high energy photons (UV, X-rays, or gamma radiation). Photoluminescence (the most often photo-fluorescence) is used both for the analysis of substances and for the detection of radiation. Notable photoluminescence appears at some, especially organic substances, called *fluorophores*. After irradiation with UV radiation, they emit light typical for a given fluorophore. If used in microscopy (excitation microscopy), various macromolecules, tissue, and cell structures can be visible. The principle of photoluminescence utilizes detectors of ionizing radiation (X-rays or gamma radiation), e.g., in sciascopy, CT, or gamma cameras.

Chemiluminescence uses the excitation of electrons due to an exothermic chemical reaction. Phosphorus luminescence is typical due to the slow oxidation of its surface. A special case is *bioluminescence*, where fluorescence occurs because of biochemical reactions. A typical case is the firefly beetle, whose buttock glows due to the oxidation of luciferin. Another example is the luminescence of rotting wood ("luminous wood") or necrotic tissue, where putrefactive bacteria emit light in the process of fermentation oxidation.

An interesting case represents *thermoluminescence*. The mechanism of this phenomenon is slightly different. Some substances, excited by ionizing radiation, enter a quasi-stable excitation state with higher energy. They can remain in this state for a long time (months, years, hundreds of years, etc.). They serve as memory elements that record and integrate irradiation in the form of energy of the excitation state. From this state, the substance can return by heating to a high temperature, which releases the accumulated energy. In this way, from the mineral fluorite, geologists determine the degree of irradiation of the rock during geological development, e.g., by nuclear events.

In biomedicine, such substances are used in personal dosimeters (dose meters—radiation cans) of health care workers who work in workplaces using ionizing radiation (radiodiagnostics, radiotherapy, nuclear medicine, etc.). The dosimeter, that the worker carries with him, is excited by radiation, and the dose information is stored. With the detection device, the dosimeter is "read" at prescribed intervals (e.g., once a month) using thermoluminescence. In biomedicine, such substances are used in the personal dosimeters of healthcare workers employed in workplaces with ionizing radiation (radiodiagnostics, radiotherapy, nuclear medicine). The dosimeter carried by the worker is excited by radiation, and the dose information is stored. The dosimeter is "read" at prescribed intervals (e.g., once a month) with a detection device using thermoluminescence.

The next form of luminescence is *radioluminescence*—luminescence due to excitation by a nuclear reaction (e.g., alpha or beta radiation). E.g., tritium enriched ZnS (the radioactive hydrogen isotope ^3H) excites the ZnS phosphor due to the beta conversion of tritium. It is used, e.g., on the hands of watches or devices working in the dark.

1.6.3.5 Semiconductor light-emitting diodes (LEDs)

Semiconductor sources LED (light emitting diode) use radiant recombination of electron-hole pairs in the PN junction.

In **Figure 11** is the energy spectrum of electrons in a P-type semiconductor with free charge carriers—holes, and N-type with free charge carriers—electrons. If the semiconductors come into contact (figure left), the chemical potential represented by the Fermi level E_F is equalized in the whole P-N system by the diffusion of electrons and holes. An insulating (non-conductive) barrier without free charge carriers is formed in the close contact space. Electrons from semiconductor N cannot get into semiconductor P and recombine with holes. But if we connect the voltage $U = E_g/e$ in the forward direction, where E_g is the width of the forbidden gap in the energy spectrum, the Fermi levels are shifted relative to each other, so that the edges of the conducting and valence bands are aligned. In this case, both electrons and the holes can freely enter the barrier and recombine there. The recombination causes the release of the energy equal to the difference $\Delta E \geq E_g$. In most cases, it transfers to the lattice (thermal transitions). In some cases, the energy is releases in the form of photons (radiant transitions), and the junction thus emits EM radiation in the frequency range around $\lambda \sim h\,c/E_g$. For $U > E_g/e$ is $\Delta E > E_g$ and the wavelength of the photons is shorter. The emitted light has a characteristic color, but it is not monochromatic. Various combinations of elements from groups II–VI (ZnS, CdS, ZnO), III–V (GaAs, GaN, GaAsP, InSb, AlGaAs), or IV–IV (SiC) are used for the PN junction production.

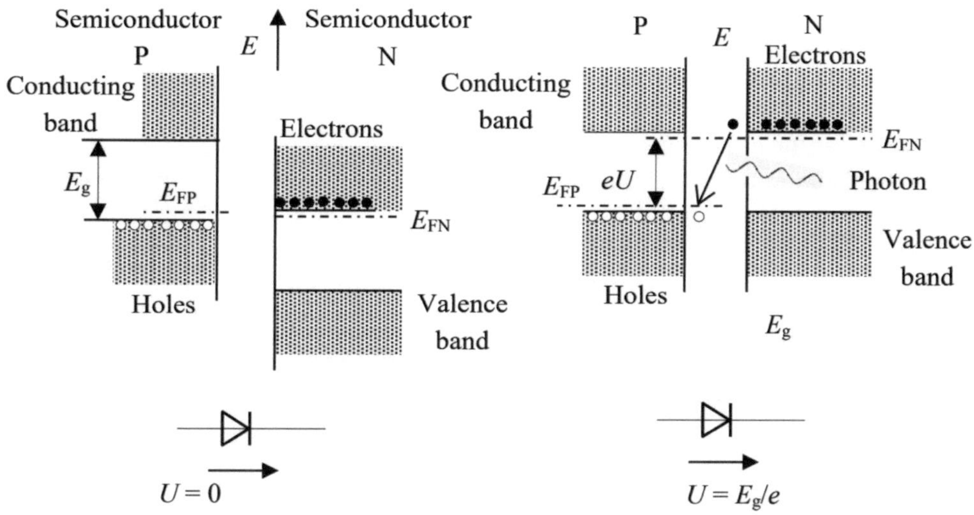

Figure 11.
Radiating PN junction—LED.

Depending on the different width E_g of the bandgap, the junction (LED) emits radiation of different colors. As we see in the **Table 4**, the LED sources cover the entire spectrum from infrared over visible to ultraviolet radiation. By combining LEDs with different colors, other colors can be reached, such as pink, purple, and especially white.

Turn in the use of white LED sources for lighting purposes (energy-saving LED bulbs) was the invention of a highly efficient blue LED based on GaN (Nobel Prize in Physics 2014) with maximum radiation at a wavelength of 465 nm. The white color is achieved by the luminophore YAG (yttrium aluminum garnet), which, after irradiation with the blue light of a GaN diode, emits broad-spectrum light in the band of 500–700 nm. The composition of the blue diode light and the phosphor light produces white light. These LEDs are used in energy-saving lighting fixtures.

Composing R-G-B (Red Green Blue) colors of different light intensities, we can create any visual color. Using LEDs with these colors, we can "mix" light with any

Light color	Wavelength λ/nm	Voltage U/V	Material
Infrared	>760	<1.63	GaAs, AlGaAs
Red	610–760	1.63–2.03	AlGaAs, GaAsP, AlGaInP, GaP
Orange	590–610	2.03–2.10	GaAsP, AlGaInP, GaP
Yellow	570–590	2.10–2.18	GaAsP, AlGaInP, GaP
Green	500–570	2.10–4.00	GaP, AlGaInP, AlGaP—traditional InGaN/GaN—pure green
Blue	450–500	2.48–3.70	ZnSe, InGaN, SiC
Violet	400–450	2.76–4.00	InGaN
UV	<400	3.0–4.1	InGaN (385–400 nm) Diamant (235 nm) BN (215 nm), AlN (210 nm) AlGaInN (up to 210 nm)

Table 4.
Various color LEDs.

other color. This system is used by LED displays (screens of TV and computers, mobile phones, etc.), which consist of a fine network of three RGB-LED radiant elements. By changing the voltage on the individual elements, the color of the image changes.

Commercially accessible RGB LEDs with four terminals are also available. They have one common terminal, and three for each RGB segment placed on one chip. It allows controlling the color of the emitted light by changing the voltage on the three terminals. They come in useful in different signal lights. As there is a direct conversion of electric energy into visible light, the LED sources have high light efficiency of 140–150 lm/W. For comparison, a vacuum bulb with tungsten filament has light efficiency of 10–12 lm/W, halogen bulb 20 lm/W, compact fluorescent lamp 50–60 lm/W, halogen lamp 100 lm/W, low-pressure sodium lamp up to 180 lm/W. The luminosity of a 5 W LED is the same as that of a standard 40 W bulb. Another parameter of the light quality is the color temperature equivalent, which corresponds to the temperature of a thermal source with the same spectrum. E.g., 6000 K corresponds to sunlight (so-called cold white with an even representation of all wavelengths). Widely used is 2700 K light, corresponding to halogen bulb (so-called warm white with reduced blue and green component).

Lighting with different spectral compositions has different effects on humans (vision, production of melatonin or vitamin D, etc.) Intensive research of LEDs currently carries out to increase the efficiency of the conversion of electricity into light and to broaden the spectrum of radiation. In addition to visible light, one uses LEDs as sources of infrared and ultraviolet radiation.

The advantage of LEDs is that they allow a point, resp. local application, e.g., local heating of tissue by IR radiation or local irradiation by UV radiation. In the **Table 4**, there are LED sources for all bands of radiation up to a UV wavelength of 210 nm. UV LEDs allow, e.g., making visible the luminescent security features of banknotes, chip cards, etc.

The photosensitivity of microorganisms is related to the absorption spectrum of DNA with a maximum around the wavelength of 260 nm. LEDs with a range of 250–270 nm are proper for disinfection and sterilization.

LEDs can have small dimensions (under 1 mm). It is advantageous in endoscopes for illumination of the examined internal organ or in laparoscopic surgery to illuminate the operating field. The integration of LED with photodetector creates an optical coupler for the galvanic separation of electronic circuits. The connection of LED to optical fiber allows leading light anywhere.

Due to incoherence, the light of the LED is proper for the transmission of energy (lighting, irradiation, heating), but it is not capable of the transmission of information. Where require coherent light, LASER is suitable as the source.

Other promising light sources include organic semiconductor light-emitting diodes—OLEDs. The semiconductor material can be individual macromolecules or polymers. They make it possible to generate low-cost diodes with low operating voltage, high contrast, and a wide range of wavelengths. Another advantage of polymer OLEDs is their easy formability and mechanical flexibility. They are thus suitable for creating displays for mobile devices, such as mobile phones, digital cameras, or televisions.

1.6.4 Sources of coherent optical radiation—LASER

If we need to utilize the wave properties of EM radiation, we use a source of coherent radiation. Because of a single source (antenna), the radiofrequency and the microwave radiations are mostly coherent. The origin of optical radiation is random spontaneous relaxation of many atoms of matter so that the resulting radiation consists of many uncoordinated or minimally coordinated elementary waves with different frequencies and phases. The resulting waving is, therefore, incoherent.

If we want to create a coherent optical wave, all excited atoms must relax together and in phase. It is achieved by *stimulated* relaxation. At first, the whole system of atoms of the substance must be excited to a higher energy quasi-stable state with a long relaxation time. After the excitation, the external resonant stimulus must induce (stimulate), at one moment, the simultaneous relaxation of all atoms. All emitted photons have properties of the stimulating one, it is, the same frequency, phase, and propagation direction. Because of many initial stimuli, elementary waves with various frequencies and directions arise. The demanded frequency and direction are selected by an optical resonator, which amplifies the resonant waves and suppresses the non-resonant ones with other frequencies and different directions. Thus, the energy of the pumped system concentrates on producing one coherent wave with a given frequency, phase, and propagation direction. This system calls LASER (Light Amplification by Stimulated Emission of Radiation).

The system takes energy continuously, and the generated waves are also taken continuously from the resonator, e.g., through a semi-transparent mirror at one of the ends of the resonator. In this case, a *continuous wave* (*continuous laser*) arises. It is about generating a narrow beam of coherent radiation with relatively low power from a few mW to hundreds of W. The continuous lasers with infrared light are used, e.g., in *laser scalpels* for soft tissue surgery. The possibility of effectively focusing a coherent beam to a diameter approximately equal to the wavelength, and the thermal effect, which causes the blood coagulation and closing the fine capillaries, is advantageous. It allows very precise, fine, and bloodless cuts. The laser can be attached to a computer-controlled manipulator and thus perform a computer-controlled operation. *Operational robots* use this option. Blue light lasers with better focusing are used for eye surgery. Blue light cannot coagulate, but this is not necessary for eye surgery, especially the cornea and lens.

The second option uses the pumping energy of a system of atoms during a longer time interval and the sudden emission of all energy E in a short pulse of coherent radiation—*pulsed laser.* If the pulse length τ is small, the power $P = E/\tau$ of the radiated pulse is very large. Thus, extreme values of radiation power are achieved, (e.g., for $E = 1$ J and $\tau = 1$ ps is $P = 1$ TW), e.g., to investigate nonlinear phenomena. In medicine, pulsed laser is use in laparoscopic *laser lithotripsy.* A series of short power pulses heat the kidney or gall stones in small points, which are mechanically disturbed due to the temperature gradient and the associated gradient of mechanical stress. After applying several series of impulses, the stone breaks down into small parts easily washed away.

Substances with a discrete spectrum of energy levels make possible a laser effect. The simplest case is a three-level system, **Figure 12***. The electrons are excited from the ground level E_1 to level E_2. The electrons immediately relax to lower levels of E_1 and E_3. The level of E_3 must be metastable, which means, electrons remain on it for a long time and accumulate there. The electrons will gradually fill the E_3 level. The excitation takes place either by irradiation with an external light source, most often a Hg gas lamp (gas and crystal lasers), or by an electric voltage (semiconductor laser). If a resonant photon with energy $E_s = E_3 - E_1$ occurs in the system, a stimulated transition of all electrons from the state E_3 to the ground state occurs. The accumulated energy radiates in the form of photons with energy $E_L = E_s = E_3 - E_1$—stimulated emission of photons with the same properties as the first initiation photon (frequency, phase, propagation direction). The laser includes a resonator with a length of N λ L (N is an integer), which is excited by resonant photons having a defined wavelength and longitudinal propagation direction. The resonator is an enclosed space bounded by two parallel mirrors M (total) and SM (semi-transparent or*

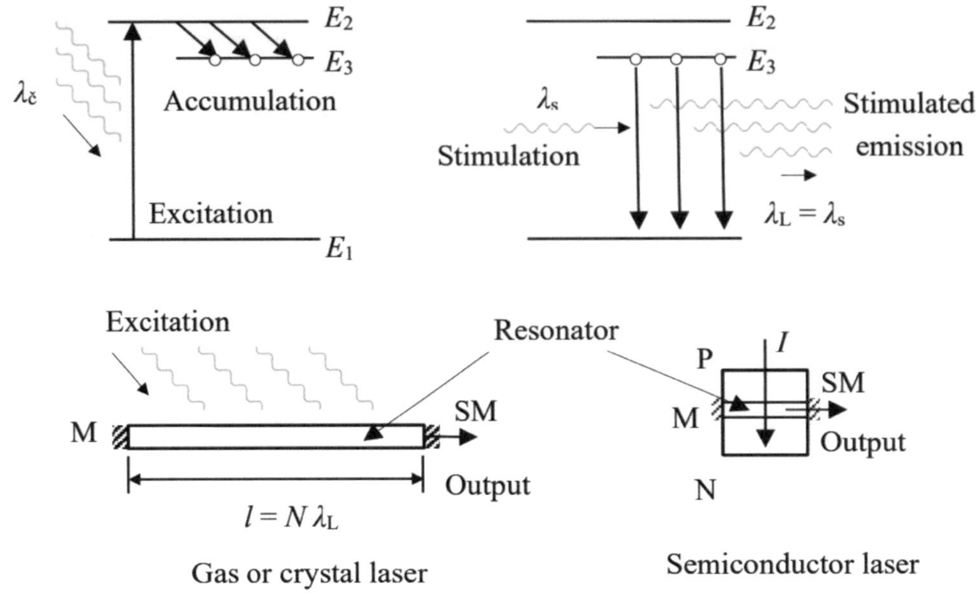

Figure 12.
Laser principle.

electronically openable in the case of a pulsed laser). Photons that do not have the exact resonant frequency and longitudinal direction will not excite the resonator.

The resonant wave reflects many times in the resonator and induces further coherent stimulated transitions to amplify the resulting wave. In a gas laser, the resonator has the shape of a tube with active gas. In a crystal laser, the resonator is the active crystal of a cylinder shape, in a semiconductor laser, the resonator represents a thin layer of the PN barrier. The coherence length of the emitted wave is many times larger than the length of the resonator. Gas lasers reach a wave coherence length of tens of centimeters to hundreds of meters, semiconductor lasers of up to 20 cm, and special fiber lasers of up to 100 km.

Note: Semiconductor lasers use a similar principle as LEDs, but used semiconductors are enriched with impurities, creating a metastable level in the forbidden band of their energy spectrum. In advance, they have a resonator, which makes the technology of laser diode production more demanding than the production of LED. Today, semiconductor laser diodes are very popular, and we can meet them, e.g., in laser pointers.

The wavelength of the laser radiation determines the active substance, i.e., the difference of energies $E_3 - E_1$ and tuning of the resonator. Some active substances have more relaxation levels, and therefore the laser effect can occur at several wavelengths. The demanded one selects the resonator by tuning from these wavelengths.

The laser light is monochromatic, and therefore a resonant absorption in different substances gets some possibilities of its application.

There is an example of the spectra of hemoglobin and water in **Figure 13**. The maximum absorption of IR radiation in water is at $\lambda \approx 3.0$ μm, which corresponds to radiation (λ = 2.94 μm) of the erbium-doped yttrium-aluminum-garnet (Er:YAG) laser. This gets possible, the surface of hard tissue correcting, e.g., in dentistry, by replacement of a drill with a painless laser. Similarly, a holmium-doped YAG (Ho:YAG) laser (λ = 2.1 μm), use in laser lithotripsy of urinary stones, where IR light is applied, using a catheter with an optical fiber through the ureter, directly into the stone.

On the contrary, the radiation of an Nd:YAG laser (λ = 1.064 μm) has a small attenuation in water and in soft tissue and thus a greater penetration depth. It is proper for the treatment of tissue in greater depth. It is a part of a laser scalpel. Radiation of the Nd:YAG with KTP laser, **Table** 5, with a wavelength λ = 532 nm,

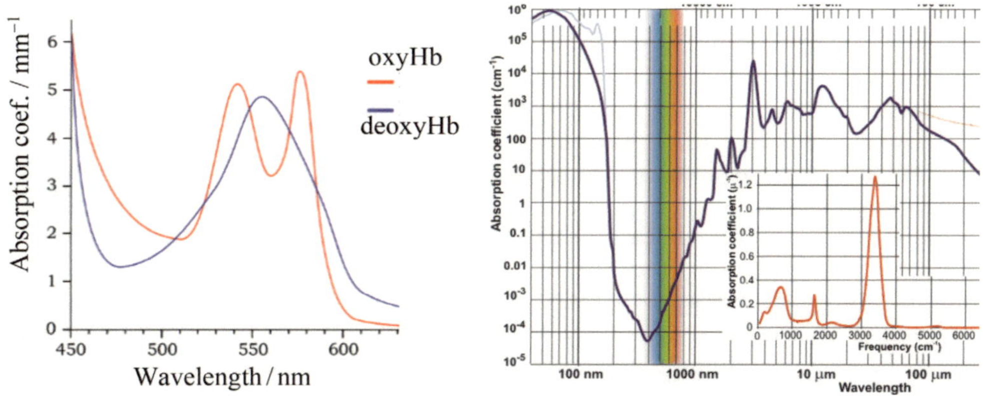

Figure 13.
Absorption spectra of hemoglobin (left) and water (right).

Material	Wavelength λ/nm	Color of the beam	Application
		Solid-state lasers	
Al_2O_3:Cr (ruby)	694.3	Red	Dermatology
Nd:YAG Nd:YVO	1064	Infrared	Surgery, laser scalpel
Nd:YVO_4 + KTP	532	Green	Treatment of angioma
Ho:YAG	2100	Infrared	Surgery, lithotripsy, stomatology
Er:YAG	2940	Infrared	Stomatology, absorbed in water
		Gas lasers	
He-Ne	633 and 543	Red, green	Holography navigation
Ar	488 and 514	Blue, green	Ophthalmology, absorbed by hemoglobin
CO_2	10,600	Infrared	Dermatology, onychomycosis, cutting laser scalpel
Excimer ArF, KrCl, KrF, XeCl, XeF	193–351	Ultraviolet	Ophthalmology, laser ablation, cornea correction
		Liquid dye lasers	
Rhodamine	570–650	Yellow to red	Dermatology, absorption by oxyhemoglobin
Coumarin	460–540	Green	Ophthalmology, surgery
		Semiconductor diode lasers	
GaAs	560 and 808	Red, infrared	Photoplethysmography
GaAlAs	670–830	Red, infrared	Telecommunication, CD players
AlGaInP	650	Red	DVD players
Ga(In)P, Ga(In)N	405 and 550	Blue, red	Blu-Ray players

YAG—Yttrium Aluminum Garnet ($Y_3Al_5O_{12}$); YVO—Yttrium Orthovanadate (YVO_4); KTP—Kalium Titanyl Phosphate ($KTiOPO_4$), nonlinear optical material used for doubling the wave frequency (half-wavelength 1064 → 532 nm).

Table 5.
Different types of lasers.

corresponds to the absorption maximum of oxyhemoglobin. It is, therefore, strongly absorbed in the blood, and is used, e.g., for the treatment of angioma (highly bloodied superficial benign tumor) by selective overheating.

Precise ophthalmology operations utilize short-wavelength lasers (green, blue, UV). An excimer laser (unstable molecules of inert gas and halogen) is used, e.g., for corneal correction, and thus correction of myopia, hyperopia, or astigmatism. Lasers with different wavelengths are widely used in dermatology. Because of the possibility to focus the collinear beam of coherent waves on the spot of the dimension of a wavelength and precisely locate the action of the laser, it is widely used in ophthalmology, neurology, or surgery. Semiconductor diode lasers represent a significant advance in laser technology. IR and red most often consist of a doped GaAs semiconductor, blue to ultraviolet on GaN, or GaP. The rate and type of doping elements can vary the wavelength over a wide range.

Since the size of the radiating surface is very small (several μm), it generates a diverging beam. It changes to a parallel beam by a small lens. Due to the small length of the resonator, the coherence length is not greater than 20 cm. The spectral width of the LED emission lines is greater than 1 nm, but it is sufficient for most applications.

The advantage of semiconductor diode lasers is their small size, which makes them suitable for portable devices like laser pointers, CDs, DVDs, and Blu-ray players, laser printers, etc. It is possible to connect the laser diode directly to an optical fiber and transmit light to any place and over a long distance. Another advantage is in the electric excitation, which allows easy modulation of the light beam by an electrical signal. They are, therefore, useful in optical communications, from simple optical couplers to long-distance transmission systems. Laser diodes are manufactured for a wide range of power from units of mW to tens of W, which provide many applications in medicine.

1.6.5 Sources of ionizing EM radiation

Ionizing by radiation causes the ionization of atoms or molecules or a change in chemical bindings. Shortwave EM radiation or radioactive particle radiation (alpha, beta, protons, neutrons) exhibits the ionizing effect. The carriers of the EM radiation energy are photons with energy $E = h\,c/\lambda$. Ionizing effects occur at energies of photons above 10 eV, chemical effects already at energies of several eV (e.g., dissociation energy of water is about 5 eV), which corresponds to EM radiation with wavelengths of approximately $\lambda < 250$ nm. This corresponds to UV-C ultraviolet radiation (100–280 nm), X-rays, and gamma radiation.

UV sources were described in the previous paragraph. E.g., an excimer laser generates the ionizing UV-C radiation.

The next section gets an overview of the sources of X-rays and gamma rays, used in medical diagnostics and therapy.

1.6.5.1 X-rays sources

X-rays represent the EM radiation with wavelengths from 10 nm up to 10 pm, i.e., with photon energy from 100 eV to 100 keV. X-rays, like optical radiation, are generated by the relaxation of electrons in atoms from higher energy levels to lower ones after the previous excitation, most often by electrons, accelerated in an electric field (accelerator). Due to the high energy of X-photons, only the atoms with a high atomic number that have sufficiently low energies of deep bonded electron states, and simultaneously hard fusible metals, can be used to generate this radiation. Tungsten is the most often used. In an accelerator with a voltage U, the electron obtains the kinetic energy $E_k = e\,U$. After impact with the tungsten target anode, the electron transfers its energy to the atoms in the surface layer. Most of the energy of the incident electrons converts into internal thermal energy so that the target heats up strongly, and into emission of the electrons from the surface layer. Some of the incident electrons cause excitation of the bound electrons to higher states. At a sufficiently high voltage U, the bound electrons are excited from deep states up to the conduction band, see **Figure 14**. Electrons from higher energy levels of the conduction band or near bound states then relax into the emptied deep states.

The maximum energy of photons is equal to the kinetic energy of incident electrons.

$$\frac{1}{2}mv^2 = eU = \frac{hc}{\lambda_{min}}, \quad \text{from where } \lambda_{min} = \frac{hc}{eU}, \tag{70}$$

where U is the accelerating voltage. E.g., for U = 40 kV is $\lambda_{min} = 31 \times 10^{-12}$ m.

The minimum wavelength can thus be varied through the accelerating voltage U.

Transitions from a wide conduction band E_c generate photons with a continuous energy spectrum, the so-called *braking radiation*, with the lower limit of the wavelength λ_{min}, **Figure 14**. Transitions from near bound levels to empty deep levels emit the so-called *characteristic radiation* with precisely defined wavelengths, which produce sharp peaks in the spectrum.

In **Figure 15(a)**, there is a classical X-rays source—a vacuum X-rays lamp. Heating filament supplied by voltage U_h heats the cathode K, which emits electrons due to thermionic emission. They move in an electric field with a voltage accelerating U to the anode A. The anode is a rotating copper disk with a layer of tungsten on an inclined surface. Disk rotation reduces overheating at the point of electron beam impact. X-rays are emitted from the point of impact of the electrons.

With the development of nanotechnology, a cathode with cold electron emission of electrons has been developed. These CNTs (Carbon Nano Tubes) cathode has very fine carbon nanotubes on the surface. After approaching a grating electrode with a positive potential (from ten to one hundred volts), a strong electric field is created on the sharp tips of the nanotubes. It causes an electron discharge (electron emission). The electrons then penetrate through holes in the grating electrode and form an electron beam. The cathode has a dimension of tenths of an mm and is relatively cold. It allows realizing miniature devices. One important invention is the

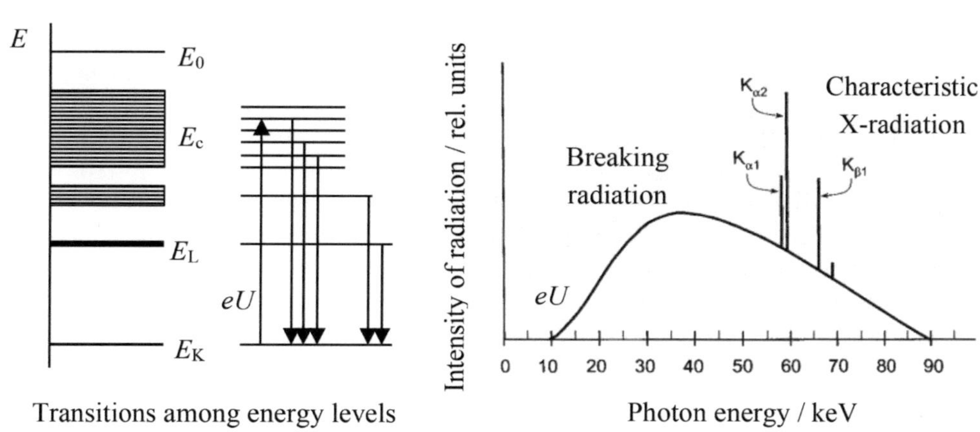

Figure 14.
Principle of rising and spectrum of X-rays.

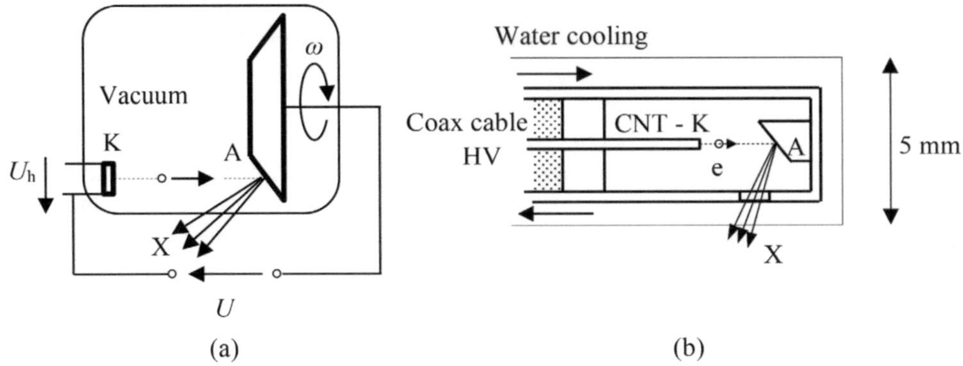

Figure 15.
X-ray sources (a) vacuum X-rays lamp, (b) micro X-ray s tube.

Micro X-rays Tube, **Figure 15(b)**. Electrons emitted from the CNT cathode electrostatically focus on the tungsten target. The voltage between cathode K and anode A supplied by the coaxial line is up to 50 kV. Accelerated electrons thus, after hitting the anode, generate X-rays, which emerge from the tube through a window. The tungsten anode warms by incident electrons, and therefore the generator is housed in an outer tube that supplies water to cool the anode. The power of emitted radiation is limited to ensure sufficient cooling. Another advantage of the CNT cathode is the possibility to control its current by the voltage at the grid with a very short time constant. It allows pulse modulation of the generated X-rays and thus to achieve a high instant radiation intensity at low average power. At a maximum cathode current of 300 μA, the microgenerator offers a dose rate of up to 0.6 Gy/min, which is sufficient for many applications. The entire X-rays probe is about 5 mm in diameter and a few centimeters long. In medicine, microgenerators are used mainly in brachytherapy (*Greek: brachys—close*) by placing the emitter directly in the place to be irradiated, e.g., tumor. The dimensions of the microgenerator allow us to place it in a catheter and insert it through a vessel, urinary, or digestive tract into the appropriate site and then turn the switch on and off for the required time.

1.6.5.2 Sources of gamma radiation

Gamma radiation is EM radiation with a photon energy of 1 MeV to 10 GeV, or with wavelengths of 10^{-12} to 10^{-15} m, which is emitted from the nuclei of atoms (nuclear radiation). Similarly, to optical radiation or X-rays, which is produced by the transition of electrons from higher energy levels to lower ones, gamma radiation is caused by the relaxation of excited nuclei. While the energies of the electron states have values from units of eV to 100 keV, and the energy of the emitted photons corresponds to this, the energy of the nucleus states has values from 100 keV up to tens of GeV. The excitation of nuclei occurs due to nuclear transformations or the impact of gamma radiation, neutron, proton, or alpha radiation on atomic nuclei. Natural sources are radioactive substances that occur in nature, such as uranium, radium, radon, etc. A significant amount of radioactive material is found in the Earth's crust, and the heat released during its transformations is one of the Earth's heat sources, together with the Sun, which maintains a friendly ambient temperature. Radioactive preparations as sources of gamma radiation are mostly artificially produced. In medicine, gamma radiation uses diagnostics because of its low attenuation in the human body. Molecules of chemicals participating in metabolic processes in the body are "labeled" with atoms of a radioactive substance (some atoms in the molecule are replaced by similar radioactive atoms that do not change their chemical properties). These molecules are called radio markers and radiopharmaceuticals. After application to the body, the radiopharmaceutical concentrates at the site where it uses the body. These sites thus appear in the increased production of gamma radiation. The gamma camera displays these places, and based on the created images, it is possible to analyze physiological processes in the body, and thus disease processes in the body. Modern nuclear imaging methods include SPECT (Single Photon Emission Tomography) and PET (Positron Emission Tomography). The discipline of nuclear medicine deals with this issue in detail.

The most often used sources of gamma radiation for SPECT are technetium ^{99m}Tc, krypton ^{81m}Kr, iodine ^{131}I. Each radioactive preparation has different energy of emitted photons, and therefore a different function in the body. The PET method uses the annihilation of positrons with electrons accompanied by the production of a pair of gamma photons. They have the same energy and propagate in opposite directions. Radioactive preparations generate positrons due to the transformation of some neutron-deficient nuclei. The proper biogenic elements are carbon ^{11}C, nitrogen ^{13}N, oxygen ^{15}O, and fluorine ^{18}F. At the conversion of the nucleus, the proton converts to a neutron and a positron. The positron is an antiparticle to an electron, and when a particle and an antiparticle meet, both annihilate and form a pair of photons.

Example 7. Gamma conversion of iodine ^{123}I nucleus.

Nuclear medicine uses unstable isotopes of nuclei of different elements as sources of gamma radiation. Isotopes of elements, which the body uses in its organs for their activities, are used for diagnostic purposes. For thyroid examination, the unstable iodine isotope ^{123}I is proper. During the nuclear transformation, the nucleus captures an electron from the lowest state of the electron shell. The transformation obeys the equation

$$^{123}_{53}\mathrm{I} + -1_0\mathrm{e} \rightarrow 52_{123}\mathrm{Te} + \gamma(0,16\ \ \mathrm{MeV}). \tag{71}$$

The reaction produces tellurium and releases a gamma photon with an energy of 160 keV, which corresponds to the wavelength.

$$\lambda = \frac{hc}{E_\mathrm{f}} \approx 7,7 \times 10^{-12}\ \mathrm{m},$$

corresponding to electromagnetic radiation from the gamma band.

Example 8. Annihilation of an electron-positron pair.

In nuclear medicine, the isotope of the fluorine atom ^{18}F, unstable with a half-life of 110 min, changes according to the equation

$$^{18}_{9}\mathrm{F} \rightarrow 8_{18}\mathrm{O} + {}^{0}_{1}\mathrm{e}^{+}. \tag{72}$$

The second particle is the positron, antiparticle, which has the same mass and opposite charge as the electron. When the positron encounters an electron while moving from the point of origin, both particles disappear—*annihilate,* producing two identical gamma photons. The reaction preserves energy and momentum, and the quantities must be considered relativists. We assume that the momentums of the particles before the collision are small and can be neglected.

$$\begin{aligned} mc^2 + mc^2 &= E_{\mathrm{f}1} + E_{\mathrm{f}2}, \\ 0 &= \mathbf{p}_{\mathrm{f}1} + \mathbf{p}_{\mathrm{f}2}. \end{aligned} \tag{73}$$

The second equation shows that the photons have the same momentum and opposite direction, i.e., they have the same energy. From the first equation we get

$$E_{\mathrm{f}} = mc^2 = \frac{hc}{\lambda}. \tag{74}$$

The energy of the photons is E_f = 512 keV and the corresponding wavelength $\lambda = 2.4 \times 10^{-12}$ m, which corresponds to gamma radiation.

1.7 Detection of electromagnetic waves

Another part of the transmission system is a detector of the radiation. Like sources, detectors depend on the function for which they are intended and the wavelength of the radiation. There are three groups of detectors—wave detectors, power detectors, and ich detect quantum detectors. In the first group are detectors, which detect the amplitude, frequency, and phase of the wave. Wave detection is possible only in the case of coherent waves. In the second group are detectors, which evaluate the energy or power of the incident radiation. They use a change of temperature of the sensor, due to the absorption of radiation. Quantum detectors use the quantum nature of radiation—photons and the energy spectrum of the detection sensor.

1.7.1 Wave detectors

Wave detectors provide information about the wave quantities—amplitude, frequency, phase, and polarization. One of the detection methods is the use of antennas and the conversion of wave quantities into voltage or current in the detection antenna. Antennas are useful mainly for radio waves and microwave ranges. Another method utilizes wave interference. This method is used mainly in the range of optical waves.

1.7.1.1 Antennas for receiving EM waves

The basic elements of antenna systems are electrical or magnetic dipole sensors. Several basic types of antennas are in **Figure 16**. The first type is a rod antenna, figure (a), in which the EM wave induces electrical voltage U. To achieve the maximum detection efficiency, the resonant mode of the antenna is tuned, i.e., the total antenna length *λ/2—the half-wave dipole*. The elementary dipole is usually a part of more complex antenna systems, where other elements serve to shape the radiation pattern of the antenna, and thus increase its gain and directivity. Figure (b) shows a Yagi antenna, used to receive a TV signal, figure (c) is a parabolic antenna for receiving astronomic signals. A similar but smaller parabolic antenna serves for telecommunication connections and the reception of TV satellite signals. Figure (d) shows a special PIFA antenna (Planar Inverse F-Antenna), used in mobile devices (mobile phones, GPS receivers, etc.).

At frequencies around 1 GHz and above, PIFA is so small that it can fit in small instruments. The example in the picture has the dimension of the width of a mobile phone. Another type is a $\lambda/4$ antenna above the conductive base plane, figure (e), where the second $\lambda/4$ part of the half-wave dipole is formed by mirroring. An example is, e.g., rod antenna (f) of WIFI communicator, or waveguide field detection probe (g). This elementary detection probe is, e.g., a part of the microwave funnel antenna (h)—the funnel adjusts the radiation pattern and impedance

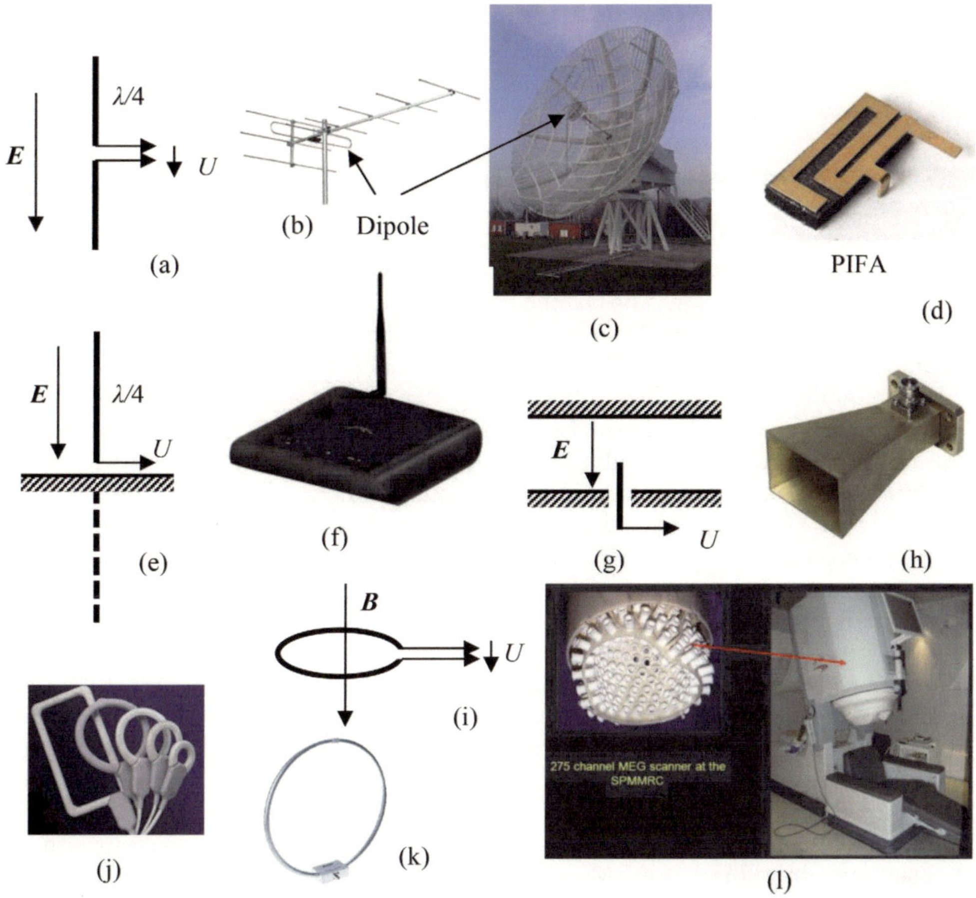

Figure 16.
Different types of antennas. (a) dipol antena, (b) Yagi antena, (c) parabolic antena, (d) PIFA antena, (e) quater wavelength antena, (f) WIFI antena, (g) waveguide antena, h) funnel antena, (i) loop antena, (j) MRI antenas, (k) frame antena, (l) MEG antena.

matching. Just behind the funnel, there is a voltage probe with a connector for joining a coaxial cable.

Another type is a loop antenna, figure (i), in which a voltage is induced, due to a change of the magnetic flux of the wave. A suitable capacitor connected to the antenna tunes resonance of the antenna, and thus maximum efficiency of detection. In figure (j) is the detection antenna of MRI (*Magnetic Resonance Imaging)* devices. Figure (k) shows a simple table frame antenna. Devices for measuring the body's magnetic manifestations, such as MKG (*Magneto Cardiography*), MMG (*Magneto Myography*), and the like, also use detection coils. Figure (l) shows a MEG (*Magneto Encephalography*) device, which serves for the examination of brain currents. The figure shows a headpiece with 275 sensors based on detection coils.

A common feature of antennas is the sensitivity to the polarization of the EM wave. The electric dipole antenna is sensitive to waves polarized in the dipole direction. Similarly, the loop antenna is sensitive to the magnetic field perpendicular to the loop.

The induced voltage U occurs at the output of the antenna. This voltage proceeds via a connecting line to the receiver, which processes it in the demanded manner. The amplitude, frequency, and phase of this voltage correspond to the same quantities of the wave. In this way, it is possible to sense the amplitude, frequency, phase, or pulse modulation of the wave, and to detect the information carried by the wave. A typical example from biomedicine is the detection of an FID signal in the magnetic resonance device.

1.7.1.2 Optical detectors

The optical radiation includes visible light, infrared, and ultraviolet radiation. There are two groups of detectors of optical radiation.

Detectors of the first group are *bolometers*. They measure the intensity of radiation using the change of temperature caused by the sensor heating due to the absorption of the radiation. The change of temperature is most often evaluated from a change of the electrical resistance of the absorbent body, which is, e.g., a thin platinum strip or semiconducting thermistor. A lens or mirror concentrates the radiation on the absorbing body. This body is thermally connected with the surrounding, thus creating its thermal equilibrium. The change of temperature, and thus of the resistance of the body, is directly proportional to the intensity of the incident radiation. The bolometer display is calibrated to directly indicate the intensity of the incident radiation. Due to the thermal inertia of the detection body, the bolometers are not suitable for monitoring faster changes in radiation intensity. The advantage of bolometers is that they are broadband, from radio waves to gamma radiation. Bolometers are used, e.g., in astronomy for the detection of stellar radiation, especially in the range of radio and infrared radiation. New types of bolometers with graphene (carbon nanostructure) as a detector are currently under development. In these bolometers, the incident radiation directly controls the electron gas without any mediation by the crystal lattice, which allows, in addition to high sensitivity and a wide sensitivity band, the short time constant of the order of up to picoseconds.

In biomedicine, bolometric, resp. calorimetric methods are used to control the exposure of infrared radiators. Measuring the intensity of X-rays or gamma radiation is used, e.g., in the calibration of therapeutic sources of ionizing radiation using phantoms. Bolometers also detect particle flow, e.g., in accelerators.

The second group can be referred to as *quantum detectors*. They use the quantum nature of radiation and the quantum nature of the energy spectrum of the detection substance. The most widely used are external or internal photoelectric effects. The first case represents vacuum phototube or photomultipliers, the second is semiconductor photoresistors, photodiodes, or phototransistors. In semiconductors, the incident radiation causes the excitation of pairs of electron-hole, which affects the electrical conductivity of the photoresistor, or the closing current of the PN passage. Due to the lower cut-off frequency of the semiconductor detector, which is given by the width of the forbidden bandgap, these detectors are not sensitive to low-frequency (thermal) noise. They are used to detect optical radiation (infrared, visible, and ultraviolet).

Special cases of semiconductor detectors are the CCD and CMOS structures. They are photodiodes, arranged in a chessboard grid on the surface of the microchip. Due to illumination, the elements of the chip accumulate the charge, which is then electrically scanned. Each element (pixel) is assigned a voltage value, which is then digitized and stored in the device's memory. There are three sub-grids on the chip, every with sensitivity to different R-G-B colors. There is imaging, due to the ratio of intensities of the light components R-G-B, any observed color. In this way, the device's memory stores complex information about the color image. Digital cameras and camcorders use these CCD or CMOS sensors. CCD sensors are most used for cameras to capture a color image in the visible region of the spectrum. CMOS sensors, which are faster and have lower noise, are mainly used for fast sensors (camcorders) and in the field of infrared (thermal) radiation imaging

DOI: http://dx.doi.org/10.5772/intechopen.101652

cameras. CMOS sensors integrated with signal amplifiers and a microprocessor are advantageous in the case of compact systems such as photo cameras in mobile phones.

1.7.2 Photomultiplier

Special electronic detectors—photomultipliers are used to detect very low-intensity optical radiation.

The principle of the photomultiplier is in **Figure 17**. The detected radiation (also the only photon) incidents on the photocathode PK. If the photon energy is greater than the edge emission energy of the electron from the photocathode, the electron is released. In an electric field with a voltage U_1 between the cathode and the first electrode D1 (dynode), the electron accelerates, and due to impact on the dynode D1, it causes the emission of several secondary electrons (secondary emission). The secondary electrons are accelerated by the voltage between the first, second, and other dynodes, and after every impact, again cause secondary emission of other upright brackets (k) electrons. In this way, the number of electrons gradually multiply, and after the impact of k^n electrons on the last electrode A (anode), arises an output current pulse in the anode resistor. This pulse is large enough to be detected by a pulse counter connected to the photomultiplier. This achieves an amplification of the number of electrons up to 108. Photomultipliers also have low noise. They are also able to detect individual photons, hitting the photocathode.

Photomultipliers are used in astronomy to detect very low radiation from distant stars, to detect very low biosignals emitted by living organisms and the like. The use of photomultipliers in ionizing radiation detectors is significant.

1.7.3 Detectors of ionizing radiation

The spectrum of electromagnetic waves also includes ionizing radiation (UV, X, gamma), which is used in radiation diagnostics (skiascopy, CT, nuclear methods—gamma camera, PET, SPECT).

For high-energy X or gamma photons, the direct photoelectric effect has low efficiency. Therefore, ionizing radiation is first transformed into an optical one. For this reason, serve *scintillation crystals*, especially Na I, Cs I, Ba F_2. After

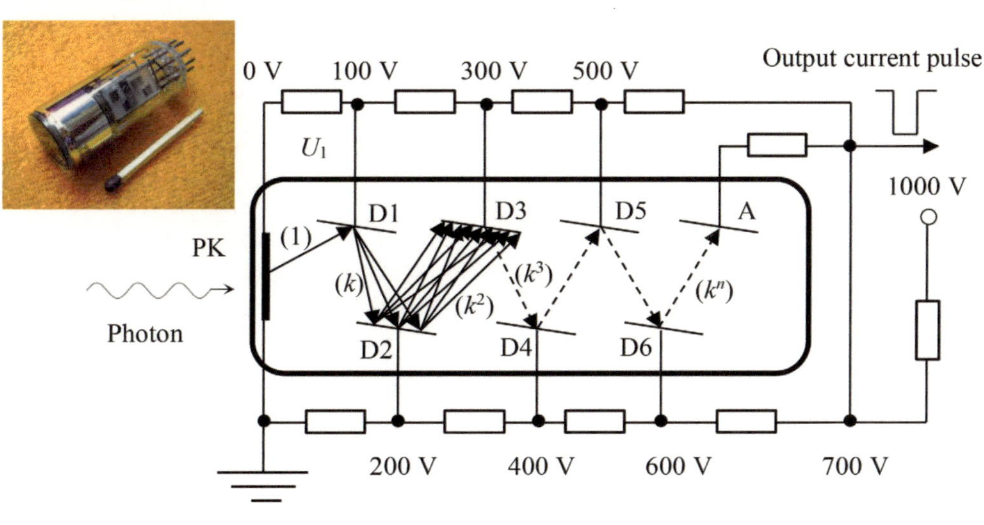

Figure 17.
Photomultiplier scheme.

irradiation with high-energy photons, electrons are excited from deep electron levels to excitation levels, from which the electrons relax to lower levels gradually (in smaller steps). It gives rise to photons with lower energy from the optical band. It represents a quantum transformation of the energy of photons from the X or γ bands to the optical one, where they can be detected by optical photodetectors. Since the probability of capturing high-energy photons is small, a sensitive detector (photomultiplier), is used to detect secondary optical photons.

Figure 18 shows an ionizing radiation detector. It consists of a matrix of individual detection cells. Each cell contains a collimator C (lead tube), which ensures that only photons 1 fall from one direction on the scintillation crystal SC. Photons 2 inclined obliquely, are captured on the walls of the tube. This ensures the directionality of the detector. The detecting cell thus determines the direction of the point of the radiation source. The cell matrix creates an area detector that scans a certain part of the body at once. Behind the scintillation crystals is a set of photomultipliers PM, from which the signals go to a computer. Scintillation detectors allow detecting X and γ rays in CT scanners, gamma cameras, PET, and SPECT scanners.

In **Figure 18** on the right, is a diagnostic *gamma camera,* which is investigating the distribution of a radioactive substance (radiopharmaceutical) in the body of the examined patient. A radiopharmaceutical is a source of radioactive gamma radiation emitted from the body. The two detection cameras are opposite each other in a rotating holder. The detection matrix only determines the direction of the place from which the radiation comes. However, if record a signal from different directions of camera rotation, it is possible to accurately determine the location of the radiation source by computer reconstruction.

In addition to scintillation detectors, ionization chambers are used to detect ionizing radiation. They utilize the ionization of the low-pressure gas in a tube, in which the release of the electron causes an electric current pulse. A typical instrument is a *Geiger-Müller counter* used for measuring the radioactivity of the environment.

The photographic dosimeter is another type of device for measuring the accumulated irradiation. The incident radiation activates the photosensitive film, and after the film developing the murkiness of the emulsion determines the radiation dose.

Another type of personal dosimeter is a *thermoluminescent dosimeter*. It is a semiconductor detector with a metastable excitation level with a long relaxation time. Due to the irradiation, electrons are excited to a metastable level and remain

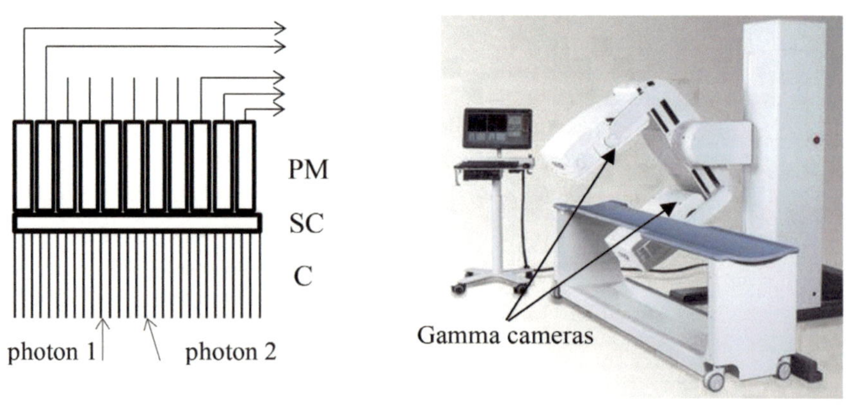

Figure 18.
Ionizing radiation detector (the principal on the left, gamma camera on the right).

there for a long time. The number of accumulated electrons is directly proportional to the irradiation. After heating the irradiated detector, the electrons relax to the ground state and emit photons with an energy equal to the energy of the electron transition. The emitted photons are detected, e.g., with a photomultiplier. The obtained photoelectric signal is directly proportional to the absorbed radiation dose. Crystals of Li F, Ca F_2, Mg Be O_4, and others for various types of ionizing radiation are proper, as materials for thermoluminescent dosimeters.

1.8 Perception of light by the human eye

An important source of information is for people the sight, which is the electromagnetic channel of direct communication between the world and a man. It involves the reception, processing, and evaluation of electromagnetic waves in the frequency range of visible light. The vision system consists of three parts. The first one is the optical processing of the incident wave, the second the detection part, and the third the processing of the detected information in the brain. In the wavelength band of approximately (380–780) nm, or the range of frequency of (385–790) THz, detects the eye EM waves (visible light) and transmits a signal through the optic nerve to the center of vision in the brain.

1.8.1 Optical system of the eye

The eye as a sensor processes light incident on the system of light-sensitive cells on the retina of the eye. The optical system of the eye ensures the creation of a real image of the observed object on the retina. The structure of the eye is in **Figure 19**. The functional parts of the optical system are the cornea, anterior chamber, lens, and vitreous body. As we can see in the picture, it is a convergent optical system, whose task is to display a beam of rays emanating from a certain point of the object to one point on the retina. The main parts important for the projection of the observed object on the retina are the lenticular anterior chamber closed from the outside by the cornea, the ocular lens with variable optical vergence by clamping on the ciliary body, and the liquid vitreous transmission medium. The total optical vergence of the eye is approximately 60 D (dioptres), of which only 20 D falls on the ocular lens. The diameter of the eyeball is 24 mm, the distance between the lens and the retina is approximately 17 mm.

When the lens muscles are completely relaxed, the lens shrinks and has maximum vergence. In this case, the object sharply displayed on the retina is at a minimum distance, called a *nearby point*. For the normal eye, it is about 10 cm. It grows with age up to 50 cm at the age of about 50 years. When tensing the lens muscles, the maximum flattening of the lens occurs. In this case, the eye focuses on the retina object at the maximum distance, called a *distant point*, ideally at infinity. Accommodation of the lens at the age of about 15 years, has a range of about 10 D. At a later age over 50 years this range is only 2 D, and at the age of 70 years, the ability to accommodate the eye completely fades. The distance of the object at which the young eye least strains by accommodation is the so-called *conventional optical distance,* approximately $l \approx 25$ cm.

If the eye is not able to focus close objects on the retina (focus is behind the retina), **Figure 19**, the eye is farsighted (hyperopic eye). This error is corrected by spectacles or contact lenses with positive optical power (converging). If the eye is short-sighted (myopic eye), the distant objects focus in front of the retina, and this error corrects diverging glasses with negative lens power. At present, there are surgical procedures, which allow modifying the lens or cornea with a laser so that it is not necessary to use glasses. Today's ophthalmic optics offer various convenient vision

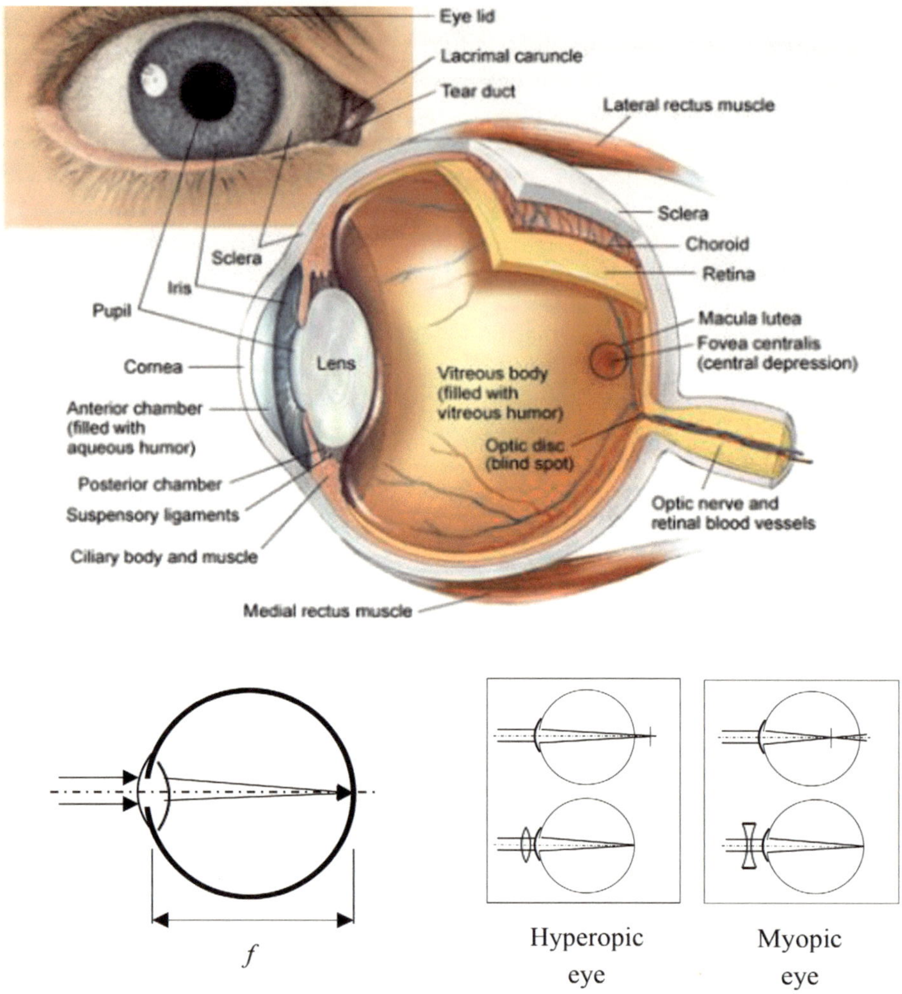

Figure 19.
Eye and optical eye defects.

correction aids, such as bifocal or multifocal spectacles, spectacles responding to light intensity (helio-variable), which are obscured by the incident radiation, spectacles with a UV filter, which protect the eyes from the harmful UV radiation, etc.

1.8.2 Light detection by eye

Light detectors are cells on the retina of the eye. There are four types of cells for vision. The rods are broadband, do not distinguish colors, and are sensitive to the wavelength band (380–650) nm with a maximum sensitivity at the wavelength of 500 nm. The cones are narrowband. There are three species with maximum sensitivity in the wavelength bands (440–450) nm (blue), (535–555) nm (green), and (570–590) nm (red). Light with wavelengths shorter than 380 nm (ultraviolet) absorbs the lens and does not hit the retina. With sufficient intensity, the eye perceives light up to a wavelength of 780 nm.

There are 5–7 million cones, and they are concentrated mainly around the yellow spot (a retina point on the optical axis of the eye). For the best color vision, you need to look directly at the object. The rods are 120 million and have the highest density at an angular distance of 25° away from the axis. For night vision, it is necessary to look at an angle of approximately 25° away from the object (so-called *side vision*) for the best sensitivity. The blind spot, where are no light-sensitive cells, is approximately 20° away from the axis towards the nose. It is the output of the optic nerve.

Color-photopic vision (cones—contain the photosensitive protein photopsin I, II, III) has a total wavelength range of (430–690) nm at the level of sensitivity drop to 1% (−20 dB) with a maximum at 555 nm (yellow-green color), **Figure 20**.

Night (black and white)—scotopic vision (rods—contain the photosensitive protein rhodopsin) has a wavelength range of (380–650) nm with a maximum at 500 nm. The eye can distinguish two colors with a wavelength difference of 1–2 nm (up to 160 colors) and up to 600 thousand shades.

As the light intensity decreases, at first the red, then blue, and finally the green cones, are gradually eliminated. Therefore, in the gloom, the scene color turns to blue-green or green.

The eye adapts to darkness in approximately 10 min (complete adaptation lasts up to 1 h). Back adaptation to light takes 2–3 min. This is the essence of the vision loss of a driver due to bright headlights at night. At low light intensity, the red cones stop working, but the green and blue remain active. If we want to illuminate something and not lose adaptation to the dark, we use red lighting.

From each cell on the retina comes a nerve fiber that conducts excitement into the brain. Close to the yellow spot, each cell has its fiber. At the edge of the retina, there are more cells connected to one fiber. Therefore, the best resolution is around the center of the retina. All fibers together form the optic nerve, which contains approximately 1 million fibers. The optic nerve originates in the eye around the blind spot, in which are no light-sensitive cells.

The angular resolution (lateral) is 1′ (angular minute) and is given by the density of the cones in the yellow spot. Due to the diffraction of light on the pupil, the resolution angle increases (**Figure 21**).

Retinal cells are characterized by the logarithmic dependence of the output signal on the intensity of illumination. Thanks to this, the eye has a huge range of brightness resolution—up to 10^{12}, i.e., 120 dB, from the smallest values of 10^{-6} cd·m^{-2} to 10^{6} cd·m^{-2}. Photopic vision requires a light intensity >3 cd·m^{-2}, scotopic <3 mcd·m^{-2}, see.

In addition to visual perception, the retina of the eye has another function. There are other Non-Images Forming Photoreceptors (NIFPs—contain the photosensitive

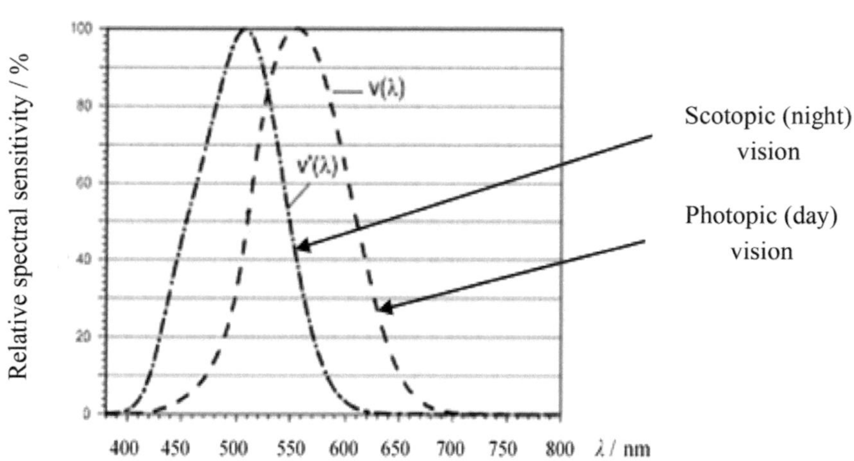

Figure 20.
The curve of relative spectral sensitivity of the eye in day and night vision.

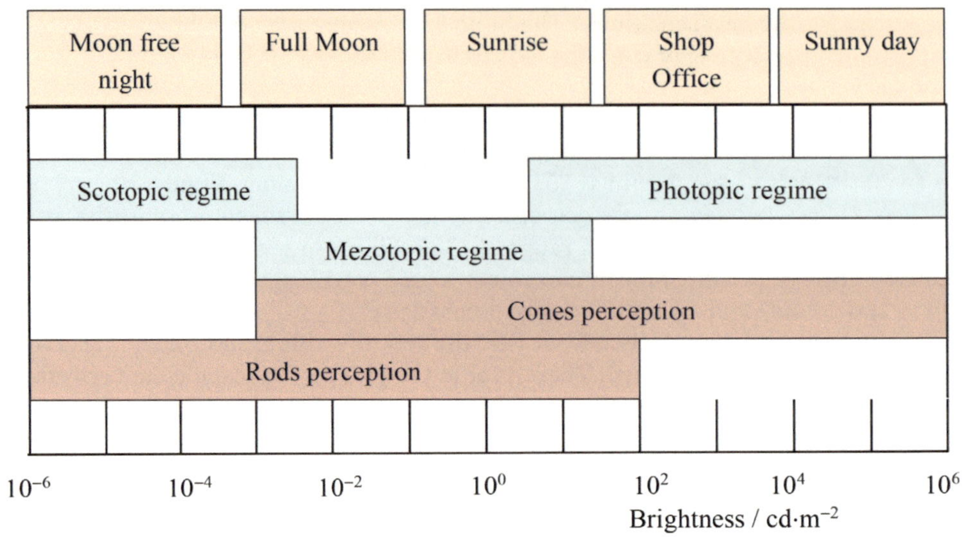

Figure 21.
Perception of objects with different brightness by different cells.

protein *melanopsin*) on the retina that does not participate in imaging. Their signals go to the pituitary gland, which controls the pineal gland, which produces melatonin, a hormone that affects sleep rhythm, and a variety of physiological functions. The spectral degree of suppression of melatonin production is shown by a graph of the *meltopic spectrum*, **Figure 22**. As we can see, blue light suppresses melatonin production the most. Melatonin regulates sleep and the sleep cycle. Sleep, e.g., does not affect red light (above 600 nm). If we do not want to disrupt melatonin production and thus sleep at night, it is advantageous to use red lighting. Blue, on the other hand, severely disrupts sleep and is used when the sleep cycle needs to be regulated. In some cars, dim interior blue lighting can be observed at night, which should have a positive effect on keeping the driver's attention while driving at night.

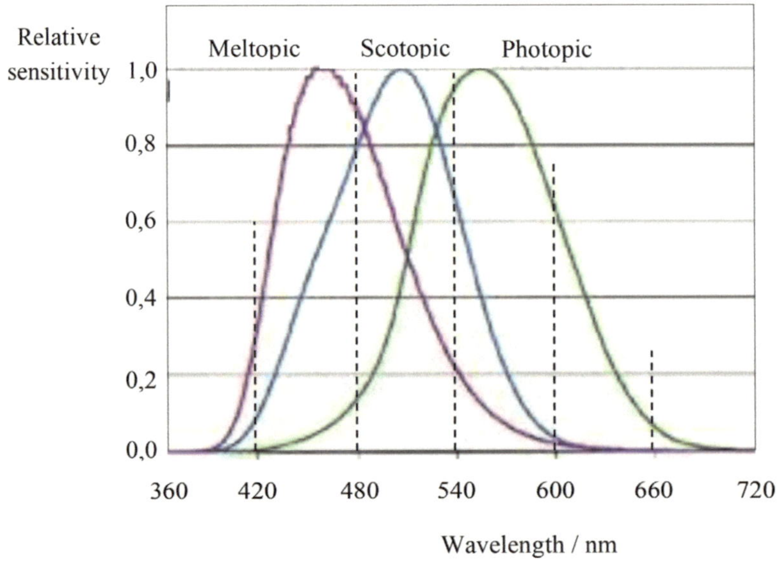

Figure 22.
Three types of eye sensitivity spectra.

1.8.3 Optic nerve signal processing in the brain

Visual perception does not arise in the eye but in the brain, where the signals of nerve fibers from both eyes terminate. After processing these signals, a spatial and color image of the object creates in the brain. During processing, the brain also uses the previous experience stored in memory and corrects some shortcomings of the received signal. For example, we can read fluently a text with errors or shuffled letters. There also arise various optical illusions. The image on the retina projected by the eye lens is inverted, but we perceive the image created in the brain as straight. There are experiments, in which the scene was turned over by special glasses. In a relatively short time, however, the normal straight view renewed again. The brain reacted and based on experience, turned over the perceived image in the brain. After taking off the glasses, one observed for some time the surroundings overturned back to the normal view.

1.8.3.1 Three-dimensional vision

One can see the scene spatially (3D) when one perceives not only its right-left sides but also its depth. This is due to a pair of eyes that are 6–7 cm apart from each other. It provides slightly different images of eyes when observing, especially near objects. The right eye sees more of the right side and left more of the left side. The synthesis of these images in the brain forms a *stereo-effect (or 3D effect)*.

To see a three-dimensional image, we must provide both eyes with corresponding images. There are several ways to do this. The first one uses the recording of both images for the left and right eye in two complementary colors and composing them into one resulting image. If looking at the resulting image by glasses with corresponding color filters for each eye, every eye perceives its image. Stereo television utilizes another system. Both images are sent alternatively with two polarizations, mutually perpendicular, and the viewer observes the TV screen by glasses with corresponding polarization filters. The next system quickly alternates both images for the right eye and the left eye on the monitor, and the observer uses electronically controlled glasses, transparency of which synchronously switch-over for the right eye and the left eye.

An example of the extraordinary ability of the brain, is the so-called *stereogram*, **Figure 23**, in which the views of both eyes are mixed into one planar image. If we look at the picture and try to accommodate the eyes to infinity, a three-dimensional object will emerge from the stereogram in a short time (you should see a wolf in the forest with spatially arranged trees in the foreground and the background). The condition is to see with both eyes, if you use glasses, also with glasses. The brain can classify seemingly chaotic pictures and create a meaningful interpretation of the signals captured by the eyes. It selects information from the image, separately for the left eye and the right eye, and creates the resulting 3D image.

1.8.3.2 Holography

In many cases, the spatial (3D) representation of objects requires, whether for scientific purposes, for demonstrations, or to archive records. 3D imaging is one of the modern trends in biomedicine.

Within 3D imaging, the name *holography* (Greek: *holos*—complete) mentions as creating a complete image of an object. 3D perception is created in the brain by processing the signals of the optic nerves of the right and left eyes, which differ slightly. If we want to display an object so that we can see it spatially, we must

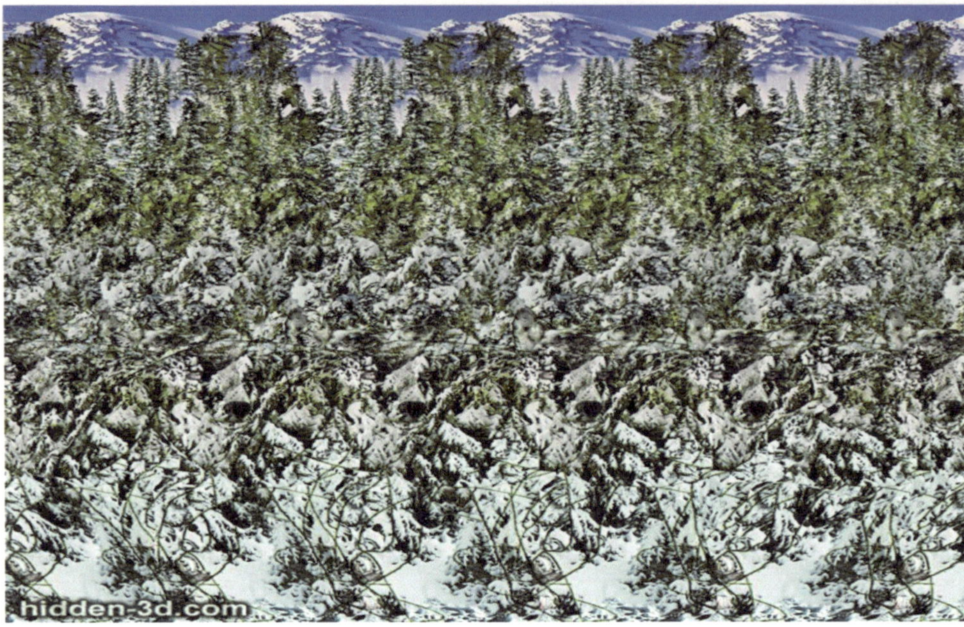

Figure 23.
Stereogram (wolf in the forest).

reproduce the original wavefield emanating from the object. The basic idea of the record is as follows, **Figure 24**.

If we illuminate the object (R1 rays) from the source S1, we see the original object, observing the reflected or scattered light (rays R2). Then we replace our eyes with a photographic plate H1. With the help of a semi-transparent mirror SM, we illuminate the plate with reference light (rays R3 emanated virtually from the virtual image VS1). The rays R2 and R3 interfere at the surface of the plate, and we record the interference maxima of light intensity by blackening the photographic emulsion. The recorded interference picture is the hologram H2. To create a static interference pattern, the light source must be coherent. The LASER is, therefore, necessary for recording and reconstruction of the hologram.

If placing the obtained hologram H2 in its original position and illuminating with the reference beam R3 the same as at recording the hologram, light diffraction on the hologram occurs. The 1st order diffraction (R4 rays) is a very reproduction of the original wavefield from the original (R2 rays). The eyes thus persist the field created by imagining an apparent image in place of the former original, as if observing a real original. Since it is a matter of creating a complete field of light (*holos*), the image has the properties of the original. It means the eyes perceive the image spatially.

The image can be viewed from different angles, as the size of the hologram plate allows. Such a hologram is often fully sufficient to replace a valuable original, e.g., exhibited in a museum, as the visitors observe it only from a limited range of angles. However, this type of hologram does not allow you to observe the back of the object. It only shows the visible front surface of the object. It also does not allow us to view the inside of the object.

Current tablets and smartphones with LCDs allow the projection of spatial images and 3D videos, using Pepper's "*Ghost effect*"—PGE, **Figure 25**. To view the subject from different sides in the plane of the screen, four images are created instead of two, which are saved in the computer's memory. LCD projects these

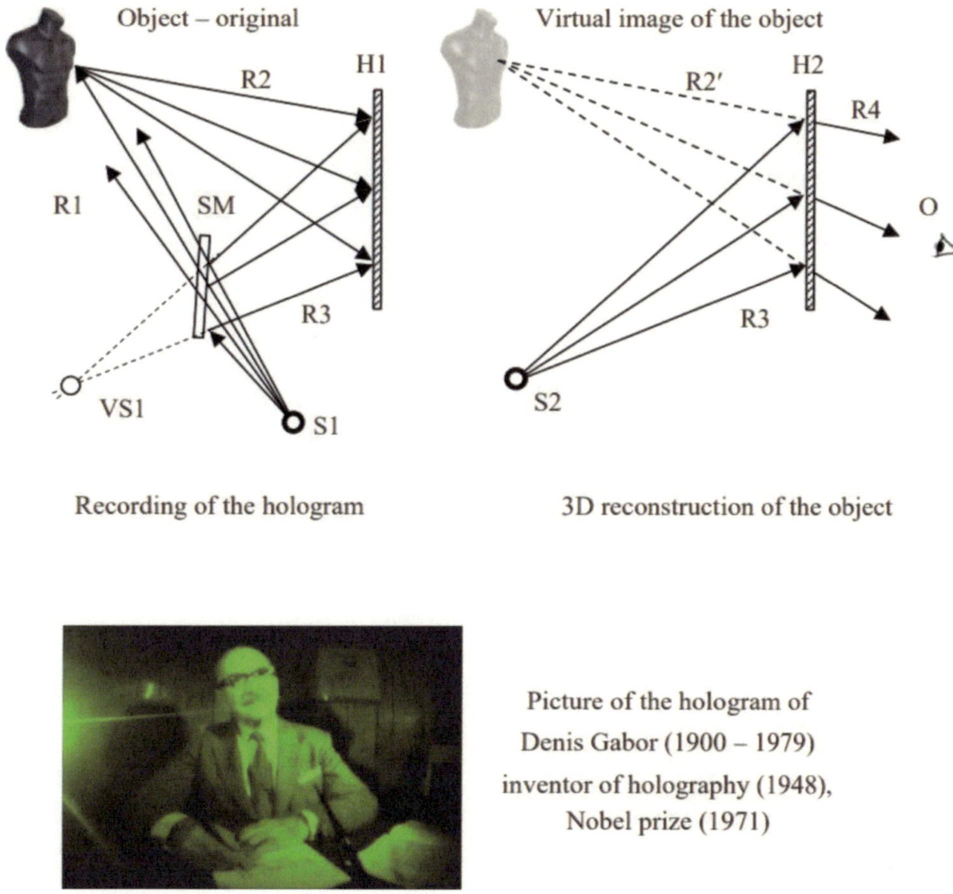

Figure 24.
Hologram recording and reconstruction.

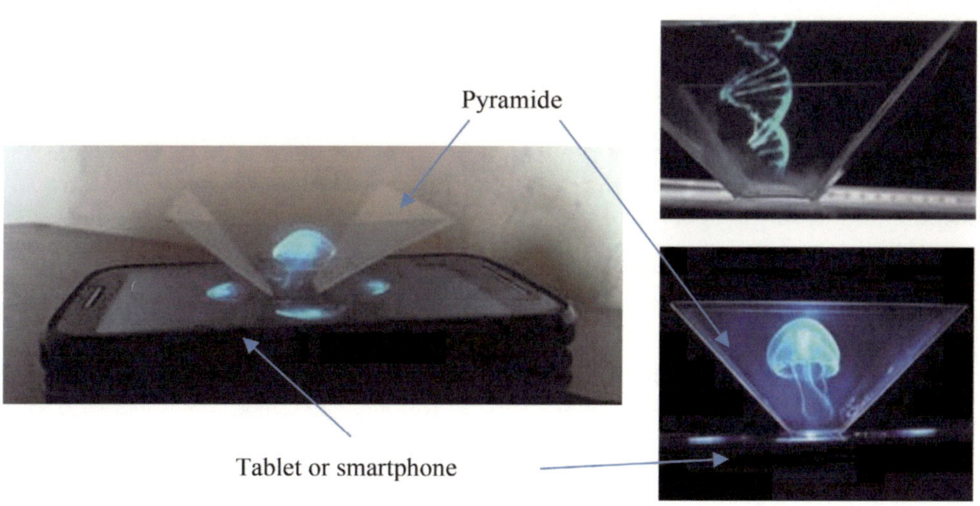

Figure 25.
Holographic display using PGE (pepper ghost effect).

images onto a pyramid, made of a special foil with an angle of inclination of 45° to the display.

The observer looks at the pyramid parallel to the plane of the display. He perceives four images created by the reflection of the displayed image on the walls of the pyramid. Each eye thus gets different images to create a stereo effect. From any angle, the observer sees the 3D image of the projected scene. The described system allows seeing a stereo video using personal electronic devices. Medicine and biochemistry use this method of spatial imaging for imaging body organs, cells, macromolecules, etc., especially for study purposes.

1.8.3.3 Virtual reality

3D vision arises if each eye receives a correspondingly different image. This also achieves using special spectacles with displays for each eye connected to a computer.

The digital model of the object is stored in the computer storage. Proper software creates signals corresponding to the demanded view of the object for each eye. One's sight then perceives a 3D image of an object, referred to as *virtual reality*. Computer software allows manipulating the object view. Virtual reality is widely used, in biomedicine, e.g., in teaching anatomy. The computer stores a model of the body with all the details, e.g., obtained from CT or MRI tomographic scanners. The software allows us to display separately individual organs, skeleton, blood circulation, muscles, etc., see.

The spectacles may be opaque, and then the observer only sees what is projected. They can also be semi-transparent, and then the observer sees the surrounded space, together with the 3D image of the object projected into this space. The spectacles have position sensors wirelessly connected to the computer so that the computer can create views from different angles and positions. Virtual reality finds application in the entertainment industry, but also in science and education. The computer allows you to create moving images, so you can project entire movies with these spectacles. Virtual reality is one of the modern trends in medicine. It especially uses databases from tomographic examinations, i.e., information databases not only about the surface but about the entire volume of the displayed object. Modern projection, as well as communication technology, enables the realization of a virtual keyboard and a "virtual cursor" with which the observer can remotely control a computer with a finger or a special pen, shoot the virtual image in various ways, make cuts, select details from the image, e.g., separate the muscles, vascular system, skeleton, select the operated organ, etc., from the body.

It is possible to connect multiple spectacles to a computer, so, e.g., the whole operating team observes the same virtual image, and during the operation, it can use the display of the operated organ, see. Virtual reality offers unsuspected possibilities, and its use will rise soon (**Figure 26**).

1.8.3.4 Tomography

Tomography is a modern method of complete 3D imaging and relates to the use of computers. The spatial object is scanned in thin layers (*Greek: tomos—layer*). The two-dimensional images (slices) thus obtained are stored in the computer's memory. Each acquired 2D image shows the entire internal structure of the object's section. For some examinations, only 2D images are sufficient, but a series of 2D images can be composed using a computer to create a 3D image of the object. This 3D image allows observing the image of the object from different sides on the

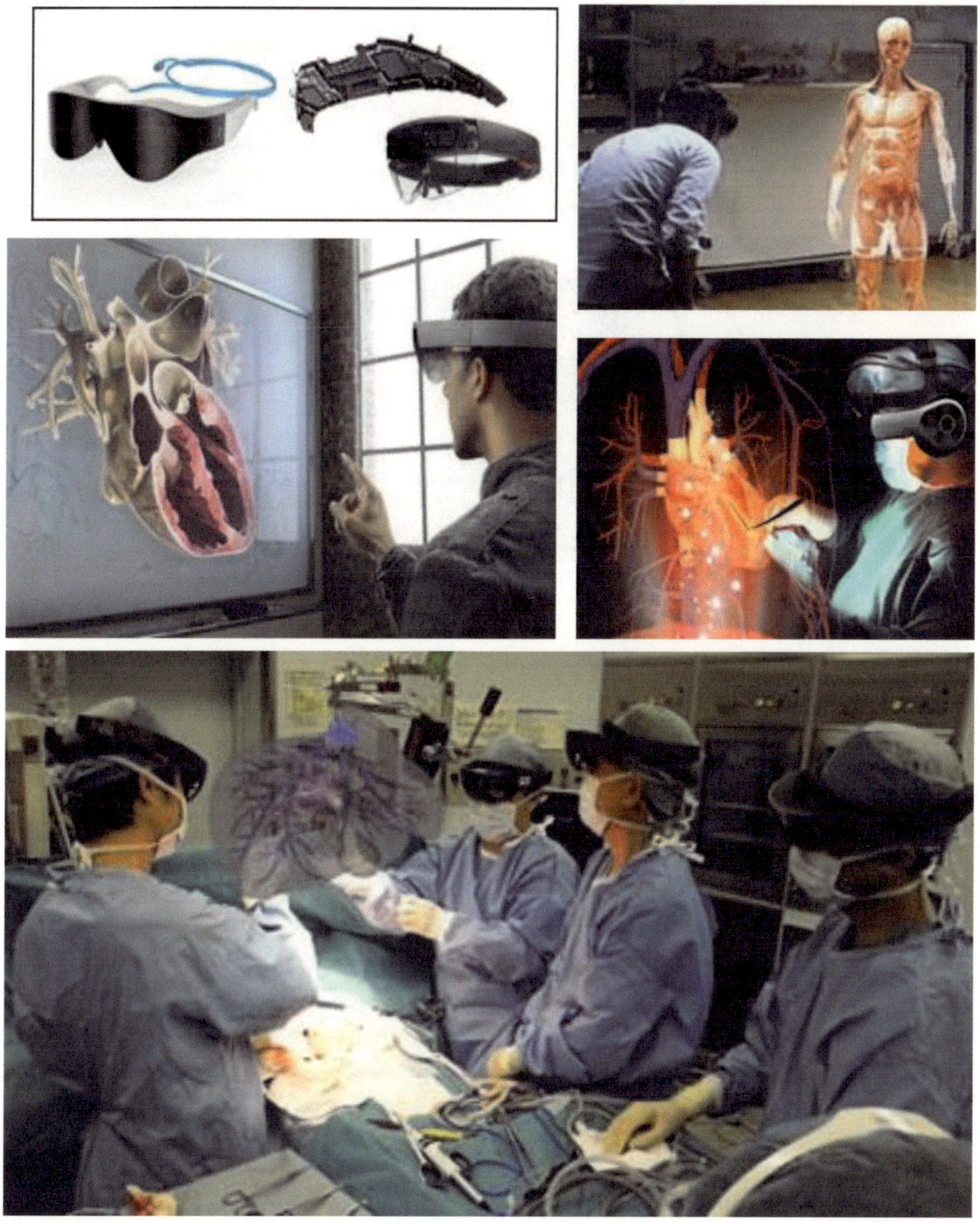

Figure 26.
Virtual reality. Examples: https://www.youtube.com/watch?v=U–m89jv8So.

screen, just like the real object. In this way, one can create a template for virtual reality. Creating a 3D image of an object layer by layer calls *tomography*. It became possible only after the development of computers with a sufficiently high operating speed and especially with huge memory capacity. The beginnings of modern computed tomography thus date back to the 1980s.

In **Figure 27** are examples of tomographic images obtained by different imaging methods.

Other tomographic images include nuclear methods using γ-irradiation, such as PET (Positron Emission Tomography) and SPECT (Single Photon Emission Computed Tomography).

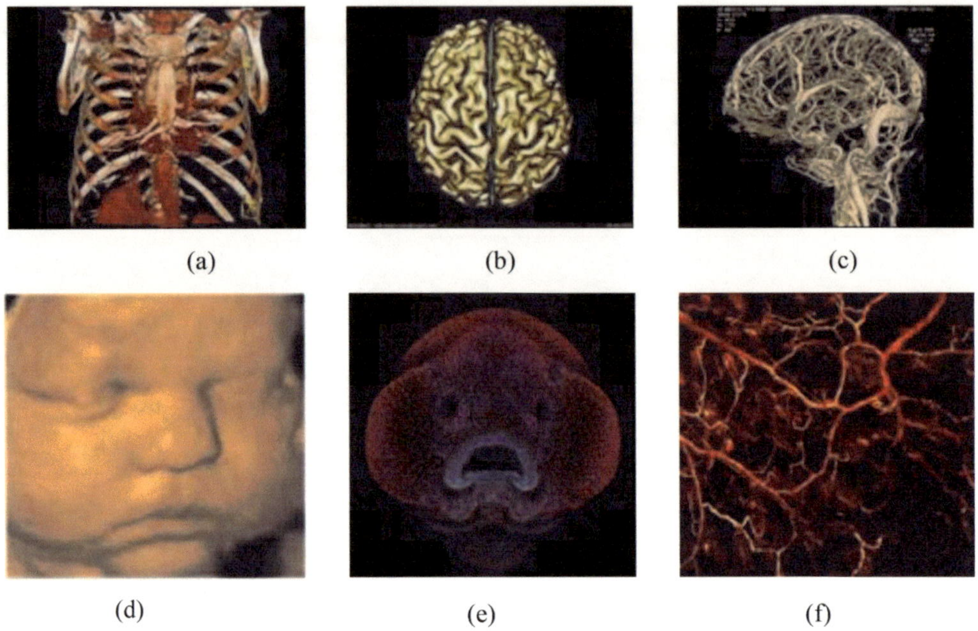

Figure 27.
Examples of tomographic images. (a) CT-Computed Tomography uses X-rays, (b) and (c) Magnetic Resonance Imaging (MRI) uses magnetic resonance imaging and RF signal FID, (d) USG (Electronic Focus Ultrasonography), (e) Confocal Laser Scanning (CLSM) Microscopy), (f) Photo Acoustic Microscopy (PAM).

1.8.4 Photometry

Most often use of light is lighting. For this reason, it is necessary to introduce physical quantities that describe the light effect of electromagnetic radiation on human vision.

In history, people used an especially made candle as the normal gauge of a point light source effect on human vision.

The accurate measurement evaluated the electromagnetic radiant power of the normal light point source of the unit luminous intensity. The light point source with the luminous intensity of 1 cd (candela) corresponds to the power of the source of thermal radiation of 1/683 W.

The current definition uses a monochromatic point source with a wavelength λ_m = 555 nm (yellow-green color), which corresponds to the maximum sensitivity of the eye in photopic (daily) vision. The luminous effect describes the quantity *luminous flux* Φ (λ), compared with the corresponding radiant flux Φ_e (λ). The unit of 1 lm (lumen) of the luminous flux, (incident on the pupil of the eye), is defined by the rate to the unit of 1 W (watt) of the radiant flux Φ_e (λ) by the relation, which respects the old definition of the candle.

$$\Phi(\lambda_m) = K_m \ \Phi_e(\lambda_m), \text{where } K_m = 683 \text{ lm W}^{-1}. \tag{75}$$

If we use monochromatic light with a different wavelength λ, the luminous effect of the radiation describes the luminous flux

$$\Phi(\lambda) = K(\lambda)\Phi_e(\lambda) = K_m \ V(\lambda) \ \Phi_e(\lambda), \tag{76}$$

where K (λ) is the *spectral sensitivity* of the eye to light of wavelength λ, and V (λ) is the *relative spectral sensitivity* to light of wavelength λ. The dependence of V (λ) on the wavelength for photopic vision is in **Figure 28**.

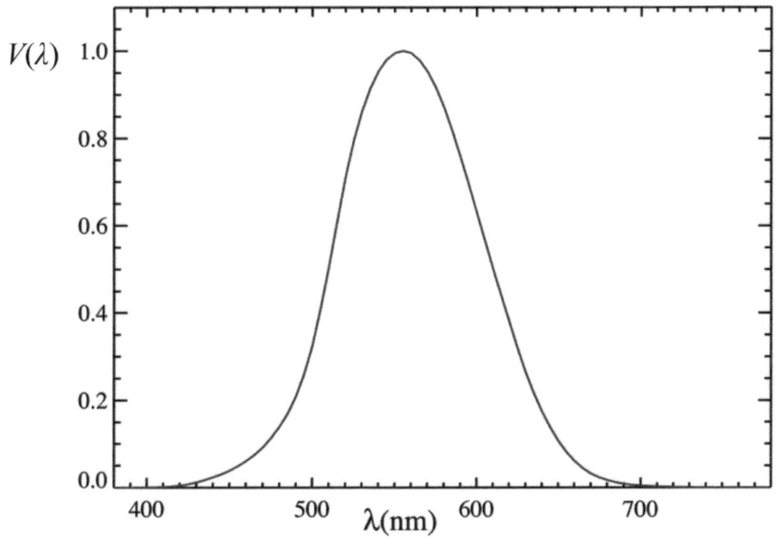

Figure 28.
Relative spectral sensitivity of the eye in photopic vision.

In the case of polychromatic light, the total light effect is equal to the integral light effect of all wavelengths

$$\Phi = K_m \int_0^\infty V(\lambda)\ \Phi_e'(\lambda)\ d\lambda, \tag{77}$$

where $\Phi_e'(\lambda) = \frac{d\Phi_e(\lambda)}{d\lambda}$ is the spectral density of the radiant flux [W m^{-1}].

The luminous intensity I of a point source is then defined by the luminous flux Φ radiated into a unit solid angle (1 sr).

$$I = \frac{d\Phi}{d\Omega}, \text{the unit } 1\text{ cd} = 1\text{ lm}\cdot\text{sr}^{-1}. \tag{78}$$

When using a lighting source, we are interested in what lighting of the object will cause the source. The quantity of *illuminance* is defined by the luminous flux incident from the source on a unit area perpendicular to the direction of light propagation

$$E = \frac{d\Phi}{dS}. \tag{79}$$

The unit of illuminance is 1 lx (lux) = 1 lm m^{-2}.

We measure the illuminance with a Lux-meter, (e.g., an application in a smartphone). It is easy to make sure that with increasing distance r from the source, the illuminance decreases, and depends on the angle ϑ of incidence of light on the surface

$$E = \frac{d\Phi}{dS} = \frac{I\,d\Omega}{r^2\,d\Omega/\cos\vartheta} = \frac{I}{r^2}\cos\vartheta. \tag{80}$$

As can be seen from (80), the illuminance decreases with the square of the distance.

When evaluating surface light sources, the brightness is described by the quantity of *luminance* (the unit 1 cd·m^{-2})

$$L = \frac{\mathrm{d}I}{\mathrm{d}S_{\mathrm{source}}}, \tag{81}$$

where d I is the luminous intensity of the elementary surface $\mathrm{d}S_{\mathrm{source}}$ of the source.

Note. 1: At present, there are modern LED lights. On the box of the LED bulb, we can read wattage 15 W, luminous flux 1320 lm, equivalent to the luminous flux of a classic bulb with a wattage of 100 W. If the bulb emitted only light with a wavelength of about 555 nm, the corresponding luminous flux would be 100 W × 683 lm/W = 6.83 × 10^4 lm. If the equivalent luminous flux is 1320 lm, the luminous efficacy of the lamp is 2%. This is because the bulb emits most of its energy in the infrared (thermal) range, while the LED bulb emits only visible light. The energy-saving when using an LED bulb instead of a conventional filament bulb is (100–15 W)/100 W = 85%.

Note. 2: The hygienic standard for workplace lighting is at least 200 lx. The classic 100 W bulb at a distance 2 m provides illumination of 35 lx. The illuminance at night at the full moon is 0.24 lx, during the day with cloudy skies up to 3000 lx and on a sunny summer day up to 100,000 lx.

Note. 3: The human eye can distinguish a source with a minimum brightness of up to 10^{-6} cd·m^{-2}.

A detailed description of photometric quantities and various light sources is provided by the physical discipline—*photometry*.

1.8.5 Colorimetry

A man distinguishes approximately 160 colors and up to 600,000 shades by photosensitive sensors for only three colors (Red-Green-Blue) and gray. All the remaining colors and shades are created by composing signals from these sensors in the brain. Just as the eye decomposes any color into three color components (signals), and the resulting color reconstructs in the brain. It is possible to create any other color from the three basic color components. This illustrates the diagram in **Figure 29**—*chromatic diagram*, or *colorimetric triangle* (*chroma lat.*—*color*). The colors perceived by the eye are closed in the area bounded by the contour line, on which there are monochromatic (rainbow) colors with the specified wavelengths from violet (340 nm) to red (700 nm). All colors from the marked area can be created by adding three basic colors.

The eyes use three monochromatic colors from the contour line. For sufficient coverage of the color scheme, however, three technical colors marked in the scheme on the vertices of the triangle R, G, B are sufficient. This covers the area of colors limited by this triangle. If we want, e.g., to create the color indicated by the point F in the diagram, the lines FR, FG, FB indicate the necessary light intensities of the primary sources to produce the desired color. It is not possible to create a color from outside the RGB triangle in this way. The diagram shows that by composing the basic colors in a suitable ratio *r: g: b*, a white color W arises. Monochromatic colors do not occur on the line BR—these represent *purple* colors and are composed of blue B and red R colors. Adding color to the base color sources is called *additive mixing.* This is, e.g., how works LED with electric color creation. Such LED contains three LEDs on one chip with three basic colors and independent power supplies. By changing the current of the individual segments, it is possible to change the color of the light in the range of the colorimetric triangle (**Figure 30**).

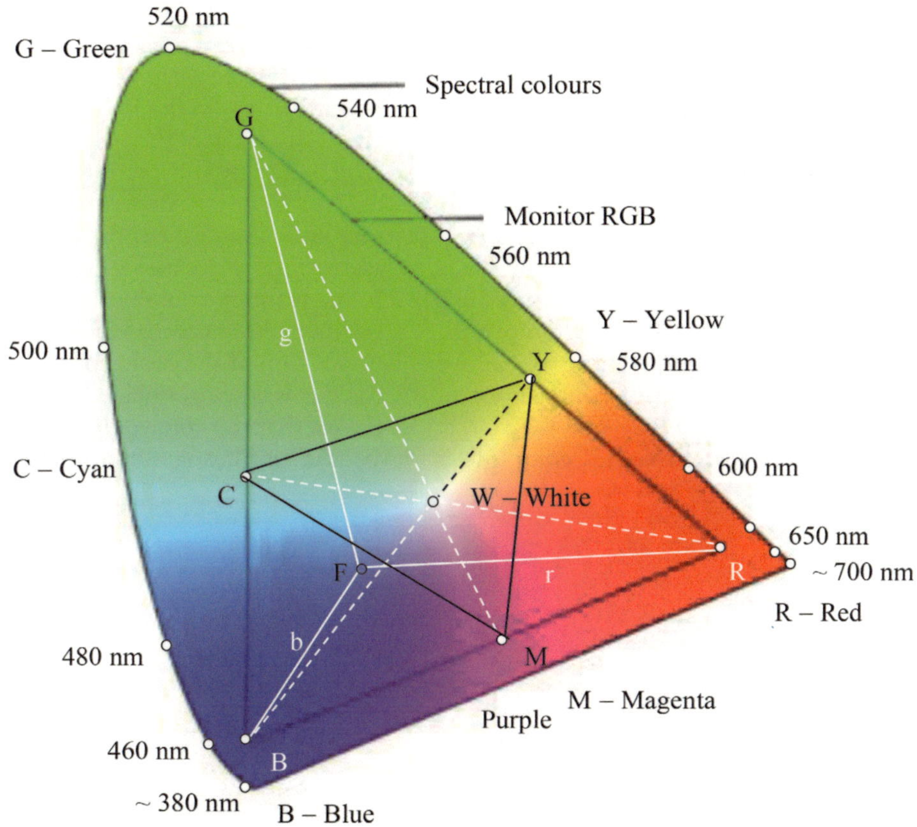

Figure 29.
Chromatic diagram (colorimetric triangle).

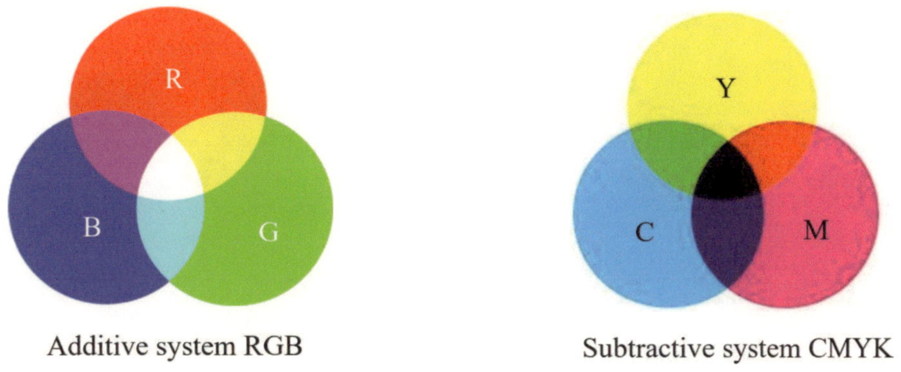

Figure 30.
Additive and subtractive color composition.

Another example is LED monitors for TVs or computers. On the monitor surface, there are three sub-grids with LEDs of three basic colors, which are powered by a digital image signal source.

For each basic color of the triangle, there is a so-called *complementary color*. By adding the basic and complementary colors in a suitable ratio, we get white. In the diagram, the base and complementary colors are represented by points on one line at the intersections with the sides of the triangle, e.g., B-Y, G-M, R-C. To blue (B) is complementary yellow (Y-Yellow = R + G), to green (G) magenta (M-Magenta = R + B) and to red (R) cyan (blue-green) (C-Cyan = B + G)). CMY points form a triangle, and by composing these colors, you can create any color within that triangle. We see that the color choice in the CMY triangle is smaller than in the RGB triangle.

The CMYK display system (Cyan-Magenta-Yellow-Black) uses the so-called subtractive folding (the resulting color is created from white by subtracting primary colors). Dyes are applied to the white background. Dyes filter out all or part of the respective base paint. By filtering out all the primary colors with the three dyes, black remains. This method is used by inkjet or laser printers. Because it is uneconomical to use three color toners to produce black, the printers contain a separate black toner used for black and white printing. A comparison of color production by both systems is in. We see that by the additive composition of the basic colors we get white, by the subtractive composition of the basic colors we get black.

A comparison of the RGB and CMY triangles shows that the color quality of the printed images is lower than the color quality of the LED or plasma monitor images.

Author details

Ivo Čáp*, Klára Čápová, Milan Smetana and Štefan Borik
Faculty of Electrical Engineering and Information Technology, University of Žilina, Slovakia

*Address all correspondence to: ivo.cap@fel.uniza.sk

References

[1] Rajeev B, editor. Handbook of Engineering Electromagnetics. Boca Raton: CRC Press; 2004. ISBN: 978-0-2030-2602-1

[2] Rajeev B, editor. Engineering Electromagnetics—Applications. Boca Raton: CRC Press; 2006. ISBN: 978-0-8493-7363-3

[3] Someda CG. Electromagnetic Waves. Boca Raton: CRC Press; 2006. ISBN: 978-0-8493-9589-5

[4] Borik S, Cap I. Non-destructive evaluation of arterial system properties using electromechanical analogies and infrared light-based diagnostic methods. Studies in Applied Electromagnetics and Mechanics. 2014;**39**:85-92

[5] Borik S et al. Photoplethysmography imaging: Camera performance evaluation by means of an optoelectronic skin perfusion phantom. Physiological Measurement. 2020;**41**(5): 054001

[6] Borik S, Cap I. Measurement and analysis possibilities of pulse wave signals. Advances in Electrical and Electronic Engineering. 2013;**11**(6): 514-521

[7] Blazek V et al. Studies in Skin Perfusion Dynamics: Photoplethysmography and Its Applications in Medical Diagnostics. Singapore: Springer; 2021

[8] Röntgen WK. Über eine neue Art von Strahlen. Annalen der Physic. Berlin 1898;**300**(1):12-17

Chapter 6

Properties and Behaviour of Waves

Ivo Čáp, Klára Čápová, Milan Smetana and Štefan Borik

1. Introduction

Waves have specific properties, which do not depend on their physical substance. It means they are common for all kinds of waves as electromagnetic, mechanical, etc. It deals mainly with such typical demonstrations as interference, diffraction, and wave displaying connected with them.

2. Wave function

The wave function is a function of space coordinates and time. It describes the wave quantity in a proper place and time, for example, $\boldsymbol{u}(r, \boldsymbol{t})$—an acoustic displacement of a mechanical wave or $\boldsymbol{E}(r, \boldsymbol{t})$ and $\boldsymbol{H}(r, \boldsymbol{t})$—intensities of electrical and magnetic components of an EM wave. Any wave propagates in space. At any point, we can define the velocity of propagation $\boldsymbol{c} = c\boldsymbol{n}^{\mathbf{0}}$, where $\boldsymbol{n}^0$ is the unit vector in the wave propagation direction.

The general form of the wave function can be expressed as

$$\mathbf{u}(\mathbf{r}, t) = \mathbf{f}\ (\mathbf{r} \pm \mathbf{c}t), \tag{1}$$

where the sign "−" stands for a wave propagating in $\boldsymbol{n}^0$ direction a "+" in the opposite direction.

2.1 Wave polarisation

The wave quantities are vector quantities, which have their direction relating to the direction of the wave propagation. If this direction is defined, we speak about a polarised wave. For example, an acoustic wave generated by a converter or EM wave generated by an antenna is polarised. One of the polarizations is a ***longitudinal polarisation***—vector of the wave quantity is parallel to the wave propagation direction, for example, sound in the air, sound or ultrasound in a liquid, ultrasound in soft tissue, etc. ***Transverse polarisation*** means direction of the wave quantity perpendicular to the propagation direction, for example, EM wave in free space, wave on an elastic string. Transverse polarisation can be ***a linear*** one if the direction of the wave quantity does not vary along with the wave, a ***circular*** one if the vector of the transverse wave quantity follows a circle or an ***elliptical*** one if the transverse wave quantity follows an ellipse. Circular or elliptical polarisation should be taken as a superposition of two harmonic linearly polarised transverse waves propagating together with mutually perpendicular polarisation and phase shift of $\pi/2$ rad. If the amplitudes of both waves are the same, the resulting polarisation is circular. In the case of different amplitudes, the polarisation is elliptical.

IntechOpen

There are also elliptically polarised waves in a plane parallel to the propagation direction. It can be considered a combination of the transversely polarised and longitudinally polarised waves. One example is the surface wave on the water. If we observe the movement of a tiny body floating on the surface of the water with the surface wave, we can see that the body oscillates in a vertical direction, but it also performs an oscillating motion in the longitudinal direction. It follows an ellipse.

If the wave is generated by many individual uncoordinated sources of polarised waves, the polarisation of the resulting wave cannot be unambiguously determined, and such a wave is called a non-polarised one. Bulk acoustic waves in gases and liquids are always longitudinally polarised because in these media the transversally polarised waves cannot propagate due to the fluidity of the medium (this does not apply to the surface waves in the liquid). If the EM wave is generated by a temperature source (hot fibre, infrared radiation of the body surface, starlight, etc.), the individual sources are single atoms of the substance that emit their waves accidentally. Each elementary wave is transversally polarised, and all polarisation directions are present equally. The resulting wave is therefore non-polarised. Typical sources of such non-polarised light are bulbs, gas discharge lamps, LEDs, etc.

Some applications require the use of polarised radiation. In this case, a source of polarised radiation, for example, LASER, can be used. Another possibility is to use a polarizer (polarising filter), a tool that suppresses (filters) one polarisation of non-polarised radiation. Polarizers use anisotropic crystals, lattice structures or reflective elements. Periodic structures (dense optical gratings) are most often used as light polarizers. Polarizers are used on glasses, cameras, or microscope lenses, polarising filters are part of LCDs (digital watches, laptops, mobile phone screens, etc.). The polarisation of light also occurs when reflected from shiny surfaces.

Reflection and transmission of light at the plane interface of two media express Fresnel's relations

$$I_{\mathrm{ro}} = I_{\mathrm{rd}} \left[\frac{n_2 \cos \alpha - n_1 \cos \beta}{n_2 \cos \alpha + n_1 \cos \beta} \right]^2 = I_{\mathrm{rd}} \left[\frac{\tan (\alpha - \beta)}{\tan (\alpha + \beta)} \right]^2 \tag{2}$$

$$I_{\mathrm{ko}} = I_{\mathrm{kd}} \left[\frac{n_1 \cos \alpha - n_2 \cos \beta}{n_1 \cos \alpha + n_2 \cos \beta} \right]^2 = I_{\mathrm{kd}} \left[\frac{\sin (\alpha - \beta)}{\sin (\alpha + \beta)} \right]^2 \tag{3}$$

$$I_{\mathrm{rp}} = I_{\mathrm{rd}} \frac{n_1}{n_2} \left[\frac{2 n_1 \cos \alpha}{n_2 \cos \alpha + n_1 \cos \beta} \right]^2 = I_{\mathrm{rd}} \frac{n_1}{n_2} \left[\frac{2 \cos \alpha \sin \beta}{\sin (\alpha + \beta) \cos (\alpha - \beta)} \right]^2 \tag{4}$$

$$I_{\mathrm{kp}} = I_{\mathrm{kd}} \frac{n_1}{n_2} \left[\frac{2 n_1 \cos \alpha}{n_1 \cos \alpha + n_2 \cos \beta} \right]^2 = I_{\mathrm{kd}} \frac{n_1}{n_2} \left[\frac{2 \sin \beta \cos \alpha}{\sin (\alpha + \beta)} \right]^2, \tag{5}$$

where index r denotes a wave polarised in the plane of incidence, index k a wave polarised perpendicularly to the plane of incidence (parallel to the plane of the interface), index d the incident wave, index "o" the reflected wave and index "p" the passing wave. The angle α is the angle of incidence (equal to the angle of reflection) and β the angle of refraction to which Snell's relation $n_1 \sin \alpha = n_2 \sin \beta$ applies.

As we can see from the relation (2), for $\alpha + \beta = \pi/2$ rad, $\tan(\alpha + \beta) \rightarrow \infty$ and $I_{\mathrm{ro}} = 0$. It means the EM wave with this polarisation is not reflected from the interface when this condition is met. From the condition $\alpha + \beta = \pi/2$ rad we get the relation

$$\frac{\sin \alpha}{\sin \beta} = \frac{\sin \alpha}{\sin \left(\frac{\pi}{2} - \alpha\right)} = \frac{\sin \alpha}{\cos \alpha} = \tan \alpha = \frac{n_2}{n_1} = \tan \alpha_{\mathrm{B}}, \tag{6}$$

where α_{B} is Brewster's angle. When light falls on the interface at the angle of incidence α_{B}, only the 'k' wave polarised perpendicularly to the plane of incidence is reflected

$$I_{\text{ko}} = I_{\text{kd}}\left[\sin^2\alpha_{\text{B}} - \cos^2\alpha_{\text{B}}\right]^2 = I_{\text{kd}}\left(\frac{n_2^2 - n_1^2}{n_2^2 + n_1^2}\right)^2. \tag{7}$$

A wave polarised parallel to the plane of incidence is not reflected.

If the *non-polarised* EM wave hits the interface at the Brewster angle of incidence, the *reflected* light is polarised perpendicularly to the plane of incidence. If proper, this polarised wave can be suppressed by the polarising filter, for example, light reflections from shiny surfaces when shooting. Similarly, unpolarized sunlight is partially polarised when scattered in the atmosphere and so the blue brightness of the sky can be partially suppressed by a polarising filter to emphasise clouds.

The incident wave with r-polarisation is reflected with the same phase as incident one when $\alpha < \alpha_{\text{B}}$ and with the opposite phase (shifted by π rad) when $\alpha > \alpha_{\text{B}}$. The wave with k-polarisation is always reflected with the opposite phase.

Light affects charged particles in biological tissue. Apart from the thermal effect, EM waves also have a direct effect on cellular structures, it can support or suppress some cellular processes. The beneficial effects of light utilise *phototherapy*. They are particularly evident when using polarised light. Polarised light has stimulation and regenerative effects and a beneficial effect on the immune system overall. It also speeds up the healing of wounds after surgery. Lasers or special lamps are used for this reason. Polarised light can also be better focused. It utilises, for example, *laser scalpel* for very fine operations in ophthalmology and neurosurgery.

2.2 Waveform coherence

In an ideal harmonic wave, the phase is defined at each place and time by the wave function $e^{j(\mathbf{k}\cdot\mathbf{r}-\omega t)}$. In actual cases, however, this phase relationship is maintained only at a certain distance l along the propagation direction. This distance is called the *length of coherence*. The concept of *coherence* expresses the fact that it is still the same wave described by the given wave function, in which there is a constant phase difference between the two points of the space in which the wave propagates. In case of harmonic wave source (powered by harmonic voltage source)—transmitting antenna, piezoelectric transducer, acoustic loudspeaker, etc. the coherence lasts for the duration Δt_{c} of the duration of the harmonic excitation signal, it is coherence length $l_{\text{c}} = c\Delta t_{\text{c}}$. The coherence length is related to the spectral width Δf of the waveform $l_{\text{c}} \approx c/(\pi\Delta f)$.

In the case of light sources, the coherence length is limited by the fact that light is generated by individual atoms of a substance. Their photon emission is more or less coordinated. In the case of temperature sources (filament lamps, gas discharge lamps, LEDs), coordination restricts to a very small space, and thus the length of coherence is very small. The large coherence length is achieved with sources that use optical resonator—lasers. Approximate values of length of coherence are filament lamp ~ 1 μm, mercury lamp ~ 10 μm, LED ~ 100 μm, semiconductor laser about 1 m, gas He-Ne laser up to 100 m, fibre laser up to 100 km.

Apart from the coherence of the waves, we also define the coherence of wave sources. The wave sources are coherent in the case of their constant phase relationship. They are then the sources of coherent waves. At the same time, there is a constant phase difference between the waves generated by such sources. For example, two loudspeakers connected to a common AC generator, or two antennas connected to a common transmitter are such coherent sources. Another example of coherent sources is an ultrasonic transducer used in ultrasonography. It is assembled from many segments powered by the same electric generator. Waves generated by two independent sources cannot fulfil the conditions of coherence. The slight difference in the frequency will earn a considerable phase mismatch. To ensure the coherence of two wave beams, they must be coupled to each other, so that the phase difference of the source signals is constant. Coherent sources can be created by letting a harmonic wave fall on two or more slits in a shielding grating. Single slits act as coherent sources for the space behind the grating (e.g., an optical grid). A similar effect is also achieved when the harmonic wave hits a suitable mirror assembly (e.g., a segmented reflector).

2.3 Plane, cylindrical, and spherical waves in lossless medium

For simplicity, consider waves in a lossless, homogeneous, isotropic, and linear medium. In the free space (outside the source), the wave equation has a form

$$\Delta \mathbf{u}(\mathbf{r},t) - \frac{1}{c^2}\frac{\partial^2 \mathbf{u}(\mathbf{r},t)}{\partial t^2} = 0, \tag{8}$$

where $\boldsymbol{u}$ is the wave quantity and c the velocity of the wave propagation, irrespective of the physical substance of the wave (mechanical or EM).

The solution is generally complicated and usually obtained by numerical methods. There are several software tools for modelling wave fields. The concrete solution of the equation depends on initial and boundary conditions. The initial conditions are determined by the time dependence of the source quantity, the boundary conditions result from the geometrical arrangement of both the source and the objects influencing the propagation of the wave.

In the following section, we will show some simple cases of wave propagation from sources with significant symmetry.

2.3.1 Plane wave

If the source is a sufficiently large and planar one that generates a wave with the same amplitude and phase over its entire surface, the wave quantities depend only on the coordinate z in the direction perpendicular to the plane of the source, $\boldsymbol{u}(z,t)$. The Laplace operator Δ is reduced only to the second derivative according to the variable z

$$\frac{\partial^2 \mathbf{u}(z,t)}{\partial z^2} - \frac{1}{c^2}\frac{\partial^2 \mathbf{u}(z,t)}{\partial t^2} = 0. \tag{9}$$

The solution of the equation has a shape of the wave function

$$\mathbf{u}(z,t) = \mathbf{f}\left(t \pm \frac{z}{c}\right), \tag{10}$$

as shown for mechanical or electromagnetic waves. A wave depending on only one spatial variable is called a *planar wave*. Its wavefronts are planes perpendicular to the direction of propagation. The quantity c is the velocity of the wave propagation, the sign "−" indicates a wave that propagates in the z-direction and "+" in the opposite direction, in other words the *forward wave* and the *backward wave*. The vector function $\mathbf{f}$ describes the waveform (impulse, harmonic, etc.).

In the case of the plane wave in a lossless medium, the shape of the wave propagating along the z-axis remains unchanged—it is not distorted. On this principle, for example, delay lines through which the time shift of the signal is realised.

A plane wave is only an idealised model of a real wave. In practical cases, the wave has a more complex spatial distribution, since the source surface is never infinitely large, which is a prerequisite for the formation of a plane wave.

2.3.2 Cylindrical wave

Simple cases of spatial two- and three-dimensional waves include cylindrical and spherical waves.

The cylindrical wave is generated by a very long rectilinear line source that generates a wave of equal amplitude and phase along its entire length. In this case, the wave quantities do not depend on the longitudinal coordinate z in the source direction and depend only on the transverse ones. In this case, it is proper to use cylindrical coordinates ρ (distance from the source axis) and φ (angle in a plane perpendicular to the source axis). Moreover, if the source is isotropic, it generates a wave equally in all directions φ, reducing the dependence of the wave quantities only on the coordinate ρ. The Laplace operator, and thus the wave equation, has then a shape

$$\left(\frac{\partial^2}{\partial\rho^2}+\frac{1}{\rho}\frac{\partial}{\partial\rho}\right)\mathbf{u}(\rho,t)-\frac{1}{c^2}\frac{\partial^2\mathbf{u}(\rho,t)}{\partial t^2}=0. \tag{11}$$

The solution of this equation depends on the specific time dependence of the wave function given by the time dependence of the source quantity. Due to the harmonic time dependence of the excitation, the solution is the Bessel functions, which for longer distances converge towards the shape

$$\mathbf{u}(\rho,t)=\mathbf{u}_0\sqrt{\frac{\rho_0}{\rho}}\sin\left[k(\rho-ct)+\psi\right]. \tag{12}$$

The direction of the vector $\boldsymbol{u}_0$ determines the polarisation direction of the wave (transverse or longitudinal), ρ_0 is the radius of the source cylinder.

As you can see, the displacement $\boldsymbol{u}$ amplitude decreases with distance ρ from the axis with $\frac{1}{\sqrt{\rho}}$ function. Since the wave intensity I is proportional to the square of the wave quantity, it decreases disproportionately with the distance from the source, $I\sim\frac{1}{\rho}$. This conclusion can also be reached by the idea that the generated power P, when propagating the wave perpendicularly to the source, is spread over an increasing cylindrical surface $S = 2\pi\rho l$, and hence the intensity $I = P/S \sim 1/\rho$.

A cylindrical electromagnetic wave occurs, for example, around the line antenna or in the transverse direction within the coaxial line or other cylindrically symmetrical structures.

2.3.3 Spherical wave

We consider a point (spherical) isotropic source that generates waves to the surrounding homogeneous and isotropic medium. Due to the source point symmetry, the generated field has also the same point symmetry. Preferably, the spherical (spherical) coordinates r, ϑ, φ is used to describe the field. If the field is isotropic (independent of the coordinates ϑ and φ), the wave equation takes the form

$$\frac{1}{r^2}\frac{\partial}{\partial r}\left(r^2\frac{\partial}{\partial r}\right)\mathbf{u}(r,t)-\frac{1}{c^2}\frac{\partial^2\mathbf{u}(r,t)}{\partial t^2}=0. \tag{13}$$

The solution to this equation has the form

$$\mathbf{u}(r,t) = \frac{\mathbf{u}_0}{r} f(r \pm ct) \text{ for } r > r_0, \tag{14}$$

where r_0 is the radius of the surface of the spherical source and $f(r - ct)$ is the non-attenuated component of the wave function, representing the wave propagating in the radial direction at the speed c. As a result, the wave amplitude decreases with a distance from the centre of symmetry proportional to $1/r$.

In the case of a harmonic wave, the solution is the wave function

$$\mathbf{u}(r,t) = \mathbf{u}_0 \frac{r_0}{r} e^{j(\omega t \pm \mathbf{k} \cdot \mathbf{r})}, \tag{15}$$

where $\boldsymbol{u}_0$ is the value of the wave quantity on the surface of the source ball with radius r_0.

Note: The correctness of solution (14) or (15) can be approved by direct substitution into the Eq. (13).

The wave intensity is proportional to the square of the wave quantity and therefore decreases with the square of the distance from the source $I \sim 1/r^2$. This dependence is also obtained from the energy considerations—if the source generates power P, it decomposes into a spherical surface with an area $S = 4\pi r^2$, and thus $I = P/S \sim 1/r^2$.

From a long-distance l (much greater than the source dimensions), each source appears to be a point source, and thus the field has the character of a point source field, it means the intensity decreases with distance according to the function $1/r^2$.

In the case of an anisotropic source, which emits different intensities in different directions (e.g., acoustic loudspeaker, directional radio transmitter), the dependence on distance $1/r^2$ remains valid, but there occurs dependence of the wave quantities on the coordinates ϑ and φ.

If we observe the wave at a long-distance r from the source and on a surface dimension of which is much less than r, the wavefronts appear to be planar (curvature of the surface is not observed in a small area). The wave thus appears a plane one in this confined space. The plane wave model, therefore, can be used in this case.

Example 1 Solar constant

The Sun emits an essential part of its energy in the form of EM radiation with a wide spectrum of frequencies. The total irradiated power gives us Stefan-Boltzmann's law for the radiation of a black body

$$P = I_0 S_0 = \sigma T_S^4 4\pi R_S^2,$$

where $\sigma = 5.67 \times 10^{-8}$ W m^{-2} K^{-4} is the Stefan-Boltzmann's constant, $T_S \approx 5778$ K temperature of the Sun surface, $R_S = 6.96 \times 10^8$ m radius of the Sun.

Numerical results are $P \approx 3.8 \times 10^{26}$ W, $I_0 \approx 63$ MW m^{-2}.

There is radiation intensity at the distance of the Earth's orbit around the Sun

$$I = \frac{P}{S} = \frac{\sigma T_S^4 4\pi R_S^2}{4\pi d_{ZS}^2} = \sigma T_S^4 \left(\frac{R_S}{d_{ZS}}\right)^2,$$

where $d_{ZS} = 1.50 \times 10^{11}$ m is the distance Earth-Sun.

After substitution, we get $I = 1.36$ kW m^{-2}, which is the so-called solar constant.

For each square meter perpendicular to the direction of radiation, this power (partially reduced by the atmosphere), which heats the Earth's surface, evaporates water and causes rain and water to supply rivers, drives atmospheric currents and thus wind, provides energy to living organisms, etc. The energy of these renewable sources, as well as direct energy, is used to generate electricity for human needs.

2.3.4 Waves propagation in waveguides

The wave may propagate in an open space or a structured transmission medium. A special case is represented by waveguides; spatial boundaries that guide the transmission of waves, and hence signal and energy of waves. The simplest case represents a homogeneous waveguide having the same properties along the entire direction of wave propagation. A classic case is a coaxial power line (coaxial cable), which is commonly used to transmit mainly a high-frequency signal. The coaxial cable has an inner conductor and an outer coaxial conductor, the space between the conductors being filled with a dielectric. Between the conductors, there is a radial electric field with an intensity $\boldsymbol{E}$ perpendicular to the conductor axis and a magnetic field with an intensity $\boldsymbol{H}$ characterised by circle induction lines in a plane perpendicular to the conductor axis. The Poynting vector thus has a wave propagation direction in the direction of the line axis. The advantage is that the EM wave remains enclosed within the cable in the dielectric so that it is not lost by dissipation into the environment, and there is no interference with the electromagnetic field of the line because the external coaxial line field is zero.

However, the waveguide does not need an inner conductor and the form of a tube with a rectangular or circular cross-section is sufficient. A waveguide performs its function if the wave is reflected from its walls without loss and remains within. It uses a full reflection of the waves at the interface of the internal and external media. The complete reflection of the EM wave occurs on a perfectly conductive wall, in which case it is the metal waveguide of the EM wave. Total reflection also occurs at the interface of dielectric media if the propagation speed c_1 in the internal medium is less than the propagation speed c_2 in the external medium, and the angle α of incidence on the interface is greater than the cut-off angle α_m of total reflection, it means $\alpha > \alpha_m = \arcsin(c_1/c_2)$, for example, optical fibres. Acoustic waveguides work in the same way.

Example 2 Conductive waveguide EM wave

A simple idea can be obtained from the EM waveguide according to **Figure 1**.

We consider two parallel planar conductive walls with a mutual distance a. Between the walls, we send out a plane EM wave at the angle α of incidence on the wall. Suppose that the wave is polarised parallel to the wall; the vector $\boldsymbol{E}$ is parallel to the wall and the vector $\boldsymbol{H}$ to the wall angle α. The plane wave propagation velocity is c. A wave vector $\boldsymbol{k}$ of magnitude $k = \omega/c$ and of an angle α with a normal line can be divided into the longitudinal component $k_{||} = k \sin \alpha$ and the transverse

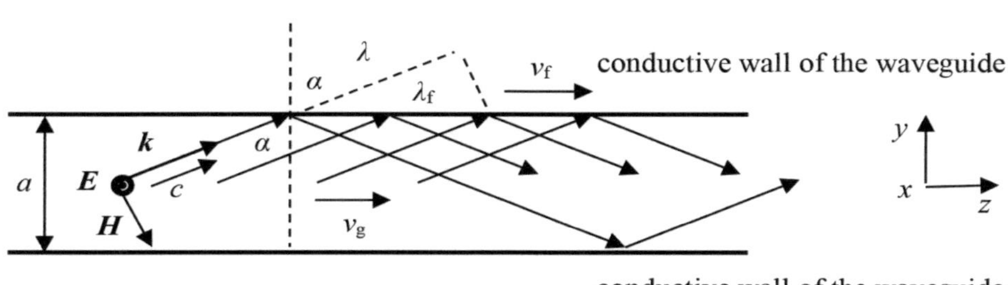

Figure 1.
Propagation of the EM wave in the waveguide.

one $k_\perp = k \cos \alpha$. Since at the conductive interface $E = 0$, there must be wave nodes on the walls; $k_\perp a = n\pi$, where $n = 1, 2, \ldots$ indicates the waveguide mode number. From there we have $ka \cos \alpha_n = n\pi$ and after substitution

$$\cos \alpha_n = n \frac{c}{2fa}, \text{ and therefore } v_{\|} = c \sin \alpha_n = c \sqrt{1 - \left(\frac{n}{2}\right)^2 \left(\frac{c}{fa}\right)^2}.$$

The condition of spreading of the n-th mode

$$f > n \frac{c}{2a} = f_{n\,\mathrm{m}} \text{ and simultaneously } f < (n+1) \frac{c}{2a} = f_{(n+1)\,\mathrm{m}}$$

(if $f > f_{(n+1)\mathrm{m}}$ the mode n changes into $n + 1$).

The phase velocity of the waveform v_f in the direction of the waveguide can be seen on the upper wall. If the wavelength is λ, the distance between the points with the phase difference of 2π on the wall is $\lambda_\mathrm{f} = \lambda/\sin \alpha$

$$\lambda_\mathrm{f} = \frac{\lambda}{\sqrt{1 - \left(\frac{f_{n\,\mathrm{m}}}{f}\right)^2}} \text{ and } v_\mathrm{f} = \lambda_\mathrm{f} f = \frac{c}{\sqrt{1 - \left(\frac{f_{n\,\mathrm{m}}}{f}\right)^2}} > c. \tag{16}$$

The group velocity of the wave progression in the z-direction is $v_\mathrm{g} = (\lambda \sin \alpha) f$. It means

$$\lambda_\mathrm{g} = \lambda \sqrt{1 - \left(\frac{f_{n\,\mathrm{m}}}{f}\right)^2} \text{ and } v_\mathrm{g} = \lambda_\mathrm{g} f = c\sqrt{1 - \left(\frac{f_{n\,\mathrm{m}}}{f}\right)^2} < c. \tag{17}$$

The velocity v_g is the velocity at which the energy, and hence the signal, propagates in the waveguide.

If the waveguide cross-section is rectangular (a, b), the same considerations apply to both transverse directions. For an EM wave that is polarised perpendicularly to the longitudinal axis (TE mode), the boundary condition applies to the wave nodes on both pairs of opposing walls. In the case of the general orientation of vector $\boldsymbol{E}$, the condition applies

$$v_{\|} = c \sin \alpha_n = c\sqrt{1 - \left(\frac{n}{2}\right)^2 \left(\frac{c}{fa}\right)^2 - \left(\frac{m}{2}\right)^2 \left(\frac{c}{fb}\right)^2}, \tag{18}$$

where n, m are integers indicating the wave mode TE_{nm}.

The condition for the transmitted wave frequency and the cut-off frequency is

$$f > \sqrt{n^2 \left(\frac{c}{2a}\right)^2 + m^2 \left(\frac{c}{2b}\right)^2} = f_{nm}. \tag{19}$$

The higher the mode numbers, the greater the geometric dispersion of the waves (as opposed to the material dispersion); it means the dependence of phase velocity on the frequency and thus distortion of the transmitted signal. Modes with low mode numbers TE_{10}, TE_{01}, TE_{11} are therefore used (both numbers n, m cannot be zero—the wave would not exist). The number of modes is limited by dimensions, or frequency using the condition for the propagation of the given mode $f > f_{nm}$.

Analogously, in the waveguide can be excited a wave that has a magnetic intensity $\boldsymbol{H}$ perpendicular to the longitudinal axis, it means transverse magnetic mode

TM. The boundary conditions are similar as for the TE mode. The waveguide can transmit TM_{nm} modes, where n, m = 1, 2, 3, ... The lowest is the TM_{11} mode.

Waveguide modes also propagate in waveguides with other cross-sections, most often circular. Similarly, like for rectangular, there exist TE_{nm} and TM_{nm} modes with similar transmission properties.

The same principle is used by optical fibres—waveguides for optical waves. Instead of a perfectly reflecting conductive wall, a total wave reflection from the dielectric interface with different refractive indices (fibre core n_1 and envelope $n_2 < n_1$) is used. Different filament modes also propagate in the fibre, like metallic waveguides.

If the cylindrical metal waveguide has an inner conductor (coaxial line), the EM wave has only a transverse character, that is, a TEM mode, which is characterised by signal propagation without distortion due to geometric dispersion. However, in the coaxial line dielectric, there are heat losses due to dielectric imperfection, and therefore the coaxial line is not used to transmit very high EM wave power when the dielectric becomes overheated. Coaxial lines are particularly advantageous for signal transmission.

2.4 Transmission of information utilising waves

The harmonic wave propagating in a medium does not transmit the information itself, but it is only an information carrier. To transmit information, the wave must be modulated by an appropriate information signal, Wyatt [1].

As an example, consider transmitting a data pulse. It can be decomposed into harmonic components using the Fourier integral. For a rectangular pulse with time length τ and carrier angular frequency ω_0 resp. frequency $f_0 = \omega_0/(2\pi)$,

$$\mathbf{u}_0(t) = U_0 \mathrm{e}^{\mathrm{j}\omega_0 t} \text{ for } -\frac{\tau}{2} \le t \le \frac{\tau}{2} \tag{20}$$

is a complex Fourier image of the pulse function

$$\mathbf{A}(\omega) = U_0 \int_{-\frac{\tau}{2}}^{\frac{\tau}{2}} \mathrm{e}^{\mathrm{j}\omega_0 t}\mathrm{e}^{-\mathrm{j}\omega t}\mathrm{d}t = \frac{2U_0}{\omega-\omega_0}\sin\frac{(\omega-\omega_0)\tau}{2} = U_0\tau\frac{\sin\frac{(\omega-\omega_0)\tau}{2}}{\frac{(\omega-\omega_0)\tau}{2}}. \tag{21}$$

This is a $\sin\alpha/\alpha$ function with a main frequency band $\Delta f = f - f_0 = 1/\tau$. To transmit a pulse with a length τ, this frequency band Δf must be transferred.

The propagation of individual harmonic components can be expressed by the wave function

$$\mathbf{u}_\omega(z,t) = \mathbf{A}(\omega)\mathrm{e}^{\mathrm{j}\,(\omega t - kz)}. \tag{22}$$

If the pulse is modulated upon a base wave with an angular frequency ω_0 and a wavenumber k_0, the current angular frequency, and the wave number can be expressed as $\omega = \omega_0 + \Delta\omega$ and $k = k_0 + \Delta k$. Thus, we get relation for the individual harmonic components

$$\mathbf{u}_\omega(z,t) = \left(U_0\tau\frac{\sin\frac{\Delta\omega\,\tau}{2}}{\frac{\Delta\omega\,\tau}{2}}\mathrm{e}^{\mathrm{j}\,(\Delta\omega t - \Delta k z)}\right)\mathrm{e}^{\mathrm{j}\,(\omega_0 t - k_0 z)}. \tag{23}$$

The carrier wave with angular frequency ω_0 propagates with phase velocity

$$c_f = \frac{\omega_0}{k_0}. \tag{24}$$

The modulation envelope is represented by the parenthesis, and thus the modulated signal propagates as a wave with parameters $\Delta\omega$ and Δk at with the velocity $c_{sign} = \Delta\omega/\Delta k$. Thus, we define a group velocity c_g for the close vicinity $d\omega$ of the basic angular frequency ω_0 as

$$c_g = \left(\frac{d\omega}{dk}\right)_{\omega_0}, \tag{25}$$

which characterises the rate of signal transmission in a medium.

If we have $c_f \neq c_g$, there occurs a signal distortion. In the mentioned case of propagation of the pulse signal, the pulse height decreases, and its width increases along the propagation path.

Note 1: In addition to the material dispersion mentioned above, a geometric dispersion, associated with the geometry of the waveguide, affects information transmission in waveguides.

Note 2: If the dispersion relationship (25) *is linear, i.e.,* c_f *is a constant independent on the angular frequency, then* $c_g = c_f$ *and the medium is non-dispersive. To minimise signal distortion, the frequency bands, in which the dispersion is minimal, are used for transmission, e.g., in optical fibres.*

2.5 Wave modulation

In the previous paragraph, we showed that waves can transmit information. For example, the sound of our voice is a superposition of single waves with frequencies from tens of Hz to several kHz. It is similar in case of the tones of musical instruments or EM waves generated by lightning during a storm.

Sometimes we need to utilise proper conditions for the propagation of waves in some range of frequency or to transmit several parallel information channels by the wave. In such a case, we use the so-called carrier wave of the required frequency ω_0 and modulate the transmitted information onto this wave. The modulation is most often amplitude or frequency one. Phase modulation is used only in special cases, for example, in MRI signal analysis. The modulation utilises control of the respective wave parameter (amplitude, frequency, or phase) by the information signal.

Suppose the signal given by its time dependence

$$\mathbf{s}(t) = \sum_{n=-N}^{N} \mathbf{S}_n e^{jn\Omega t}, \tag{26}$$

where $\mathbf{S}_{mn}$ are phasors and $-N\Omega$, ... $-\Omega$, 0, Ω, 2Ω, ..., $N\Omega$ angular frequencies of spectral components of the signal. The frequency range is $\Delta\Omega = 2N\Omega$.

2.5.1 Amplitude modulation: AM

The wave with amplitude modulation (AM) represents the relationship

$$\mathbf{u}(x,t) = [U_0 + \mathbf{s}(t)]\ e^{j(\omega_0 t - k_0 x)} = U_0 e^{j(\omega_0 t - k_0 x)} + \sum_{-N}^{N} \mathbf{S}_n e^{j[(\omega_0 + n\Omega)t - k_n x]}, \tag{27}$$

where it applies to phasors $\mathbf{S}_n = \mathbf{S}^*_{-n}$ of harmonic components. From here, we can see that the modulated wave contains frequency components from $(\omega_0 - N\Omega)$

to (ω_0 + $N\Omega$). The frequency bandwidth is thus twice the cut-off frequency $N\Omega$ of the modulation signal.

If two independent information channels are to be transmitted, their carrier frequencies ω_{01} and ω_{02} must be separated from each other by more than $N_1\Omega_1 + N_2\,\Omega_2$, so that the signals do not interfere with one another.

The wave amplitude changes with modulation. Since the frequency component with the carrier frequency ω_0 contains no information, it is often suppressed to reduce the energy of the transmitted (and generated) waves.

AM is used to transmit radio broadcasts on long, medium, and short waves. The officially agreed bandwidth of the radio station is 9 kHz so that the maximum frequency of the modulation signal spectrum is 4.5 kHz. This is enough for clear speech transmission but not enough for high-quality music transmission.

A special case is pulse amplitude modulation. It is used mainly for digital signal transmission. Pulsed AM is used, for example, when sampling an analogue signal. The bandwidth of the EM wave required to transmit pulses with a length τ is $\Delta f \sim 1/\tau$. For 1 ns pulse transmission, a channel width of the order of 1 GHz is required. Since $\Delta f \ll f_0$ is required, microwaves are used for high-frequency data transmission, for example, transmission by satellite with frequencies of the order of 100 GHz, or terrestrial fibre-optic links with IR wavelength of about 1.6 μm (~150 THz).

The advantage of amplitude modulation is the relative simplicity of modulators and demodulators. The main disadvantage is the liability to interferences and a higher signal-to-noise ratio.

2.5.2 Frequency modulation: FM

In VHF and UHF radio and TV channels with a carrier frequency of about 100 MHz, there is enough space for a wider band (for radio 40 kHz, for TV 7–8 MHz) that provides high-quality audio and video transmission. The fast transfer is also required for the transmission of large data files in telemedicine (e.g., CT and MRI images, online video transfer of the medical operation, etc.).

Concerning transmission better security (suppression of signal error and interference) and reduction of the signal to noise ratio, frequency modulation of the waves is used. Frequency modulation consists of the control of the frequency of the wave by the modulation signal. The amplitude and thus the power remains constant (as opposed to AM when the power fluctuates and is thus more susceptible to interference).

The frequency modulated wave can be described by function

$$\mathbf{u}(x,t) = U_0 \mathrm{e}^{\mathrm{j}\,[(\omega_0 + m\,u(t))\,t - k_\omega x]} = U_0 \;\; \exp \;\; \mathrm{j}\left[\left(\omega_0 + m\sum_{-N}^{N} \mathbf{S}_n \mathrm{e}^{\mathrm{j}\,n\,\Omega t}\right) - k_\omega x\right], \tag{28}$$

which can be expressed as a series of Bessel functions, where the spectral components of the wave are the same as in the case of AM.

Pulse FM used in data transmission, consists of a change of frequency at the time pulse duration. Since this change is limited in time, the same condition as AM applies to bandwidth $\Delta f \sim 1/\tau$.

2.6 Material dispersion of the wave

The wave velocity depends on the parameters of the medium, depending on the frequency of the wave. This phenomenon is called material dispersion. As shown in the previous paragraph, $c_f \neq c_g$ applies to the dispersive medium, that is, the velocity of information propagation is less than the phase velocity of the wave. The material dispersion is most often manifested in light waves. The dispersion prism is used in spectrometers to decompose white light into individual monochromatic components. The dispersion of light in water causes the formation of a rainbow due to the internal reflection of the light in the raindrops. The material dispersion also contributes to the distortion of infrared waves transmitted by optical fibres.

The material dispersion appears significantly at a large relative bandwidth $\Delta f/f_0$ of the transmitted wave. Therefore, for a given bandwidth Δf, the maximum carrier frequency f_0 is chosen.

The material dispersion in the case of the transmission of (pulse) data information in the optical fibres is reduced by selecting a frequency domain with minimal material dispersion, for example, in glass fibres around $\lambda \sim 1.6$ μm.

3. Ray optics

For the wave at a great distance from the source, that is, at the distance much greater than the dimensions of the source (so-called far Fraunhofer region), the ray representation of the wave can be used.

A ray is a line along which a wave passes. In addition to the rays, there are defined wavefronts. They represent the surfaces of the constant phase, in the case of a harmonic wave, and the surfaces that the wave reaches over some time, in the case of pulse or other waves. The wavefronts and rays are orthogonal to each other. At any point, the beams are perpendicular to the wavefronts.

Wave propagation obeys two basic principles, the Fermat principle, and the Huygens principle, which follow from the basic wave equations.

3.1 Fermat's principle

Fermat's principle says that the wave propagates from point A to point B along a spatial curve at which the time t_{AB} required to overcome the path l_{AB} is minimal

$$t_{AB} = \int_{l_{AB}} \frac{dl}{c} - \text{minimal}, \quad \text{or} \quad \delta\left(\int_{l_{AB}} \frac{dl}{c}\right) = 0, \tag{29}$$

where the symbol δ represents a variation of the respective functional (expression in parentheses).

For EM waves, phase velocity c can be expressed using refractive index n

$$t_{AB} = \frac{1}{c_0}\int_{l_{AB}} n dl - \text{minimal}, \quad \text{or} \quad \delta \int_{l_{AB}} n dl = \delta l_{opt} = 0,$$

where $l_{opt} = \int_{l_{AB}} n\, dl$ is *optical path length*.

Fermat's principle then says that EM waves propagate from point A to point B along the shortest optical path.

Example 3 Reflection and refraction of waves on the plane boundary of two homogeneous media

It follows from the Fermat's principle that in a homogeneous medium, where c is constant, the shortest wave path is the abscissa. Hence the notion that the waves

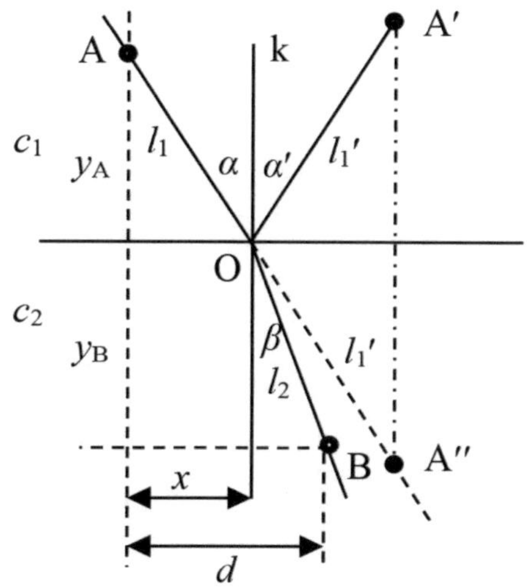

Figure 2.
Reflection and transition of wave through an interface.

propagate straightforwardly. However, this applies only to a homogeneous medium. In a non-homogeneous medium, the rays are curved.

At **Figure 2** there is a ray going out from point A and reflected to point A′ and refracted to point B.

The curvature of the optical beam in a non-homogeneous medium utilises, e.g., GRIN lens, see Section 6.2.2.

The ray OA′ has the same length as its mirror image OA″. As the ray travels in the same medium, the shortest wave path is equal to the shortest geometric path whose length corresponds to the length of the abscissa between points A and A″. The point of reflection O lies on the line AA″so that the angles $\alpha' = \alpha$. This is the law of reflection, which states that the ray incident, reflected, and the line perpendicular to the interface lie at one plane perpendicular to the interface and the angle of incidence α is equal to the angle of reflection α'.

Consider now the transition to the second environment from point A to point B. We denote the distances x and d, as shown. We are looking for a minimum of expression

$$t_{AB} = \frac{l_1}{c_1} + \frac{l_2}{c_2}, \text{where } l_1 = \sqrt{x^2 + y_A^2}, \text{and } l_2 = \sqrt{(d-x)^2 + y_B^2}. \tag{30}$$

We express the relation for t_{AB} as a function of the variable x, which indicates the position of the point O

$$t_{AB} = \frac{\sqrt{x^2 + y_A^2}}{c_1} + \frac{\sqrt{(d-x)^2 + y_B^2}}{c_2}.$$

We obtain the minimum t_{AB} using the zero value of the derivative according to the variable x:

$$\frac{dt_{AB}}{dx} = \frac{2x}{2c_1\sqrt{x^2 + y_A^2}} - \frac{2(d-x)}{2c_2\sqrt{(d-x)^2 + y_B^2}} = \frac{\sin\alpha}{c_1} - \frac{\sin\beta}{c_2} = 0,$$

from where we get Snell's refraction law

$$\frac{\sin \beta}{\sin \alpha} = \frac{c_2}{c_1}, \text{ or for light } \frac{\sin \beta}{\sin \alpha} = \frac{n_1}{n_2}. \tag{31}$$

Example 4 Total reflection
We express the relation for the angles of incidence and refraction in the form

$$\sin \beta = \frac{c_2}{c_1} \sin \alpha \leq 1.$$

From this inequality, we get the condition of the refraction of the beam

$$\sin \alpha \leq \frac{c_1}{c_2}, \text{or } \sin \alpha \leq \frac{n_2}{n_1}.$$

For $c_1 > c_2$, or $n_2 > n_1$, there is no restriction on the angle α of incidence. If $c_1 < c_2$, or $n_2 < n_1$ there exists a limit angle α_m given by the relation

$$\sin \alpha_m = \frac{c_1}{c_2}, \text{or } \sin \alpha_m = \frac{n_2}{n_1}, \tag{32}$$

where the refraction of the ray occurs when the condition $\alpha < \alpha_m$ is fulfilled.

For the angles of incidence $\alpha > \alpha_m$, the refraction cannot occur, and therefore the incident wave is only reflected and does not pass into the second medium—this phenomenon calls total reflection.

The total reflection phenomenon is used, for example, in optical fibres, or generally in waveguides. If the refractive index n of the optical fibre is greater than the refractive index n_0 of the surrounding medium, $n > n_0$, and the light enters the fibre at an angle $\alpha > \alpha_m$ relative to the normal to the cylindrical surface of the fibre, it spreads inside the fibre without losing energy by irradiation into the surroundings.

In biomedical applications, optical fibres are used in laser lithotripsy, laser scalpel, endoscopy, and the like.

Example 5 Optical fibre

Many applications use waves led in optical fibre. These are mainly signal transmission (e.g., optical computer networks), illumination of inaccessible areas (e.g., an internal organ in the body using an endoscope), the transmission of radiation power (e.g., in laser lithotripsy). The essence of the optical fibre transmission is that the wave is completely reflected from the fibre walls and cannot escape from the fibre. This creates an optical waveguide. The basic condition is that the wave must strike the fibre wall at an angle of incidence $\alpha > \alpha_m$, greater than the total reflection one. The transition of the wave along the fibre is in **Figure 3**.

The beam of parallel rays is centred by the lens S on the inlet surface of the cylindrical filament, the angle of incidence on the filament front being $\beta < \beta_0$. From

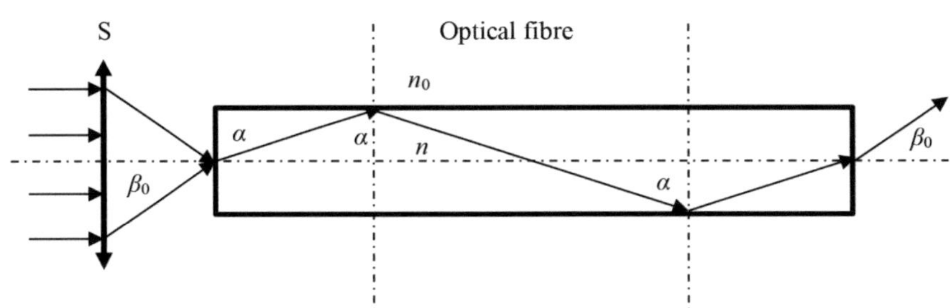

Figure 3.
Transition of light along with an optical fibre.

the surrounding medium with refractive index n_0 the light refracts into the fibre environment with refractive index $n > n_0$ at the refracting angle $\pi/2 - \alpha$, for which the refractive law $\sin(\pi/2 - \alpha) = \cos\alpha = n_0/n \sin\beta$. The angle α is the angle of incidence on the fibre wall and must be $\alpha > \alpha_m$, where $\sin\alpha_m = n_0/n$. Thus, we obtain a condition for the cut-off angle β_m: $\cos\alpha_m = \frac{n_0}{n} \sin\beta_m$, from where

$$\sin\beta_m = \frac{n}{n_0}\cos\alpha_m = \frac{n}{n_0}\sqrt{1-\sin^2\alpha_m} = \sqrt{\left(\frac{n}{n_0}\right)^2 - 1}. \tag{33}$$

If $\beta_0 < \beta_m$, the entire beam enters the fibre and travels through the filament along its axis. At the other end, it gets out at the same angle β.

The wave proceeds along the fibre axis at a phase velocity $v_f = \frac{c}{\sin\alpha}$ and group velocity $v_g = c \sin\alpha$, which depends on the angle α, or β. As a result, rays incident at different angles interferes with each other, thereby suppressing some directions and strengthening some others. Thus, only some modes are effectively propagated in the fibre, like the metallic waveguide, see Example 2. The interference of modes distorts the transmitted signal. A more detailed analysis suggests that the number of modes depends on the ratio of fibre diameter to wavelength. The single-mode fibre that is mostly used to transmit information (e.g., data transmission over a computer network) has a diameter of (6–7) λ, that is, for IR radiation with $\lambda = 1.3$ μm, the core diameter of the filament is (8.5–9.5) μm. In the case of energy transfer only, thicker multimode fibres with a diameter of up to 0.1 mm or more can be used, depending on the application.

The optical cable consists of many fibres. In endoscopes, an optical cable is used to transfer the image so that the image produced by the lens of the objective is projected onto a bundle of optical fibres, each transmitting 1 pixel of the image. The cable consisting of 100,000 fibres with a diameter of 5 μm (for a light wavelength of about 500 nm) has a diameter of approximately 1.5 mm. After leaving the cable, the light strikes the detector (CCD chip).

3.2 Huygens and Huygens-Fresnel principle

The propagation of waves in space is described by the *Huygens principle*. Huygens had the following idea:

If the wave reaches a certain wavefront, each point of the wavefront becomes a point source for the next part of the space. The following wavefront is then the contour surface of the wavefronts of these elementary spherical waves.

In this way, we can construct one wavefront after another and gradually depict the whole wave field. The procedure is shown in **Figure 4**. In the figure, three wavefronts correspond to times t_0, $t_0 + \Delta t$, and $t_0 + 2\Delta t$. Between the wavefronts are drawn elementary spherical waves originated in individual points of the previous wavefront.

In the figure, the elementary wavefronts do not have the same radius, which relates to different velocities of wave propagation in different places of the non-homogeneous medium. The rays are orthogonal to the wavefronts. We can see that in a non-homogeneous medium, the rays decline towards parts of the space with the lower velocity of propagation, lower right part in the figure.

Fresnel extended Huygens' idea to add a quantitative dimension. The wave quantity at a given point P of the following wave is a superposition of individual waves of elementary sources in the points M of the previous wavefront S, for illustration, see **Figure 5**.

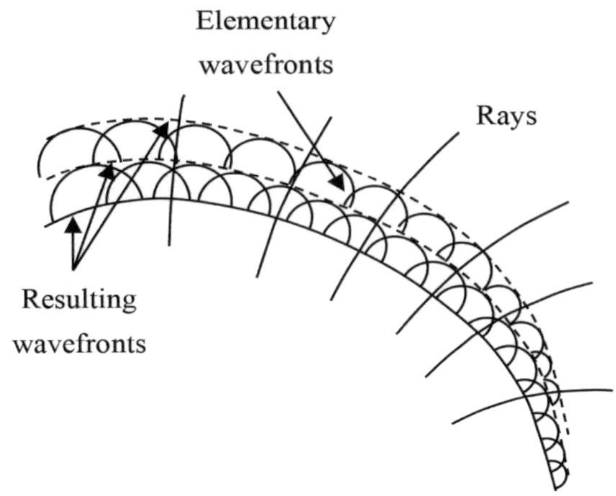

Figure 4.
Illustration of the Huygens principle.

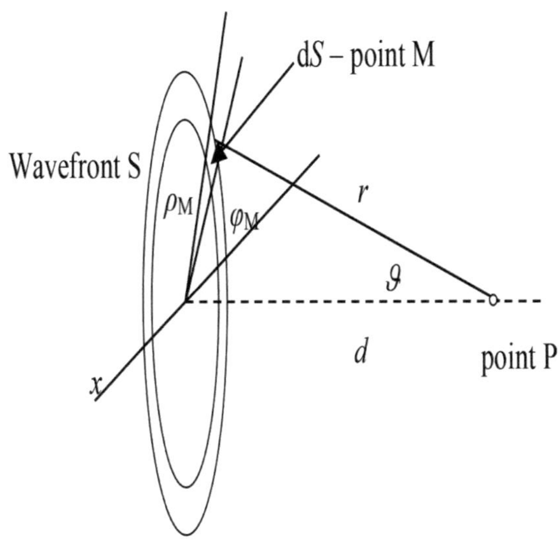

Figure 5.
Propagation of the plane wave.

$$\mathbf{u}(\mathrm{P}) = -\frac{jk}{2\pi} \iint_S \mathbf{u}_0(\mathrm{M}) \frac{\exp(\mathrm{j}\mathbf{k}\cdot\mathbf{r})}{r} \cos\vartheta \ \mathrm{d}S, \tag{34}$$

where $\boldsymbol{k}$ is the wave vector, $\boldsymbol{r} = \boldsymbol{r}_{\mathrm{P}} - \boldsymbol{r}_{\mathrm{M}}$ the position vector of the point P originating from the point M and ϑ the angle between the vector $\boldsymbol{r}$ and the normal to the wavefront at point M. The constant before the integral was formed by matching this approach to the proper solution of the wave equation, see the following Example 6.

Example 6 Plane wave and the Huygens-Fresnel (H-F) principle

As an illustration of the application of the H-F principle, let us give an example whose result we know. Consider a plane wavefront of a plane wave as a source (points M) and examine the further propagation of the wave—to the point P at a distance d from the wavefront, **Figure 5**. We divide the wavefront into elementary annular rings with radius ρ_{M} and width $\mathrm{d}\rho_{\mathrm{M}}$, and then into angular segments $\mathrm{d}\varphi_{\mathrm{M}}$. Source elementary area $\mathrm{d}S = \mathrm{d}\rho_{\mathrm{M}}(\rho_{\mathrm{M}}\mathrm{d}\varphi_{\mathrm{M}})$, and $\cos\vartheta = d/r$.

The H-F integral then has an expression

$$\mathbf{u}(\mathrm{P}) = -\frac{\mathrm{j}k}{2\pi}\,\mathbf{u}_0 \int_0^{2\pi}\int_0^{\infty} \frac{\exp(\mathrm{j}kr)}{r}\,\frac{d}{r}\,\rho_\mathrm{M}\,\mathrm{d}\rho_\mathrm{M}\,\mathrm{d}\varphi_\mathrm{M} = -\mathrm{j}k\,\mathbf{u}_0\,d\int_0^{\infty}\frac{\exp(\mathrm{j}kr)}{r^2}\rho_\mathrm{M}\,\mathrm{d}\rho_\mathrm{M}.$$

Since $r^2 = d^2 + \rho_\mathrm{M}^2$, by differentiation, we get $r\mathrm{d}r = \rho_\mathrm{M}\mathrm{d}\rho_\mathrm{M}$ and adjust the integral to form

$$\mathbf{u}(\mathrm{P}) = -\mathrm{j}k\,\mathbf{u}_0\,d\int_d^{\infty}\frac{\exp(\mathrm{j}kr)}{r}\mathrm{d}r = -\mathrm{j}k\,\mathbf{u}_0\,d\int_{kd}^{\infty}\left(\frac{\cos kr}{kr} + \mathrm{j}\,\frac{\sin kr}{kr}\right)\mathrm{d}(kr). \quad (35)$$

If $kd > 2\pi$, that is, in the distance $d > \lambda$, we can use the approximation of functions *integral sine* and *integral cosine*

$$\int_x^{\infty}\frac{\sin x}{x}\mathrm{d}x \approx \frac{\cos x}{x} \quad \text{and} \quad \int_x^{\infty}\frac{\cos x}{x}\,\mathrm{d}x \approx -\frac{\sin x}{x}$$

and we adjust the H-F integral to this shape

$$\mathbf{u}(\mathrm{P}) = -\mathrm{j}k\,\mathbf{u}_0\,d\left(-\frac{\sin kd}{kd} + \mathrm{j}\frac{\cos kd}{kd}\right) = \mathbf{u}_0\,\mathrm{e}^{\mathrm{j}kd}, \quad (36)$$

which is a complex function of the plane shifted by d.

From the initial planar wavefront, we get the following parallel planar wavefront, which corresponds to the propagation of the plane wave in space.

This example has shown that (34) correctly describes the wave propagation and the construction of the next wavefront, which is more than λ away from the previous one.

The Huygens-Fresnel principle will be used in the next section to explain the diffraction phenomenon.

4. Wave interference

If several waves propagate in a linear medium, they compose—*linearly interfere* with each other. The resulting waveform is the vector sum of the waveforms of the individual waves $\mathbf{u} = \sum_{i=1}^{n}\mathbf{u}_i$, where n is the number of interfering waves. We obtain significant results if the individual waves are coherent with each other, that is, have a defined phase relation expressed by their wave functions. Interference may result in amplification of the wave (*constructive interference*) or mutual suppression (*destructive interference*).

4.1 Constructive and destructive interference

Let us consider two plane harmonic waves with the same polarisation, and the same frequency, which propagates in the same direction and the phase difference φ between them. The resulting wave is

$$\mathbf{u}(z,t) = \mathbf{u}_1(z,t) + \mathbf{u}_2(z,t) = \mathbf{u}_1\;\mathrm{e}^{\mathrm{j}(\omega t - kz)} + \mathbf{u}_2\;\mathrm{e}^{\mathrm{j}(\omega t - kz + \varphi)}. \quad (37)$$

We set the relationship to shape

$$\mathbf{u} = \mathbf{u}_1 \, e^{j(\omega t - kz)} \left[1 + \frac{u_2}{u_1} \, e^{j\varphi}\right] = \mathbf{u}_1 \, e^{j(\omega t - kz)} \left[\left(1 + \frac{u_2}{u_1} \, \cos\varphi\right) + j \, \sin\varphi\right]$$

The resulting wave has the wave properties of the original waves, the amplitude

$$u = u_1 \sqrt{\left(1 + \frac{u_2}{u_1} \, \cos\varphi\right)^2 + \sin^2\varphi} \tag{38}$$

and phase shift for the wave $\boldsymbol{u}_1$

$$\psi = \arctan \frac{\sin\varphi}{1 + \frac{u_2}{u_1} \, \cos\varphi}. \tag{39}$$

If the waves have the same amplitude $u_1 = u_2$, we get the amplitude and phase shift of the resulting wave

$$u = u_1 \sqrt{(1 + \cos\varphi)^2 + \sin^2\varphi} = u_1 \sqrt{2(1 + \cos\varphi)} = 2u_1 \left| \cos \frac{\varphi}{2} \right|, \tag{40}$$

and

$$\psi = \arctan \frac{\sin\varphi}{1 + \cos\varphi}.$$

Under constructive interference $\varphi = 2n\pi$, it means, the shift by $\Delta z = n\lambda$, where $n = 0, 1, 2, \ldots$ (even multiple π or half-wave). Then we obtain

$$u = 2u_1, \text{and } \psi = 0.$$

The resulting wave has twice the amplitude and the same phase as the original waves.

Under destructive interference $\varphi = (2n + 1)\pi$, it means, $\Delta z = (2n + 1)\lambda/2$ (odd multiple π or half-wave). Then we obtain

$$u = 0, \text{and } \psi\text{—has no sense.}$$

In the first case, the wave is amplified to double the amplitude, in the second one the waves are mutually suppressed.

Example 7 Reflection of waves from thin film

A typical interference phenomenon is the reflection of the wave from a thin layer of substance. Consider the perpendicular impact of the wave from the medium with propagation velocity c_1 on the layer with the propagation velocity c_2. Let us suppose wave impedances $Z_1 < Z_2 < Z_3$, for example, light falling from the air onto the reflective layer on the glasses.

The incident wave is reflected from the first interface backward with the opposite phase, that is, $\Delta\varphi_1 = \pi$ rad and the layer penetrates without phase change. From the second interface, the wave is reflected again with a phase change $\Delta\varphi_2 = \pi$ rad. After passing through the layer forward and backward, a phase shift $\Delta\varphi_3 = k2d$ occurs at the wave reflected from the second interface, where d is the layer thickness, and $k = 2\pi/\lambda = (2\pi/\lambda_1)(c_1/c_2)$. This wave then passes through the first interface out of the layer without changing the phase and interferes with the first reflected wave.

DOI: http://dx.doi.org/10.5772/intechopen.101653

The interference is constructive when $\Delta\varphi = \Delta\varphi_1 - (\Delta\varphi_2 + \Delta\varphi_3) = 2n\pi$, from where we get the condition for layer thickness

$$d_{\mathrm{k}} = n\ \frac{\lambda_1}{2}\frac{c_2}{c_1} = n\ \frac{\lambda_2}{2}. \tag{41}$$

If the layer has a thickness d_{k}, it reflects the maximum extent, and it means that wave penetrates the layer and therefore enters the third medium to a minimum extent. This principle is used in the production of reflective layers, for example, UV interference filters on lenses of glasses or optical instruments.

As we can see from the result, constructive reflection depends on the wavelength. If white light falls on the layer, only a certain colour is reflected. If the layer thickness changes, the colour of the reflected light changes as well. This is used, for example, for measuring the thickness of thin films. If there is a thin oil layer on a surface of the water, which does not have the same thickness everywhere, different colour patterns are formed because of interference reflection. We can see it on water puddles. The effect is most noticeable when $n = 1$.

Destructive interference occurs when $\Delta\varphi = (2n + 1)\pi$, from where we get layer thickness

$$d_{\mathrm{d}} = (2n+1)\frac{\lambda_1}{4}\frac{c_2}{c_1} = (2n+1)\frac{\lambda_2}{4}. \tag{42}$$

A layer of a thickness dd reflects minimally, and thus maximally transmits. This is used to form anti-reflective layers, which we use to get the maximum of the incident light. They are used, for example, for glasses to increase the brightness of the observed objects, for telescope lenses, etc.

As we can see, the layer is anti-reflective only for certain wavelengths, but for other wavelengths, it should be reflective. The thickness of the layer can be set to wavelength according to our demand to support or suppress the light transmission. Since the wavelength of yellow light is about twice the wavelength of ultraviolet one, the layer can be reflective for the UV light and at the same time transparent for a yellow one.

4.2 Wave beats

In another case, consider two harmonic waves with the same direction of polarisation and the same amplitude, which propagate in the same direction and whose angular frequencies differ by a small difference $\Delta\omega = \omega_1 - \omega_2$. By folding both waves, we get a wave field

$$\mathbf{u}(z,t) = u\ \left\{ \mathrm{e}^{\mathrm{j}\ \left[\left(\omega_0 + \frac{\Delta\omega}{2}\right)t - \left(k_0 + \frac{\Delta k}{2}\right)z\right]} + \mathrm{e}^{\mathrm{j}\ \left[\left(\omega_0 - \frac{\Delta\omega}{2}\right)t - \left(k_0 - \frac{\Delta k}{2}\right)z\right]} \right\}.$$

We adjust the resulting wave function to shape

$$\mathbf{u}(z,t) = \left[2\ u\ \cos\ \left(\frac{\Delta\omega}{2}t - \frac{\Delta k}{2}z\right)\right]\ \mathrm{e}^{\mathrm{j}\ (\omega_0 t - k_0 z)}\ . \tag{43}$$

The composition of waves results in a wave that represents a carrier wave with a mean angular frequency of ω_0 and a corresponding wavenumber k_0, whose phase velocity $c_{\mathrm{f}} = \omega_0/k_0$, with the modulation envelope described in square brackets. A modulation envelope is a wave with a frequency of $\Delta\omega/2$ and a wavenumber of $\Delta k/2$ that proceeds with a group velocity of $c_{\mathrm{g}} = \Delta\omega/\Delta k$.

Wave intensity is

$$I \propto |\mathbf{u}(x,t)|^2 = 4\ u^2 \cos^2\left(\frac{\Delta\omega}{2}t - \frac{\Delta k}{2}x\right) = 2\ u^2\ [1 + \cos\ (\Delta\omega t - \Delta k x)]. \tag{44}$$

The wave intensity I represents a wave with an angular frequency $\Delta\omega$ that travels in space at c_g. At a given point in the wave field, the intensity varies with an angular frequency $\Delta\omega = |\omega_1 - \omega_2|$ between zero and a maximum value proportional to u^2. This variation of the wave intensity is called *wave beats*.

Note: Beats are used, e.g., when tuning musical instruments. If the tone frequency approaches the tuning fork frequency, the beats gradually disappear. Similarly, in the "octave" music interval where $\omega_2 = 2\omega_1$, *the angular frequency of the beats is* $\Delta\omega = \omega_1$ *and thus beats fuse with a wave of lower frequency. Wave beats are therefore not observed. This serves to check the correct tuning of the octave interval.*

Example 8 Stereo sound reproduction

The preferred way of listening to recorded music is stereophonic reproduction. The record is scanned by two microphones located at an appropriate distance. The recording is then played back from two parallel speakers whose distance is d.

The listener P moves along a line parallel to the speaker apertures at a distance r, **Figure 6**. The distance of P from the centre is indicated by x.

Suppose that the electric current through the loudspeakers has the same frequency and phase. Both speakers thus generate coherent waves with the same amplitude and phase. The waves from both speakers are composed at the listener position P

$$\mathbf{u}(\mathrm{P}) = -\frac{\mathrm{j}k}{2\pi}u_0 S\left(\frac{\mathrm{e}^{-\mathrm{j}kr_1}}{r_1}\cos\vartheta_1 + \frac{\mathrm{e}^{-\mathrm{j}kr_2}}{r_2}\cos\vartheta_2\right), \tag{45}$$

where $\cos\vartheta_{1,2} = r/r_{1,2}$.

The sound intensity in the point P of the listener is

$$I(\mathrm{P}) = I_0\frac{S^2r^2}{\lambda^2 r_1^4}\left[1 + \left(\frac{r_1}{r_2}\right)^4 + 2\frac{r_1^2}{r_2^2}\cos k(r_2 - r_1)\right], \tag{46}$$

where $r_{1,2} = \sqrt{r^2 + \left(x \mp \frac{d}{2}\right)^2}$.

The dependence of the relative sound intensity in front of a pair of speakers is shown in the graph at **Figure 7**. For the clearness of the illustration, the plots for two different frequencies are drawn. We can see that in some places the sound of some frequency is not heard. Thus, the spectral composition of the music you listen to depends significantly on the position P of the listener. It results in the change of

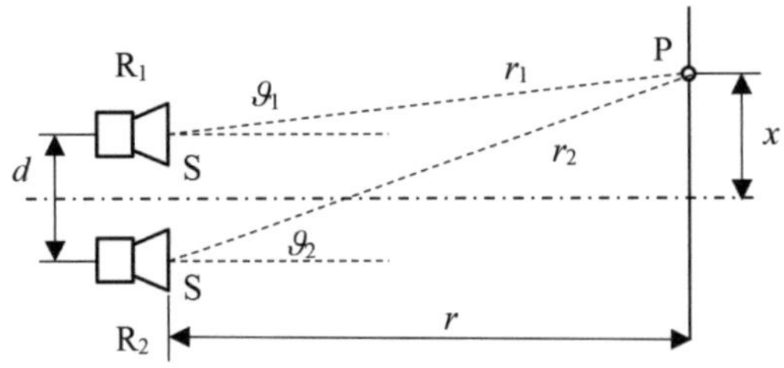

Figure 6.
Interference of sound of two loudspeakers.

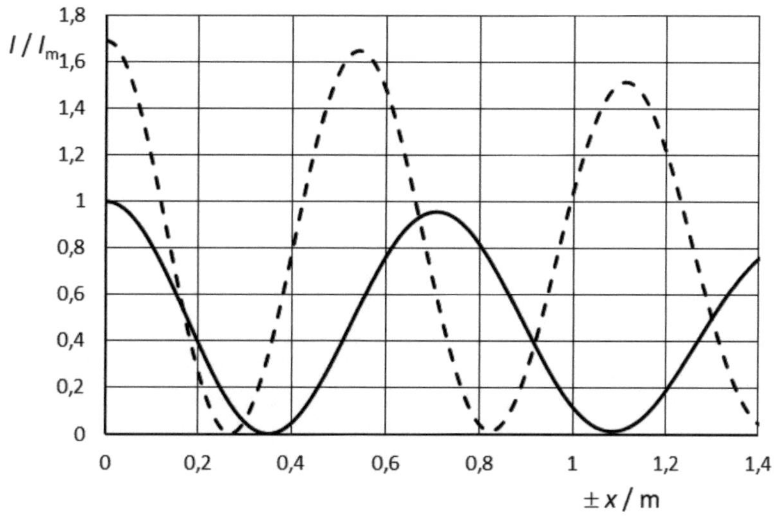

Figure 7.
Result of two speakers' interference for f_1 = *1.0 kHz (solid line) and 1.3 kHz (dashed line) relative to the maximum intensity.*

tone colour, and thus the whole harmony of the music. The only place where we do not hear this distortion is on the axis of the system $x = 0$. It is advisable, for a quality experience of recorded music, to sit in the axis of a pair of speakers.

Suppression of these negative phenomena in two-source stereo is solved by a set of more speakers, for example, a quadraphonic system.

4.3 Standing waves and resonators

Consider two harmonic plane waves with the same polarisation and frequency that propagate in opposite directions. The resulting wave is the superposition of both waves

$$\mathbf{u} = \mathbf{u}_1 + \mathbf{u}_2 = u_1 e^{j(\omega t - kz)} + u_2 e^{j(\omega t + kz)}.$$

The term can be broken down into two parts

$$\begin{aligned}\mathbf{u} &= (u_1 - u_2)\ e^{j(\omega t - kz)} + u_2 \left[e^{j(\omega t - kz)} + e^{j(\omega t + kz)}\right] \\ &= (u_1 - u_2)\ e^{j(\omega t - kz)} + 2u_2\ \cos\,(kz)\, e^{j\omega t}.\end{aligned} \tag{47}$$

The resulting wave has two different components. The first one is a moving wave that propagates in the z-direction and has an amplitude equal to the difference of amplitudes of both waves. The second component represents oscillations with frequency ω and amplitude $u(z) = 2u_2 \cos(kz)$ dependent on the coordinate z. It is a *standing wave*.

If the amplitudes of the two waves propagating against each other are the same, a pure standing wave occurs

$$\mathbf{u} = 2u_1 \cos\,(kz)\, e^{j\omega t}. \tag{48}$$

Points where $kz_u = n\pi$, resp. $z_u = n(\lambda/2)$, where $n = 0, 1, 2, \ldots$ is $u_u = 0$. The amplitude of the oscillations is zero and these points are called *nodes of the standing wave*.

Conversely, points where $kz_k = (2n + 1)\pi/2$, resp. $z_k = (2n + 1)\lambda/4$, the maximum amplitude $u_k = 2u_1$. These points are called *antinodes of the standing wave*.

Standing wave or partially standing wave arises when the wave is reflected from the interface of two media by the composition of both direct and reflected waves.

The relation (22) shows that the maximum displacement is $u_1 + u_2$ and the minimum displacement $|u_1 - u_2|$.

The quantity

$$SWR = \frac{u_1 + u_2}{|u_1 - u_2|} \tag{49}$$

defines the standing wave ratio—*SWR*. $SWR = 1$ is a purely moving wave, $SWR \to \infty$ is a purely standing wave. *SWR* is mainly used to evaluate signal reflections on lines or the reflectance of various acoustic structures.

The principle of standing wave formation is used in resonators. One example of a resonator is the reflection of the wave from the thin film described above. The resonator may be used as a wave amplifier. Multiple wave reflections, inside the resonator, can cause its amplification, like resonance in a serial RLC electrical circuit, wherein the resonance state the voltage at the capacitor is Q times a voltage of the source. Q is the quality factor (in the low-loss circuit $Q \gg 1$). Similarly, in the wave resonator, the intensity of the wave in the resonator is many times greater than the intensity of the coming wave, resp. of the wave generated near the node. A typical example is creating a sound on a piano string—the hammer gently strikes the string near the knot (point of string fixation). The string sounds only with tones corresponding to the resonance condition (basic and higher harmonic frequencies). It is like the air column of the wind musical instrument, where the tongue vibrates the air near the knot, and the entire column sounds with multiple intensities.

Example 9 Standing wave on the string—vocal cords

The vibration of vocal cords whose frequency determines the tone of the voice can be modelled with a simple model of standing wave on the string. The string (the musical instrument) is fixed at the endpoints, which cannot move. They represent, therefore, standing wave nodes. For the standing wave then applies

$$l = n\,\frac{\lambda}{2} = n\,\frac{c}{2f} = \frac{n}{2f}\,\sqrt{\frac{F}{\mu}}, \text{and } f_n = \left(\frac{1}{2l}\,\sqrt{\frac{F}{\mu}}\right)n = nf_1 \tag{50}$$

On the string, there arise standing waves with discrete frequency spectrum f_n. The term in parentheses represents the base frequency f_1, which determines the base pitch of the tone. Other higher harmonics change the colour of the tone (different contents of higher harmonics cause different colours of the same tone at different musical instruments). Wave velocity on the string depends on the force F tensioning the string and the linear weight $\mu = m/l$ of the string (see chapter Mechanical waves). We can tune the resonance frequency, and therefore the pitch of the tone, changing values of F, μ and l.

The vocal cords are the muscle bundles between which there is a gap. As the air flows through the gap, the vocal cord muscles tremble, the fundamental frequency of oscillations being dependent on the thickness of the vocal cords, and the force that strains the vocal cords. Children and women have vocal cords thinner, so they have a higher voice frequency. In men in adolescence, the vocal cords coarsen (mutation), and the voice becomes deeper. You can control the pitch of a tone by changing the vocal cord tension, so you can intonate when singing (intonation—pitch control).

Example 10 Standing wave in a tube—ear canal

The outer ear canal is an acoustic resonator that increases the sensitivity of hearing at the middle frequency of audible sound (about 3 kHz). The incident longitudinally polarised wave is reflected on the eardrum and interferes with the wave passing directly. This creates a standing wave and resonantly amplifies the sound.

A simple model idea is provided by the description of the standing wave in the air column in the canal. If the tube is closed at the end, there is a standing wave node at the end, there is an anti-node in the open mouth. The length of the ear canal thus represents a quarter of the wavelength.

$$l = \frac{\lambda}{4} = \frac{c}{4f}, \text{resp. } f = \frac{c}{4l}. \tag{51}$$

Substituting the values of $c \approx 330\ \text{m·s}^{-1}$ and the length of the ear canal $l \approx 2.5$ cm, we obtain a resonant frequency $f \approx 3.3$ kHz. It is known from audiometric measurements that the maximum sensitivity of the auditory organ is around this frequency.

Example 11 Ultrasonic transducer

To generate ultrasound, for example, in sonography or lithotripsy, piezoelectric transducers are used. The ultrasonic transducer is a plate of an anisotropic piezoelectric material with suitable orientation and electrodes on its surface. When the AC voltage is applied, the mechanical stress in the plate changes alternately, and thus the deformation (plate thickness slightly alternately increases and decreases) generates oscillations that represent a standing wave in the plate. If the wave impedance of the outer medium is less than the impedance of the plate, there occurs reflection of the wave on the surfaces of the plate and the standing wave arises in the plate. Thus, resonance occurs when the plate thickness is approximately equal to half the wavelength. For values used in sonography, for example, $f = 5.0$ MHz, and ultrasonic velocity in ceramic piezoelectric $c \approx 3.4\ \text{km s}^{-1}$, we obtain plate resonance thickness $d \approx \lambda/2 = c/(2f) \approx 0.34$ mm.

Example 12 Infrasound in the room

The danger for a human is represented by vibrations with frequencies below the audible limit of $f = 15$ Hz, referred to as infrasound. The walls of rooms, especially concrete structures, vibrate due to the transmission of vibrations from the ground or the operation of machines in the building. The oscillations of the subsoil, unless we consider an earthquake, come mostly from traffic. Wall oscillations generate acoustic waves in the room, which can be amplified by wave resonance. High impedance concrete walls represent almost ideal reflective surfaces and are nodes of rising standing waves. The basic resonant frequency corresponds to the condition $l = \lambda/2$.

For a room with a length of $l = 10$ m and a sound velocity $c = 330\ \text{m s}^{-1}$, the base frequency of the standing wave is $f_1 = c/2l \approx 16.5$ Hz. The maximum oscillation is in the centre of the room. If in the office working place, for example, in the middle of the room, acoustic vibrations can harm the health of a person. To reduce the risk of low-frequency vibrations, it is possible to treat the walls with an anti-reflective cover.

5. Diffraction

Wave diffraction is a phenomenon that is sometimes referred to as wave bending and, in simplified terms, can be characterised as wave propagation beyond an obstacle. When interpreting the phenomenon, we will use the Huygens-Fresnel principle.

5.1 Radiation of the planar source

Planar sources are often used to generate waves, for example, piezoelectric plates for generating ultrasound, reflectors of sources of EM radiation, or funnel antennas of microwaves. The planar source can also be an aperture in a screen, which is hit by a plane wave—the aperture becomes a planar source for additional space.

5.1.1 Long rectangular strip source

Thin strip transducers, especially ultrasonic ones, are often used. Such a source may be also a slot that is hit by a plane wave, for example, the light.

Using the Huygens-Fresnel principle, the strip of width a is divided into elementary sources, elementary strips of width dx, **Figure 8**.

The interference of cylindrical waves of elementary sources is expressed as

$$\mathbf{u}(\mathrm{P}) = -\frac{\mathrm{j}}{\sqrt{\lambda}}\, u_0(\mathrm{M}) \int_{-a/2}^{a/2} \frac{\exp(\mathrm{j}\mathbf{k}\cdot\mathbf{r})}{\sqrt{r}} \cos\varphi \; dx. \tag{52}$$

Consider a wavefield at a distance $r \gg a$ (Fraunhofer region—distant field) for which we get vectors $\boldsymbol{r}$ and $\boldsymbol{r}_0$ to be parallel and $\cos\varphi$ constant.

The wave function argument is expressed

$$\mathrm{j}\boldsymbol{k}\cdot\boldsymbol{r} = \mathrm{j}\boldsymbol{k}\cdot\boldsymbol{r}_0 - \mathrm{j}kx\,\sin\varphi$$

and after calculation of the integral, we obtain

$$\mathbf{u}(\mathrm{P}) = -\frac{\mathrm{j}a}{\sqrt{\lambda r}}\, u_0\, \cos\varphi\; \mathrm{e}^{\mathrm{j}\,\mathbf{k}\cdot\mathbf{r}_0}\, \frac{\sin\left(\frac{ka}{2}\sin\varphi\right)}{\left(\frac{ka}{2}\sin\varphi\right)}. \tag{53}$$

The wave propagates from the elementary source as a cylindrical one in all directions, but the wave is not isotropic and has a distinct directional pattern depending on the angle φ under which we observe the radiation.

The wave intensity is

$$Z\,\omega^2 u^2(\mathrm{P}) = \frac{a^2}{\lambda r}\, Z\,\omega^2 u_0^2\, \cos^2\varphi\;\; \mathrm{F}(\alpha), \text{resp. } I = I_0\,\frac{a^2}{\lambda r}\, \cos^2\varphi\;\mathrm{F}(\alpha), \tag{54}$$

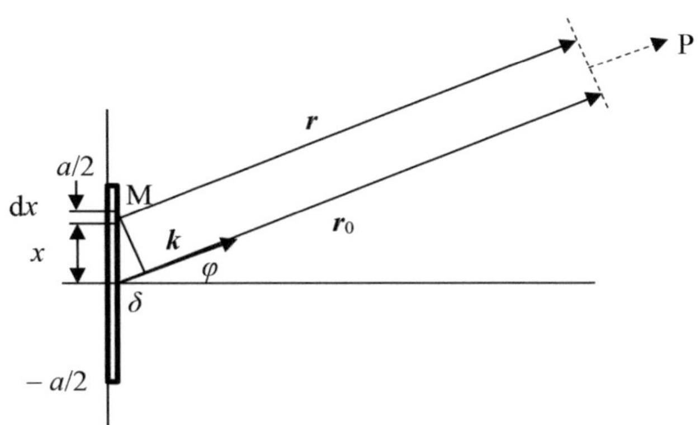

Figure 8.
Diffraction on the strip.

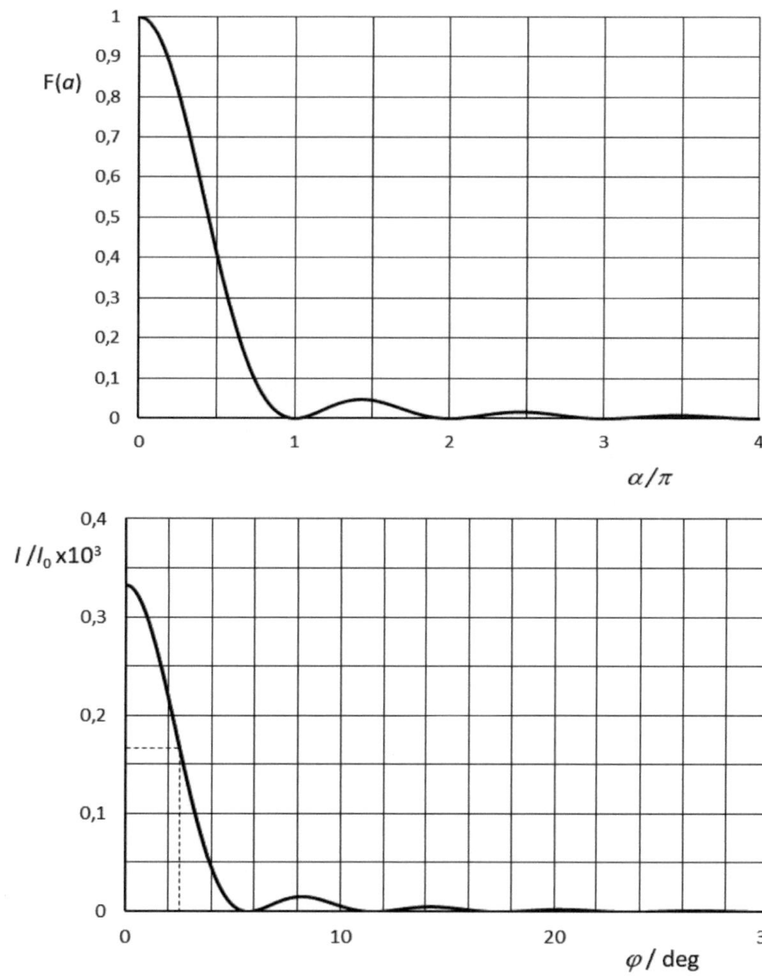

Figure 9.
Graph of the function F(α) = (sin α/α)² versus α/π (upper), and directional radiation characteristic of the strip source (λ = 500 nm, a/λ = 10, r = 15 cm)—lower one.

where $F(\alpha) = \left(\frac{\sin\alpha}{\alpha}\right)^2$, and $\alpha = \frac{ka}{2}\sin\varphi = \pi\frac{a}{\lambda}\sin\varphi$.

In the graphs in **Figure 9**, we see the diffraction function $F(\alpha)$, and the directional radiation characteristic I/I_0, from which we can see to which angles φ the source emits the radiation. The main lobe is significant. Its width is determined at the level of intensity decrease to 50% of the maximum value. The characteristic width in the figure is $\Delta\varphi \approx 5°$. While the cos φ function changes only slowly and monotonically from the unit value in a straight line perpendicular to the surface of the plate, to zero in a direction parallel to the plate. The profile of the diffraction pattern is mainly described by the function $F(\alpha)$.

The maxima of the function $F(\alpha)$ determine the directions in which the radiation has a local maximum. As we see in the picture, the maximum of the 0th order is the biggest one, others are significantly lower. The maximum of the 1st order, for $\alpha/\pi \approx 1.4$, is only 5% of the main maximum.

The value $\alpha/\pi = 1$ (minimum of function) corresponds to the geometric angle $\varphi_{\min 1}$, for which we have

$$\alpha = \frac{ka}{2}\sin\varphi_{\min 1} = \pi, \text{or } \sin\varphi_{\min 1} = \frac{\lambda}{a}. \quad (55)$$

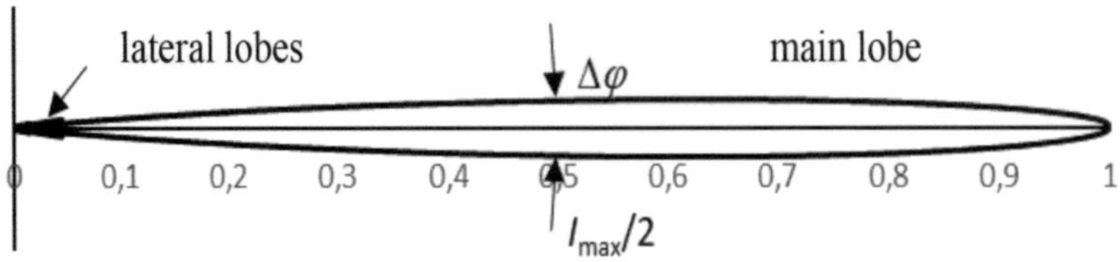

Figure 10.
Radiation characteristic in the polar coordinates for a/λ = 10.

In **Figure 10**, the radiation characteristic of a strip with $a/\lambda = 10$ is plotted in the polar coordinates I/I_0 versus φ.

The width $\Delta\varphi$ of the main lobe is determined at the level of intensity decrease −3 dB (50%). If $\cos^2\varphi \approx 1$ for narrow characteristics $\Delta\varphi \ll 1$, the decrease is determined by the function F(α). For the intensity decrease to 50%, applies the equation

$$\left(\frac{\sin\alpha}{\alpha}\right)^2 = \left(\frac{\sin\left(\pi\frac{a}{\lambda}\sin\varphi\right)}{\pi\frac{a}{\lambda}\sin\varphi}\right)^2 = \frac{1}{2}, \text{resp.} \quad \sin x = \frac{x}{\sqrt{2}}. \tag{56}$$

It results in the numerical solution $x \approx 1.39$.

The width of the main lobe is then

$$\Delta\varphi = 2\arcsin\left(0.44\ \frac{\lambda}{a}\right). \tag{57}$$

For the characteristic at **Figure 10** (λ/a = 1/10) we get $\Delta\varphi \approx 5.0°$.

For a wide strip with $a \gg \lambda$, we can use an approximate relation

$$\Delta\varphi \approx 0.88\frac{\lambda}{a}. \tag{58}$$

If we want to achieve a narrow characteristic, for example, in sonographic imaging, we must choose a small ratio λ/a. For f = 5 MHz, and c = 1500 m s^{-1} is λ = 300 μm. To generate a beam with divergence $\Delta\varphi$ = 1°, a plate with a width $a \approx 1.5$ cm is required. This dimension is too large. Therefore, a narrowing of the radiation characteristic we obtain using a set of parallel strips (lattice) as described in the following paragraph.

The above-described diffraction occurs at a distance $r \gg a$. In the near, the so-called Fresnel region, the wave advances as a beam with a transverse profile corresponding to the shape of the transducer. It proceeds in a direction perpendicular to the transducer, **Figure 11**.

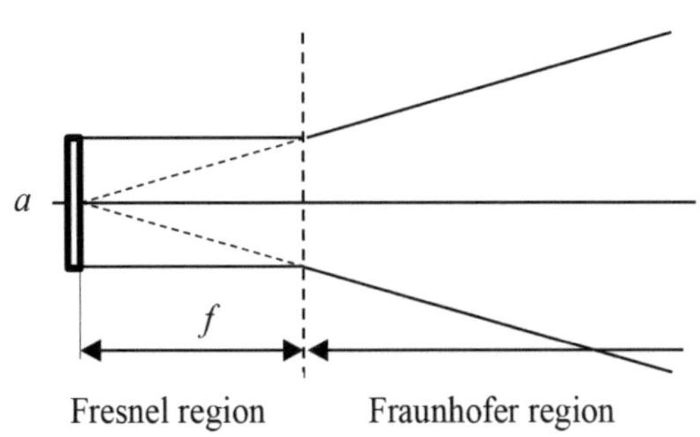

Figure 11.
Near and distant region of the transducer.

Only from a distance f occurs the divergence of the wave due to diffraction. We have

$$\frac{a}{2f} = \tan\varphi_{\mathrm{m}} = \frac{\sin\varphi_{\mathrm{m}}}{\sqrt{1-\sin^2\varphi_{\mathrm{m}}}} = \frac{0.44\,\frac{\lambda}{a}}{\sqrt{1-\left(0.44\,\frac{\lambda}{a}\right)^2}},$$

from where

$$\frac{f}{\lambda} = \frac{1}{2}\,\frac{a}{\lambda}\sqrt{\left(\frac{1}{0.44}\times\frac{a}{\lambda}\right)^2 - 1}. \tag{59}$$

For λ = 300 μm and a = 1.5 cm is $f/\lambda \approx 2.8 \times 10^3$ and $f \approx 84$ cm. In this case, which corresponds to the ultrasound frequency of sonography, the length of the Fresnel region f is greater than the depth of the organs of the body. The lateral resolution of 1.5 cm is unacceptably high for imaging. It is, therefore, necessary to narrow the wave beam. For a thin strip, $a = \lambda = 0.3$ mm $f/\lambda \approx 1.0$ and hence $f \approx 0.3$ mm. However, the beam divergence in the distant region is $\Delta\varphi \approx 52°$, which is too large to display. This problem is solved by a structured grid transducer, see Chapter 3.

5.1.2 Rectangular and circular planar source

To illustrate the diffraction effect, there are shown, in **Figure 12**, diffraction patterns formed on the projection screen after irradiation of a rectangular aperture (left image) and a circular aperture (right image) with a plane wave of the laser beam. The series of bright points on the horizontal axis (left) corresponds to the diffraction maxima according to **Figure 9**. The rectangular source can be taken as the combination of two mutually perpendicular strips. Each side induces diffraction in a direction perpendicular to the respective side with parameter α according to (54) to side a or equally β to side b. The resulting diffraction pattern of the rectangular (or square) source is shown in **Figure 12** left. The length of the side of the rectangular source can be calculated by measuring the distance of the maximums on the screen.

In the case of a circular source, the Huygens-Fresnel integral has a form

$$\mathbf{u}(\mathrm{P}) = -\frac{\mathrm{j}k}{2\pi}\iint_S u_0(\mathrm{M})\,\frac{\exp\left[\mathrm{j}k\left(r-\frac{x}{r}\xi-\frac{y}{r}\eta\right)\right]}{r}\,\cos\vartheta\;\mathrm{d}\xi\,\mathrm{d}\eta, \tag{60}$$

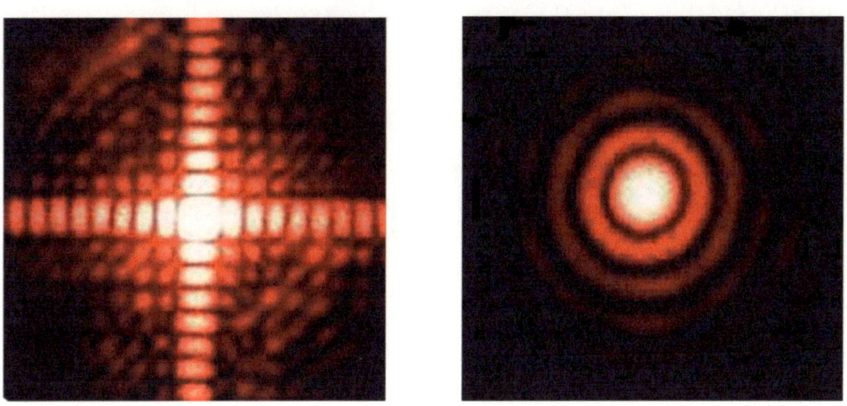

Figure 12.
Diffraction patterns of the square and circular sources of light.

where x, y are coordinates of the point P on the screen, ξ and η coordinates of the point M on the surface of the source, r is the mutual distance of points M and P.

Considering $r \gg R$, where R is the radius of the circular source, the distance r can be considered independent of the position of the point M of the source and hence taken from the integral. Since the system is axially symmetrical, it is preferable to use polar coordinates

$$x = r \sin\vartheta \ \cos\alpha, \quad y = r \sin\vartheta \ \sin\alpha, \quad \xi = \rho \ \sin\beta, \quad \eta = \rho \ \cos\beta,$$

and the surface element of the source $\mathrm{d}S = \mathrm{d}\xi \ \mathrm{d}\eta = \rho \ \mathrm{d}\beta \ \mathrm{d}\rho$.

$$\mathbf{u}(\mathrm{P}) = -\frac{\mathrm{j}k}{2\pi} u_0 \frac{\mathrm{e}^{\mathrm{j}kr}}{r} \cos\vartheta \int_0^R \int_0^{2\pi} \mathrm{e}^{-\mathrm{j}k\rho\sin\vartheta \ \cos(\beta-\alpha)} \rho \, \mathrm{d}\beta \ \mathrm{d}\rho. \tag{61}$$

By solving this integral we get

$$\mathbf{u}(\mathrm{P}) = -\frac{\mathrm{j}k}{2\pi} u_0 \frac{\mathrm{e}^{\mathrm{j}kr}}{r} \cos\vartheta \ 2\pi \int_0^R \mathrm{J}_0(k\rho \sin\vartheta) \ \mathrm{d}\rho,$$

where $\mathrm{J}_0(x)$ is the Bessel function of the 0th order. After its integration we have

$$\mathbf{u}(\mathrm{P}) = -\mathrm{j} \frac{2\pi R^2}{\lambda} u_0 \frac{\mathrm{e}^{\mathrm{j}kr}}{r} \cos\vartheta \frac{\mathrm{J}_1(kR\sin\vartheta)}{kR\sin\vartheta}, \tag{62}$$

where $\mathrm{J}_1(x)$ is the Bessel function of the 1st order. We get the wave intensity as a function of the angle ϑ relating to the axis of the transducer

$$I = I_0 \left(\frac{2\pi R^2 \cos\vartheta}{\lambda r} \right)^2 \mathrm{F}(\gamma), \tag{63}$$

where $\mathrm{F}(\gamma) = \left[\frac{\mathrm{J}_1(\gamma)}{\gamma}\right]^2$, and $\gamma = kR \sin\vartheta = \frac{2\pi}{\lambda} R \ \sin\vartheta$.

In **Figure 13** (right) we see the irradiation characteristics. At 50% of the maximum, the width of the main lobe is $\Delta\vartheta \approx 2.9°$. In this case, the diffraction pattern forms circular traces, **Figure 12** (right).

The central bright circle is called the Airi disk. It is surrounded by a circle of zero intensity $\mathrm{F}(\gamma)$ and thus $\mathrm{J}_1(\gamma) = 0$ for $\gamma \approx 3.832$, which corresponds to the angular radius

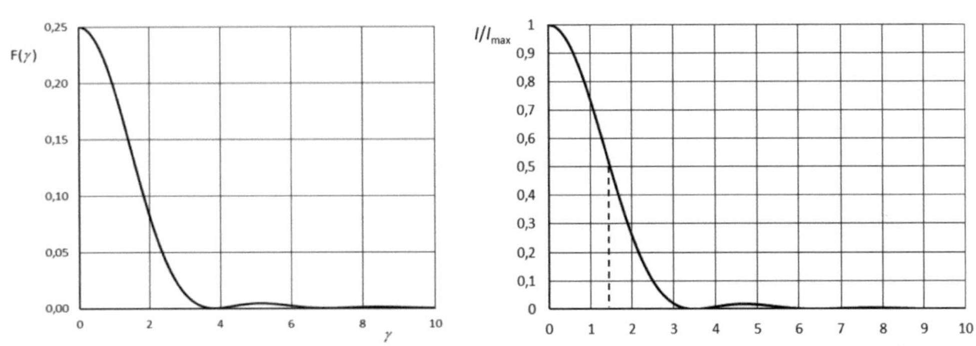

Figure 13.
Plot of F(γ) versus parameter γ—left, and relative intensity versus angle ϑ for λ = 500 nm, R/λ = 10—right.

$$\vartheta_{1\ \min} = \arcsin\left(\frac{1.22\ \lambda}{2R}\right). \tag{64}$$

For the values in **Figure 13** is $\vartheta_{1\ \min} \approx 3.5°$.

The results indicate that the angular diameter of the Airi disk and thus the scattering angle of the radiated wave decreases as the diameter of the source increases.

Again, the result is valid in the far Fraunhofer region $r \gg R$. In the near Fresnel region, the beam has a diameter of the transducer.

5.2 Structured plane sources

5.2.1 System of parallel strip sources with the same phase

Consider a simple transducer structure consisting of a grid of N parallel equal strips (according to). As in the previous paragraph, we observe the angular dependence of the radiation intensity. The distance between the centres of the strips is d and their width a. The resulting wave is a superposition of the waves emitted by the individual strips, see (25), using a phase shift resulting from the unequal ray length from the individual strips

$$\mathbf{u}(\mathrm{P}) = \sum_{n=1}^{N} \mathbf{u}_n = -\frac{\mathrm{j}\,a}{\sqrt{\lambda r}}\ u_0\ \cos\varphi\ \mathrm{e}^{\mathrm{j}\,\mathbf{k}\cdot\mathbf{r}_0}\ \frac{\sin\alpha}{\alpha} \sum_{n=1}^{N} \mathrm{e}^{-\mathrm{j}\,k\,n\,d\ \sin\varphi}. \tag{65}$$

If we express the sum of the geometric progression, we get

$$\mathbf{u}(\mathrm{P}) = -\frac{\mathrm{j}\,a}{\sqrt{\lambda r}}\ u_0\ \cos\varphi\ \mathrm{e}^{\mathrm{j}k\ r}\mathrm{e}^{-\mathrm{j}\ (N+1)\frac{kd}{2}\sin\varphi}\ \frac{\sin\alpha}{\alpha}\ \frac{\sin\left(N\frac{kd}{2}\ \sin\varphi\right)}{\sin\left(\frac{kd}{2}\ \sin\varphi\right)} \tag{66}$$

and radiation intensity

$$I = I_0\ \frac{a^2}{\lambda r}\ \cos^2\varphi\ \left(\frac{\sin\alpha}{\alpha}\right)^2 \left(\frac{\sin N\beta}{\sin\beta}\right)^2 = I_{\max}\ \mathrm{F}(\alpha)\ \mathrm{G}(N,\beta), \tag{67}$$

where $\alpha = \frac{ka}{2}\ \sin\varphi$ and $\beta = \frac{kd}{2}\ \sin\varphi$.

The function $\mathrm{F}(\alpha)$ describes the diffraction on a single strip and the function G (N, β) is the so-called lattice diffraction function. The width of the strip a shall be chosen so that its radiation characteristic is sufficiently wide. The lattice function G (N, β) is periodic with period π. For values $\beta_n = n\pi$, where $n = 0, 1, 2, \ldots$ the function acquires the maximum value of $\mathrm{G}(N, \beta_n) = N^2$. For the angle φ_n of the diffraction maximum, we get the relation

$$\sin\ \phi_n = n\frac{\lambda}{d}. \tag{68}$$

For the width of this maximum, we have $\Delta\beta = \pi/N$, and when converted to the angular width

$$\Delta\varphi = 2\ \arcsin\left(\frac{1}{N}\ \frac{\lambda}{2d}\right). \tag{69}$$

For small values of angular width, we get approximate relation

$$\Delta\phi \approx \frac{1}{N}\frac{\lambda}{d}. \tag{70}$$

The relation (68) shows that the original beam of incident waves is divided into individual diffraction beams deviated from the original direction by angles φ_n. The angle φ_n depends on the wavelength of the wave.

Example 13 Diffraction grating spectroscope

A diffraction grating is used to separate the wave components of different wavelengths from one another. If white light falls on the grating, it is broken into individual colour components. The first diffraction maximum is used for the decomposition of light (λ = 400–600 nm). For λ = 400 nm, we choose the ratio $\lambda/d \approx 0.57$, so that $2\lambda/d > 0$ and thus the second maximum does not arise. The grating period is d = 700 nm and strip separation a = 350 nm. The range of diffraction angles is from φ_{1f} (400 nm-violet) = 35° to φ_{1r} (700 nm-red) = 59°.

For grating with N = 5000 strips, that is, the total width of the structure D = 3.5 mm, for λ = 520 nm (green), the diffraction maximum width $\Delta\varphi \approx 1.5 \times 10^{-4}$ rad.

The diffraction grating can distinguish wavelengths with the difference $\delta\lambda = \lambda_1 - \lambda_2$, for which the difference in angles of the maxima is $\delta\varphi \sim \Delta\varphi$. From the relation (32) we get for the 1st order maximum for λ = 500 nm (green) φ_{1g} = 44°.

$$\delta(\sin\varphi_1) = \cos\varphi_1\ \delta\varphi = \frac{\lambda}{d}\frac{\delta\lambda}{\lambda} = \sin\varphi_1\frac{\delta\lambda}{\lambda},$$

from where $\dfrac{\delta\lambda}{\lambda} = \dfrac{\Delta\varphi}{\tan\varphi_1}$.

For the given values $\delta\lambda/\lambda \approx 1.6 \times 10^{-4}$ and wavelengths resolution $\delta\lambda \approx 0.1$ nm.

In the light spectrum of the sodium lamp that emits yellow light, there is an emission double line (doublet) with wavelengths λ_1 = 588.9 nm and λ_2 = 589.6 nm. The difference $\delta\lambda$ = 0.7 nm, and therefore the doublet is distinguished by the diffraction grating (*note: we do not distinguish them with the naked eyes*). Analysis of the radiation spectra is called spectroscopy. Based on the spectrum analysis, we can investigate the properties of the radiation source, for example, chemical composition. Thus, we can analyse the composition of stars using spectral analysis of the light coming from them. The spectrum of radiation is also modified as it passes through the material. In this way, we can analyse the properties of the material, for example, to determine the chemical composition of human body fluids (cerebrospinal fluid, blood, plasma, etc.). In haematology, the blood fat content before blood donation is determined by spectral analysis.

Example 14 Diffraction grating monochromator

In some applications, monochromatic radiation (single wavelength) is required. In such a case, the light with the desired wavelength can be obtained using its selection from intense white light, for example, of halogen lamp, by a diffraction grating monochromator.

The principle is the same as in the previous example. The white light is dispersed by the diffraction grating into individual colour components, and the desired wavelength is selected using a slit-shaped aperture. In addition to the transmission grating, a reflective one is often used as well. It consists of parallel strips with a reflective surface that is illuminated by white light. The individual strips thus represent, in reflected light, a set of parallel wave sources, which interfere with each other as in the case of a transmission grating.

The arrangement of the monochromator is in **Figure 14**. The white light source and the aperture are fixed. The reflective grating is deflected so that light with the desired wavelength λ passes through the aperture gap. The deflection of the grating is usually done by a micrometre screw calibrated at wavelengths.

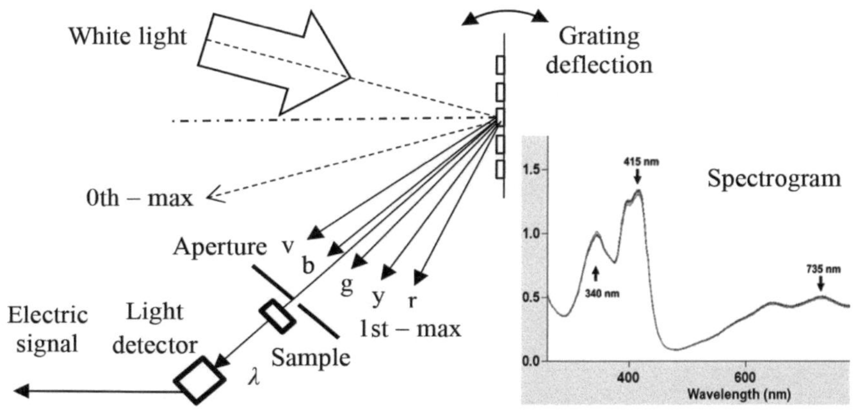

Figure 14.
Monochromator with reflection grating.

In spectrometers, the sample to be examined is placed behind the aperture. Its absorbance is determined from the signal of the detector versus wavelength (deflection of the grating). The result is recorded in a spectrogram, a picture on the right, from which it is possible to determine the presence of certain substances in the sample, for example, the haemoglobin spectrum or the fat content in the blood.

From the results (69), resp. (70), transducers with multiple periodic structures have a significantly narrower radiation pattern than a single strip source. If the aim is to concentrate the wave power to a small scattering angle $\Delta\varphi$, it is required that no non-zero order diffraction maxima occur, in order not to dissipate the wave energy. This is achieved when $\lambda/d > 1$. If λ/d is approximately equal to one, the width of the radiation beam is approximately $1/N$ in radians.

Example 15 Sonographic probe

A structured transducer consisting of more parallel piezoelectric strips is used as the ultrasonographic probe. In the case of N = 64 strips with a width of a = 0.1 mm and a spacing d = 0.2 mm at 5 MHz and ultrasonic speed c = 1500 m·s^{-1} (λ = 0.3 mm and λ/d = 1.5 > 1) radiation characteristic width $\Delta\varphi \approx 1.3°$.

Such a structured transducer has a sufficiently high angular resolution.

5.2.2 Electronic deviation of the radiated wave

Many applications require changing the direction of radiation, for example, radars, or ultrasonography. This can be achieved by a mechanical deviation of the antenna, for example, swinging, or rotating radar antennas, or USG probes with a mechanical deviation of the ultrasonic transducer.

The controlled deviation of the radiation characteristic can also be achieved electronically. In the previous case of structured multistrip transducer, all strips generated their waves with the same phase on their surface. If, however, the individual strips are excited, so that the phase shift ψ of the excitation of adjacent strips is constant, the resulting wave is formed by superposition of the waves of the individual strips, **Figure 15** on the left, and we have

$$\begin{aligned} \mathbf{u}(z,t) &= \sum_1^N \mathbf{u}_n = \sum_1^N u_{mn}\ \mathrm{e}^{\mathrm{j}\ (\omega t - k r_0 + k n d \sin\phi + n\psi)} \frac{\sin\alpha}{\alpha} = \\ &= u_\mathrm{m}\ \mathrm{e}^{\mathrm{j}\ (\omega t - k r_0)}\ e^{j(k\ d \sin\phi + \psi)\frac{N-1}{2}}\ \frac{\sin\alpha}{\alpha}\ \frac{\sin\ N\gamma}{\sin\ \gamma}\ , \end{aligned} \tag{71}$$

where $\gamma = \frac{kd}{2}\sin\ \phi + \frac{\psi}{2}$.

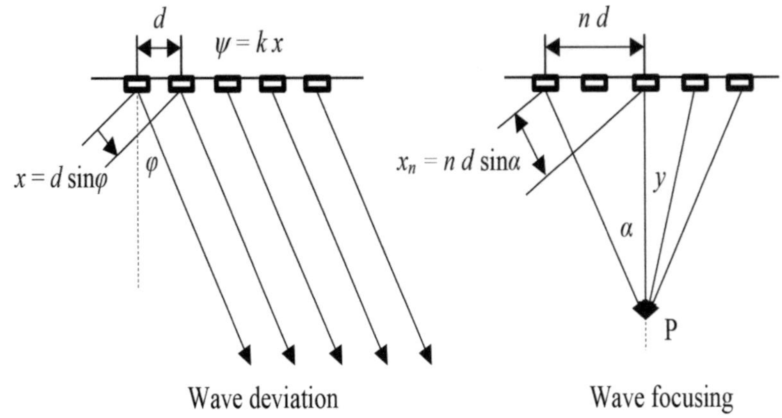

Figure 15.
Electronic deviation and focusing of wave.

The main maxima correspond to γ = 0, $\pm\pi$, $\pm 2\pi$, ..., from we get

$$\sin\phi = \frac{\lambda}{d}\left(n - \frac{\psi}{2\pi}\right), n = 0, \pm 1, \pm 2, ...$$

If $\lambda/d \gg 1$ and $\psi/2\pi \ll 1$, the relation has only one real solution for n = 0. The deviation angle is then

$$\varphi = -\arcsin\frac{\lambda}{d}\frac{\psi}{2\pi} \approx -\frac{\psi}{kd}. \tag{72}$$

Due to varying the phase shift ψ between the exciting signal of the strips, we can electronically deviate the radiated wave by an angle φ, **Figure 15** on the left. Thus, by periodic changing the phase difference ψ using the electrical supply of the strips, the generated wave continuously deviates. This method of electronic deviation of the ultrasonic beam is used in sectoral ultrasonography. To create a typical sectoral image of the internal organs, the elder probes used mechanical beam deviation. It had, however, some disadvantages. The probes for electronic deviation have no moving parts, and therefore the beam deflection can be faster than in the case of the mechanical ones.

5.2.3 Electronic focusing of the radiated wave

To achieve the necessary resolution of the ultrasonographic image of the tissue at the desired depth, it is necessary to focus the wave to that depth. The elder method used an acoustic lens on the surface of the ultrasonic transducer. The current method consists of focusing the wave electronically. It is achieved by a suitable phase shift of the individual waves radiated by the strips of the transducer, **Figure 15** on the right.

The individual waves from the strips are concentrated in the focus P when they encounter in the same phase, and constructive interference occurs.

The path of the n-th individual wave is longer than the distance from the middle wave by $x = nd\sin\alpha$, which corresponds to the phase shift ψ_n, by which its exciting signal needs to be back phase-shifted,

$$\psi_n = kx_n = nkd \sin \alpha = \frac{2\pi}{\lambda} nd\sqrt{(nd)^2 + y^2}. \tag{73}$$

If the electrical exciting signals of the individual strips are programmed so that their phase decreases gradually according to (73), the resulting wave concentrates in the focus P at a depth y from the transducer. Changing the value of the y parameter in the phase shift calculation can change the focusing depth of the wave.

Different generated beam profiling can be achieved through digital processing of the exciting signal. The digital control of phase shifts of the individual elements of the transducer using a computer is considerably simpler than the analogue solution.

6. Wave imaging

Waves, both mechanical or electromagnetic, occur in a wide range of phenomena and applications. One of the technical and natural phenomena is the transmission of information. We can see objects by vision or perceive sound through hearing. The basis of human perception of the waves is processing many signals provided to the brain by biological sensors, which are light-sensitive cells on the retina of the eye or cells of the cochlea sensitive to vibrations in the inner ear. Paired sensor organs (a pair of eyes, a pair of ears) provide the brain with information to create a stereo effect. In space, we orient ourselves by sight and hearing. The essence of sensory perception is the detection of the spatial–temporal distribution of the respective wave, which is created by its source and carries information about the properties of the source. By detecting this field, we infer the configuration of the waveform and create such an image of the source (optical, acoustic, etc.). The observed image is formed in our brain. The projection of an object into the structure of brain cells represents a certain transformation by which the object is transmitted to the brain cell's structure using neural signals. From the created image in the brain, we infer the position, arrangement, and other observed properties of the object. But the image in the brain only shows the perceived waves field. Between the object and the human sensors, the perceived field may be modified by many obstacles. It means, the image created in the brain need not match the object faithfully, for example, if we look into a crooked mirror the image created in the brain does not match the real object (we do not believe our eyes). In the perception of vision, the waves emanating from the observed object are modified before their impact on the eye retina cells by the eye lens and cornea. On the retina, the incident wave creates a two-dimensional image of a three-dimensional object. For example, kilometres large object is displayed as a centimetre image on the retina, and then it is sensed by sensory cells.

The brain has a memory, and it stores received images. Human memory is subjective so that various methods of wave-field recording are used for objective image preservation. If not only the amplitude but also the phase information is recorded, we get a complete record—a hologram. But two-dimensional recording only amplitude information is much simpler and widely used, for example, an ordinary photo. A suitable combination of amplitude records can create a spatial impression, for example, an acoustic stereo effect using headphones with a separate signal for the right and left ear, or optical by creating separate two-dimensional images for the right and left eye (e.g., using stereo glasses). However, this stereo effect is incomplete because it provides a spatial view from only one direction. Full digital image recording, tomography, is allowed by computer memory which can store a series of two-dimensional images of thin slices (*Greek: tomos—slice*) of the object with different values z of the third spatial dimension.

Wave imaging follows three basic goals. The first is to make the observed object visible or audible to the human senses, for example, observation of infrared, X-ray, ultrasound, or infrasound and ultrasound, or other waves "invisible" to humans. The second one is to allow observation of very distant, very large or very small objects, observation of very fast or very slow events, etc. The third goal is to record images for both analysis and archiving purposes. In addition to artistic recordings (paintings, sculptures), there are recordings on storage media, which may be chemical emulsions (classical photography), mechanical, magnetic or optical sound recordings (turntables, magnetic tape, magnetic disc, optical disc) or digital recording in computer memory. Records can be temporary (short term) or permanent (long term).

Short-term recording (computer display, microscope or telescope image, computer RAM recording, etc.) serves mainly to analyse the current structure and properties of the observed object, for example, observation of tissue by a microscope, observation of internal organs by an endoscope, etc. The long-term records are mainly used for archiving, for example, photo albums, X-rays images, etc. A modern and very economical way of archiving is archiving in digital form on various storage media. Digital archiving saves considerable space in healthcare facilities instead of storing printed reports or photographic images. Also, archived digital records allow rapid search and operative communication using communication networks.

The basis of imaging is to create a readable image, either for the observer's eye or for the respective recording medium. Wave imaging, except for volumetric holography, is two-dimensional (eye retina, film, camera CMOS or CCD chip, tissue tomography slice). The wave imaging aims to display the object as accurately as possible on the surface of the recording medium. For this purpose, serve the individual elements of the display systems, such as mirrors and lenses, or different complex systems, for example, optical, and acoustic microscopes, telescopes, photographic objectives.

6.1 Elements of display systems

6.1.1 Mirrors

One group of display system elements are mirrors. The mirror may be planar or curved. In **Figure 16** are several types of used mirrors.

(a) The planar mirror creates an image virtual, straight, and right-left inverted (that is why persons know themselves differently from a mirror and a photograph). When properly positioned, a planar mirror allows looking around the corner (known application is a periscope). (b) The 3D corner reflector consists of three mutually perpendicular planar mirrors forming a "corner". At the present 2D figure, only a pair of mirrors is shown. The ray of wave incident at any angle on one mirror is reflected from the other one exactly in the opposite direction. The principle of the 3D corner reflector is the same. It is used, for example, in roadside reflecting pieces, or in the safety reflecting elements, where the light of a vehicle headlamp is always reflected towards the driver. (c) Curved concave mirror (usually spherical or parabolic in more demanding applications). The beam of rays parallel to the optical axis incidents in the mirror and is reflected the focal point F located at the centre of the distance between the top of the mirror and the curvature centre. It is used in medicine, for example, as an ORL mirror that the doctor puts on the head. It concentrates the light from the lamp on the examined place, usually an ear. The doctor looks at the place through the aperture A at the top of the mirror. In advance, the mirror shields the disturbing direct light falling

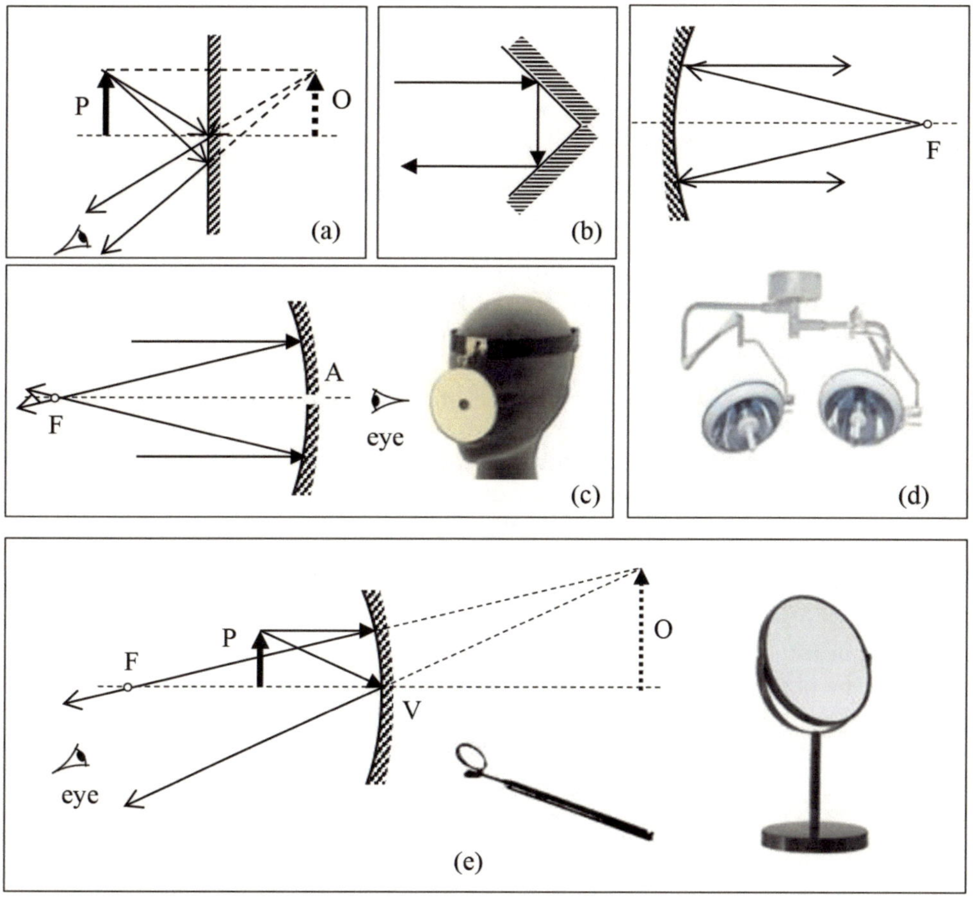

Figure 16.
Different types of mirrors.

into the doctor's eye, thus increasing the contrast of the object under investigation. If a detector is placed in the focus of the concave mirror, the energy of radiation striking the entire surface of the mirror (parabolic antennas) is concentrated there. The larger the mirror radius, the stronger the signal is detected. This principle is used, for example, at antennas for satellite reception or microwave radio transmission of a digital signal. Similarly, the principle also uses a parabolic antenna to receive mechanical waves of distant acoustic sources. (d) If a point source of the wave is placed in focal point F, the wave, when reflected from the concave mirror (reflector), forms a parallel beam of rays. It is used, for example, when illuminating the operating field during surgery or dental procedures. By changing the position of the source on the axis, a slightly diverging or converging beam of radiation is achieved. (e) The curved concave mirror is also used to display the object. If the object P is placed between the focus F and the top V of the mirror, a direct and enlarged virtual image is produced, with a greater distance from the mirror. This is used, for example, as dental mirrors for the diagnosis of teeth or cosmetic mirrors. These principles are common to any wave, regardless of its physical nature, whether mechanical (sound, ultrasound) or electromagnetic (light, infrared radiation, radio waves, etc.).

Note: In addition to parabolic mirrors, which focus a beam of parallel rays into the focus of a parabola and vice versa, there are also elliptical mirrors (rotating ellipsoid-shaped mirror surfaces) that concentrate rays radiated from a point source located in one focus into the second one. There are various architectural structures, such as halls, with vaulted walls and ceilings, which consist of ellipsoidal areas. There exist so-called "corners of lovers". If one person is in one corner (focus) and quietly speaks in a noisy room, the other person in the other corner (focus) can hear what the first person is, while other people outside the place hear nothing.

6.1.2 Lenses

Unlike mirrors, which use reflection, lenses use a transition through the material of the lens with a refractive index different from the refractive index of their surroundings. The basic types of lenses are shown in **Figure 17** with the indicated passage of the light rays through the lenses.

Lenses in the figure have refractive index $n > n_0$, where n_0 is the refractive index of their surroundings.

(a) The converging (positive) lens concentrates a beam of rays parallel to the axis into the image focus F′ and forms a diverging beam behind the focus like a point source located in the focus. The intensity of the wave in the focus is greater, the larger the area of the lens from which it gathers incident rays. Like an optical lens, an acoustic lens works by concentrating an incident ultrasonic or sound wave into the focal plane. Acoustic lenses have been used in ultrasonography to focus the ultrasonic beam. Today they are replaced by digital focusing. (b) If we place a point source in the object focus F of the lens, for example, halogen bulb, the lens forms a parallel beam of rays similar to a spherical mirror (while in the case of a mirror the source shields part of the reflected beam, this does not occur when the lens is used). It is used in projection devices as a condenser. (c) The figure shows the display of points lying outside the lens axis. If the object is located at a distance $a > f$, where f is

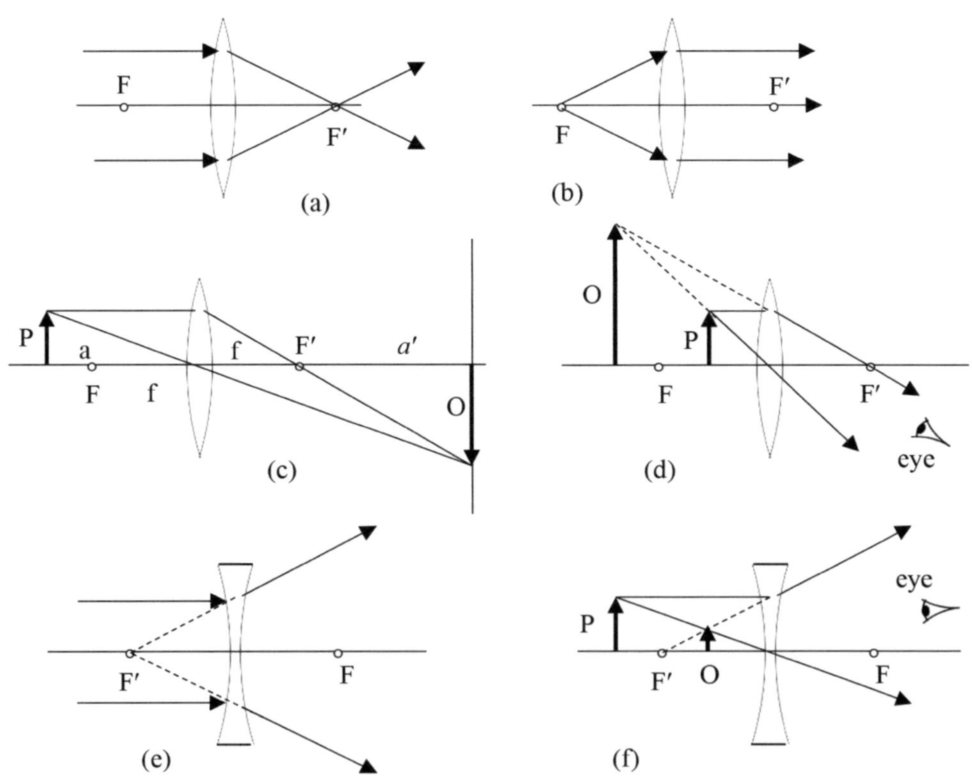

Figure 17.
Converging and diverging lens (P-object, O-image).

the focal length of the lens (inverse value $D = 1/f$ is the optical power and is given in dioptres, denoted D), a real and inverted image occurs in the image plane. It can be recorded with a suitable storage medium. This is used by photographic cameras, which focus incident rays on the detection surface (film, CCD, or CMOS chips) in the image plane, where creates an image of the object. The lens of the eye also concentrates the light incident on the pupil to a point on the retina of the eye and creates there an image of the observed object. We see from the figure that the image distance needs to be adjusted to the proper position to sharpen the image, for example, by moving the lens (focusing on the camera) or changing the optical power of the lens (eye accommodation). (d) If the object is between the object focus F and the lens, a direct, apparent, and magnified image occurs at a greater distance and can be observed with the eye. This is the principle of a magnifying glass for observing small objects. (e) The diverging (negative) lens scatters the incident beam as if the rays were coming from a point source located in the image focus F′. Thus, for example, create a wave field of the point source from the laser beam of parallel rays. (f) Displaying by a diverging lens is indicated in the figure. The object placed in front of the lens creates a virtual, direct, and reduced image that can be directly observed with the eye.

Lenses (glasses, contact lenses) are used to correct long-sightedness (positive lenses) or short-sightedness (negative lenses) if the eye lens is not capable of the necessary accommodation.

Note: If the inequality $n < n_0$ applies, the function of the lenses will be reversed (e.g., an air bubble in the glass or the water). The positive lens acts as a negative one and vice versa.

6.2 Imaging systems

Various imaging systems are assembled from the individual optical elements to display the object for observing it by a human eye with sufficient resolution or an image recording by a proper device (photograph, file on a memory disk). Imaging systems allow observing very distant objects (binoculars—telescopes) or very small objects (microscopes). The displaying system can be supplemented, for example, by diffraction grating for spectral analysis of the incident radiation. See also Splinter [2].

6.2.1 Photographic camera and projector

The simplest optical system is a photo camera, projector, or the human eye. The principle of the camera is in **Figure 17** on the left. The device objective can be a single lens or a set of lenses. Due to the dispersion of light in the lens material and correction of this undesirable phenomenon, complex objectives composed of several lenses (converging and diverging) of different materials are created for cameras to correct these defects. The camera objective at all is a converging system that concentrates the rays from the object on a recording medium (photographic film or plate or detecting sensor—CCD or CMOS chip) to create an image. As shown in the section on lenses, a distant object creates an image in the focal plane of the lens. The focal length f is indicated on the objective. For conventional cameras with a width of 35 mm recording field is $f \approx 50$ mm. If we want to enlarge the displayed field, we use a wide-angle objective with a focal length of about 28 mm.

To display distant objects a telephoto lens with a focal length of up to 400 mm is used, which has a small viewing angle but displays very distant objects on the recording medium. Optical devices also use lenses with variable focal lengths, zooms, which allow using both a wide-angle and a telephoto lens when retuning. The zoom can be optical (optical zoom) when the focal length of the imaging system changes, or electronic (digital zoom), when the selection of image points on the recording medium is electronically changed. By selecting the material of the elementary parts of the optical system and the detecting medium, it is possible to realise cameras for displaying visible light (VL)—photo cameras, or cameras for displaying infrared radiation (IR)—thermographic cameras. The IR camera works on the same principle as a VL camera, only the elements of the optical system must be transparent for infrared radiation and opaque for visible light (e.g., monocrystalline germanium), and the detector must be sensitive to IR radiation. CMOS detectors have the best features (sensitivity, noise) for it. IR cameras are used in thermographic diagnostics, whether technical or medical.

Projector, **Figure 18** on the right, is used to project film slides or digital recordings on a screen. The current modern tool is a digital data projector. The projector contains an intense light source (usually a halogen lamp). The diverging beam of the point source is changed to a collinear beam using a condenser (positive lens). The light hits a film or digital recording and projects it onto the screen using an objective. Projectors are used to present movies, images, or digital recordings from a variety of storage media.

6.2.2 GRIN lens

In an optically or acoustically inhomogeneous medium, the rays of the waves are curved. It is used in various technical applications. The optical inhomogeneity of the medium is used, for example, in optical fibres or GRIN lenses.

Example 16 Curvature of the acoustic beam in the surface layer of water in the sea

In the sea, the chemical composition and pressure of the saltwater change with depth. This affects the velocity of sound propagation in water. At steady conditions, the velocity of sound in saltwater decreases approximately linearly to a depth of about h_1 = 500 m and then increases again with the same gradient. At the surface, the velocity of sound in water is c_0 = 1500 m s^{-1} and at depth h_1 = 500 m is c_1 = 1480 m s^{-1}. Velocity gradient $k = \mathrm{d}c/\mathrm{d}h = 4.0 \times 10^{-2}$ (m s^{-1}) m^{-1}.

We show that the sound beams are curved and have the shape of a circular arc, **Figure 19**. The figure on the right shows the elementary section of the beam with the radius of curvature R in a thin layer with a thickness dh. When the wave velocity c changes, the angle α to the normal to the water level changes as well. According to Snell's law of refraction, we have

$$\frac{\sin\alpha}{c} = \frac{\sin\alpha_1}{c_1} = \text{constant, or after differentiation} \qquad (74)$$

$$-\frac{\sin\alpha}{c^2}\mathrm{d}c + \frac{1}{c}\ \cos\alpha\ \mathrm{d}\alpha = 0.$$

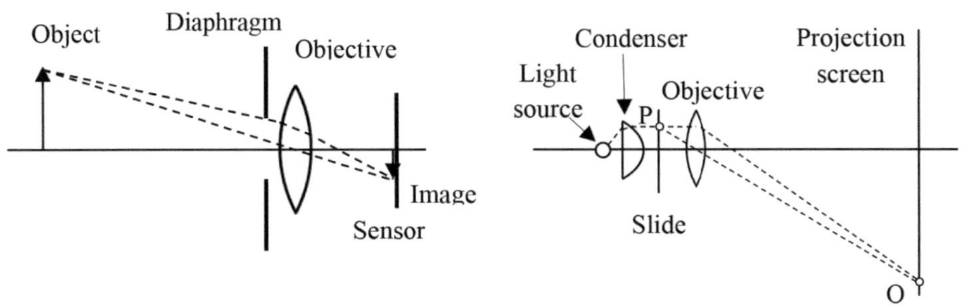

Figure 18.
Camera (left) and projector (right).

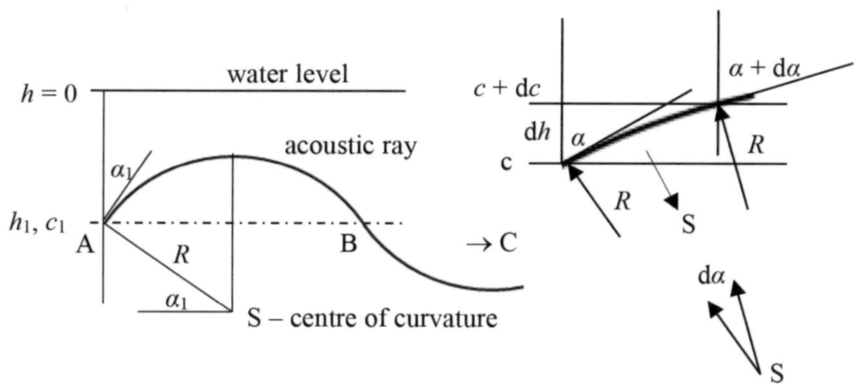

Figure 19.
Curvature of the acoustic ray in inhomogeneous sea water.

The length of the elementary section of the ray can be expressed by $R d\alpha$ or $dh/\cos\alpha$. After being replaced by refraction law, we get

$$\frac{1}{R} = \frac{\sin\alpha}{c}\frac{dc}{dh} = \frac{k}{c_1}\sin\alpha_1, \text{ which is constant.} \tag{75}$$

The beam is, therefore, a curve with a constant curvature, that is, circular arc. If an acoustic wave is emitted from a source at point A, it propagates along a circular ray to point B at the same depth h_1. The horizontal distance x_{AB} is

$$x_{AB} = \frac{2c_1}{k\tan\alpha_1}, \tag{76}$$

then it continues along a next circular arc to point C at the depth h_1, etc. It represents a waveguide through which the wave propagates. However, this applies only in the plane perpendicular to the water level. In other directions, this circular curvature does not apply, because in them the velocity gradient is zero.

Note: We observe a similar phenomenon with light in a medium with an inhomogeneous distribution of the refractive index. Like in the example, light propagates in a gradient optical fibre whose refractive index is greatest at the centre of the fibre and decreases towards its surface. If light enters the fibre with a sufficiently small angle α1, the light beam is curved and does not leave the fibre, i.e., propagates in the fibre without attenuation associated with radiation.

Elements of optical systems with a modulated refractive index, are mainly used in micro-optical applications. As mentioned, the basic element with a transversally modulated refractive index is an optical fibre.

Another element, especially of endoscopic imaging systems, is the GRIN lens (Gradient Refraction Index). The principle of focusing is indicated in **Figure 20**, like Example 16. In the middle is a sample of a GRIN lens with its typical dimensions. On the right is a sample of the endoscope tip.

GRIN lenses are particularly advantageous in that they have very small dimensions and do not require any specially shaped surface like conventional lenses. By suitable profiling of the refractive index, a special shaping of the optical beam can be achieved. **Figure 20** indicates the use of GRIN technology to implement a converging lens. This application is mainly used as an end optical element of endoscopes.

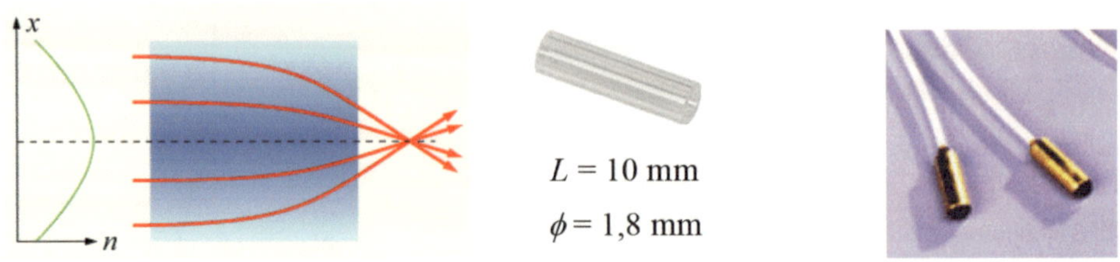

Figure 20.
GRIN lens.

6.2.3 Endoscopy

The endoscope is an optical imaging device that allows investigating internal organs inaccessible to direct observation. The endoscope is a cable that is inserted into the examined area. It contains illumination of the investigated area and a camera for its displaying. Typical applications are gastroscopy (endoscope inserted into the oesophagus), colonoscope (endoscope applied through the rectum to the large intestine), and the like. In the endoscope, the GRIN lens has two different functions. They are used as collimators to illuminate the field of view. A laser beam propagates through the optical fibre, and the GRIN lens extends it into a diverging light beam. The second function is in getting the image, where it has the same function as the camera objective.

The GRIN lens displays the subject in the image plane, from which it is captured. Two techniques are used. Most endoscopes are fiberscopes that introduce images into the optical fibre bundle (about 100,000 fibres with a diameter of several μm) in the image plane, and the fibres guide the light of the individual pixels of the image to a detection device at the outer end of the endoscope. The second option is to use a CCD sensor that transforms the image in the image plane into an electrical signal. Fiberscopes have a smaller head and a higher signal-to-noise ratio. They are mainly used in laparoscopic operations and endoscopy of fine structures (in angiography, neurology, etc.). The CCD chip has larger dimensions and a lower quality signal, but it allows an electric connection with an output. It is used, for example, in endoscopic capsules, **Figure 21**. The capsule with a diameter of about 10 mm contains an optical system with a GRIN lens and LED illumination around the circumference (see the front view of the capsule). The image is captured using a CCD, and the electric signal is

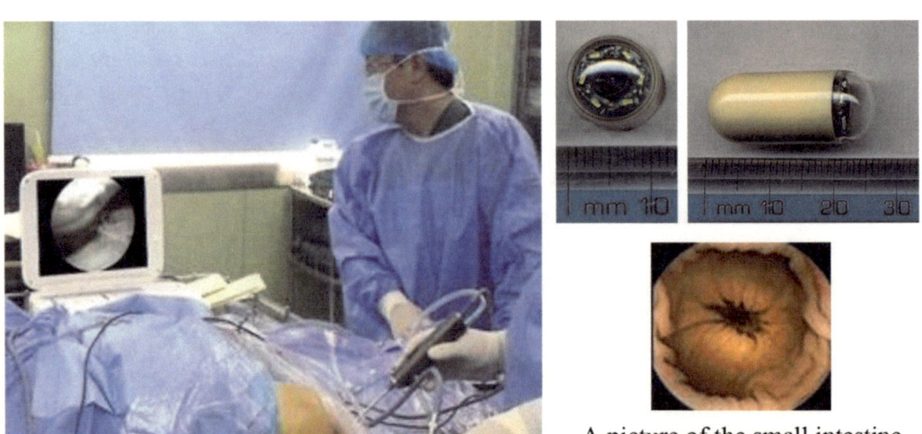

Figure 21.
Endoscopy (on the left a classic endoscope during laparoscopic surgery, on the right a wireless endoscopic probe and an image of the small intestine created by this probe).

transmitted via Bluetooth to an external sensor on the body surface. The capsule has an internal power supply. It is used to investigate the small intestine, which cannot be reached by a standard endoscopic probe, gastroscopy of the stomach and duodenum, or colonoscopy of the large intestine. After swallowing, the probe moves through the digestive tract and transmits images of the intestinal wall.

6.2.4 Optical system of the telescope

A telescope is an optical system that is mainly used to image distant objects or to expand or compress a wave beam.

The basic set of the telescope consists of two lenses, where the image focus F_1' of the first lens (objective) is identical with the object focus F_2 of the second lens (eyepiece). Lens telescope has an objective converging lens. The first Galileo telescope used an eyepiece the diverging lens, **Figure 22a**. The focal length f_1 of the objective was greater than the focal length f_2 of the eyepiece.

Then the angle φ_1 of view of the distant object is smaller than the view angle φ_2 at which we observe the object through the telescope. We see, there occurs an angular magnification. A small field of view expands, and so it is possible to observe details that cannot be seen by the naked eyes. As can be seen from the image, Galileo's telescope creates a direct image. When observing, for example, stars, or in compression of the wave beam, the inversion of the image does not matter, and a Kepler telescope with an eyepiece converging lens can be used, **Figure 22b**. This telescope has better optical properties but is structurally longer and produces an inverted image. An increase in the angular magnifying is in **Figure 23c**.

The disadvantage of lens binoculars is the loss of part of the power of the incident radiation by reflection at the lens-air interfaces. This is solved by mirror telescopes, in which the objective lens is replaced by a hollow mirror (Newton's or Cassegrain's telescope). The intensity of the image depends on the aperture of the lens $S_1 = \frac{\pi d_1^2}{4}$, which catches the power $P_1 = S_1 I_1$. If we do not consider losses, this power is then radiated by an eyepiece with area $S_2 = \frac{\pi d_2^2}{4}$, **Figure 22d**.

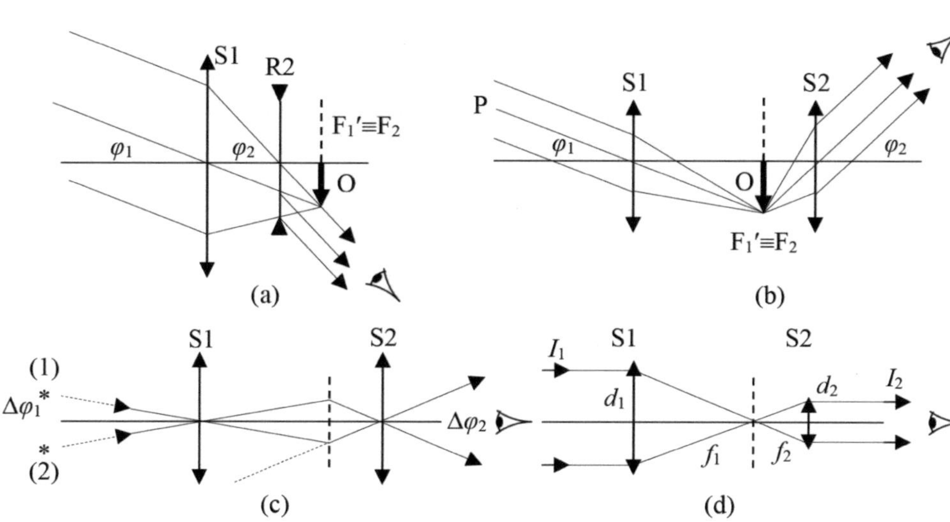

Figure 22.
Display the telescope function.

The intensity of the compressed beam

$$I_2 = \frac{P_1}{S_2} = I_1 \frac{d_1^2}{d_2^2} = I_1 \left(\frac{f_1}{f_2}\right)^2.$$

For d_2 = 8 mm (the eyepiece diameter corresponds to the size of the pupil of the eye) and d_1 = 50 mm (ordinary hunting telescope) is $I_2/I_1 = 40$, that is, increases the intensity of the incident light 40 times. In the dark, details visible through the binocular are invisible to the naked eyes. In mirror telescopes, apertures with a diameter of several meters (the largest astronomical telescopes) can be realised, and thus observe distant objects on the edge of the Universe.

Binoculars are also used together with a recording device mounted behind the eyepiece instead of the eye, or with a Doppler analyser, which allows determining the speed of movement of the observed object. Such a device uses, for example, police to measure speed and record road vehicles. The camera (photo or video) with a telephoto objective also performs a similar function.

6.2.5 Optical system of the microscope

Unlike the telescope, the microscope is used to image very small and near objects. We will explain the principle of the optical microscope, but the same principle uses infrared or acoustic one.

The microscope, **Figure 23**, consists of two converging lenses S1 and S2. There is an optical interval Δ between the image focus F_1' of the objective S1 and the object focus F_2 of the eyepiece S2. Subject P is in front of the focus F_1 of the objective. The lens S1 forms a real image O, and the focal plane of the eyepiece (F_2) is adjusted into this image plane. The eyepiece then forms a beam of parallel rays, which form an angle of view φ_2 to the optical axis. From the conventional distance of view l_k = 25 cm, the same object can be seen at a viewing angle φ_1. The angular magnification of the microscope is defined as $z = \varphi_2/\varphi_1 \gg 1$. A red blood cell with size d = 7.2 μm is observed from the distance l_k at an angle $\varphi_1 \approx 0.1'$ (angular minutes). The resolution of the eye is 1′, that is, the blood cell cannot be seen with the naked eyes. Using a microscope with magnification z = 100, the angle of view is $\varphi_2 \approx 10'$, that is, the shape of the blood cell is visible under a microscope. Optical microscopes have a magnification z up to 2000. Despite the high magnification, objects of the order of less than the wavelength of light cannot be observed due to diffraction. An increase in the cut-off resolution is achieved by shortening the wavelength (minimum wavelength of light is approximately

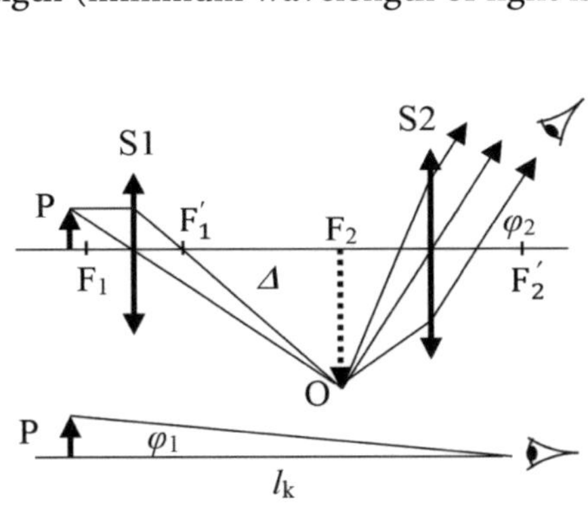

Figure 23.
Principle of microscope imaging.

DOI: http://dx.doi.org/10.5772/intechopen.101653

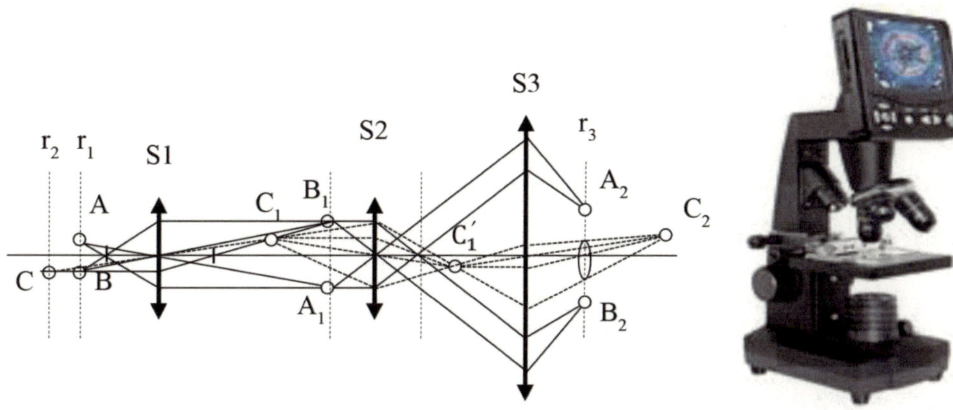

Figure 24.
Imaging by a microscope and depth of field.

350 nm). Extremely high resolution is achieved using an electron microscope, which achieves a resolution of up to 10^{-9} m, that is, allows to display viruses (15–300 nm), macromolecules, and the like. Top electron microscopes achieve magnification up to 10^6 and resolution up to 0.5 nm. Although the electron microscope image is in principle like that of a scanning optical microscope, the function of the apparatus, which uses an electron beam instead of an optical one, is considerably more complicated.

Conventional microscopes are used to image only thin planar (2D) samples. The image of the volume (3D) sample is blurred. **Figure 24** is the construction of images of objects that lie in different places and object planes r_1 and r_2. Let us first consider two objects A, B in one object plane r_1 the microscope is focused on. If we observe the course of the characteristic rays, objective S1 creates real images A_1, B_1 in the focal plane of the eyepiece. Behind the eyepiece, beams of parallel rays at different angles concerning the axis correspond to each of the objects. There is another imaging lens behind the eyepiece, either the lens of the eye in the case of visual observation or the camera lens if the image is recorded on a recording medium. In modern digital microscopes, the recording medium is a CCD chip. We can see that the lens S3 focuses the rays sharply to the points A_2, B_2 in the only image plane r3.

Even in this simple figure, we see that the distance A_2B_2 is greater than that of AB. The image is then projected on the LCD screen, or the digital recording is transferred to a computer. The advantage of a digital microscope is that it allows the image to be saved to disk, archived, or further processed.

Consider now point C, which is in another plane r_2 of the 3D object. If we observe the course of the characteristic rays, we see that the objective S1 creates a real image C_1, which is displayed by the eyepiece to a point C_1' at the intersection of the converging rays. The lens S3 then creates an image C_2 behind the detection plane. The beam pointing to point C_2 covers the trace indicated by a little ellipse in the detection plane. Object C thus does not create a sharp point image in the detection plane, but a wider track. Points that are in an object plane other than r_1 thus cover the resulting image in the detection plane with such surface tracks and blur the image.

Thus, a conventional microscope is not suitable for imaging 3D objects. However, it is suitable for imaging thin planar slices or liquid samples placed between two microscope slides, for example, in the investigations of various histological findings, blood particles, movement of sperm in the semen, the occurrence of chromosomes in cells in genetic tests, etc. Conventional optical microscopes are used in precision surgery, ophthalmology, neurology, dentistry, and the like.

6.2.6 Confocal microscope

A digital confocal microscope (CLSM—Confocal Laser Scanning Microscopy) is used to observe 3D objects. The scheme of the microscope is in **Figure 25a**. There is displayed only point A of the object plane. The overall image of a given sample plane is obtained by scanning the sample in two x, y directions perpendicular to the system axis. The confocal microscope displays only the points of the object plane on which the microscope is focused. Points from other planes of the object are suppressed and do not blur the resulting image (like a conventional microscope). In **Figure 25** are, for comparison, images of a defect on the skin surface: (b) from a conventional microscope and (c) from a confocal microscope focused on different planes of the object. It can be seen from the images that the confocal microscope images are significantly sharper than the image (b). By moving the sample in the z-direction, we get images of different planes of the sample layer by layer. By combining these images in a computer, a 3D image of the object can be created. It is an optical tomography. An example of a 3D image of cancer cells is shown in **Figure 25d**. A confocal microscope is standard equipment in the pathology department and the biochemical laboratory.

The principle of imaging is in **Figure 25a**. The laser beam of parallel beams is focused by the lens L1 on a small aperture of the screen S1, thus creating a point source of coherent light. The diverging beam is reflected by the semi-transparent mirror SM onto the lens L2. It focuses the rays to point A in the object plane. At point A, the light is reflected or scattered, and the rays going back from this point of the object incident on the lens L2 are returned to the semi-transparent mirror SM. Some of the light reflects towards the laser, but now we are interested in the light passing through the semi-transparent mirror.

At the same distance from the SM as the screen S1, there is a screen S2 with a small hole in the straight direction. Since the beams from point A are focused on the centre of its aperture, only the light from point A passes through the aperture to the lens L3 of the recording detector. The magnitude of the detector signal is directly

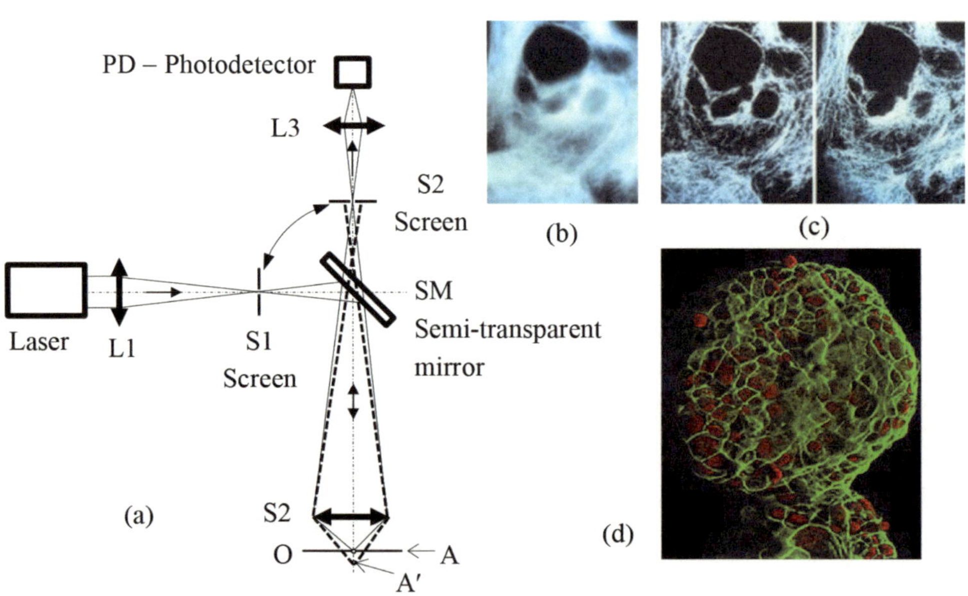

Figure 25.
Confocal microscope.

proportional to the reflectivity of point A of the object. By moving the sample (scanning), the detector signal is changed, which is digitised and recorded.

The laser light incident on the sample illuminates also points outside point A. The light emanating from point A′ at another depth also hits the lens L2 but forms a converging beam (dashed in the figure) that is not focused on the small aperture S2. It does not, therefore, pass through the aperture. The light emanating from a depth other than the depth of point A thus does not affect the detector signal and, therefore, cannot blur the image of the O plane. Similarly, the points in the plane O sideways from point A form an emanating beam, which is deflected by direction and thus also does not pass through the aperture S2. The detector signal thus corresponds only to point A of the displayed sample and its very close surroundings. The created digital image is, therefore, very sharp.

6.2.7 Microscope with phase contrast

The subjects of observation are often samples, especially in biochemistry and biology, which contain transparent objects like cells, small microorganisms, etc. A standard microscope evaluates the intensity (amplitude) of light, and this is not affected by transparent objects. Such objects are very faintly visible in the sample image, **Figure 26a**. However, the investigated objects have a different refractive index than the surrounding medium. As light passes through the sample, a different phase shift of the light beam occurs. If such a beam can interfere with a suitably arranged reference beam, the light may be increased or reduced depending on whether the interference is constructive or destructive. Thus, the phase shift caused by the different refractive index of the object is converted into amplitude information visible in the resulting image. In this way, originally invisible objects become visible—phase contrast is achieved, **Figure 26b**. The phase-contrast microscopes belong to the fundamental equipment of laboratories working with biological samples (pathology, biochemistry, etc.)

6.2.8 Fluorescence microscope

The fluorescence microscope is used to image organic and inorganic components of samples that are characterised by fluorescence. It uses the excitation of the fluorescent components of the object by ultraviolet radiation and detects the visible light that the substances emit when relaxed. The construction of the fluorescence microscope is like that of a conventional one. It is only extended by a source of UV radiation, **Figure 27**. The light from the UV lamp passes through the filter F1. UV

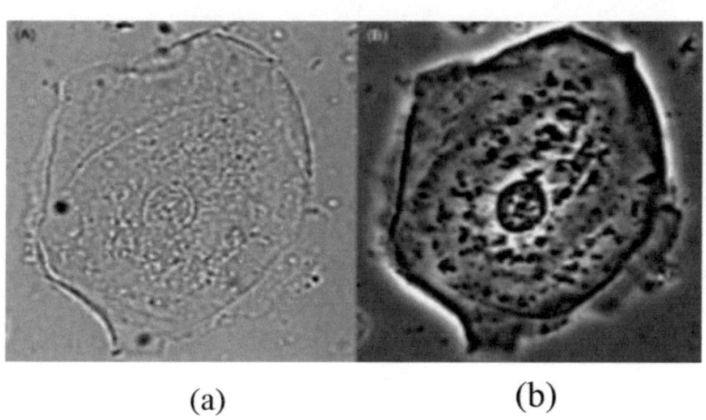

Figure 26.
Image of a transparent sample created by (a) amplitude sensitive microscope, (b) phase-contrast microscope.

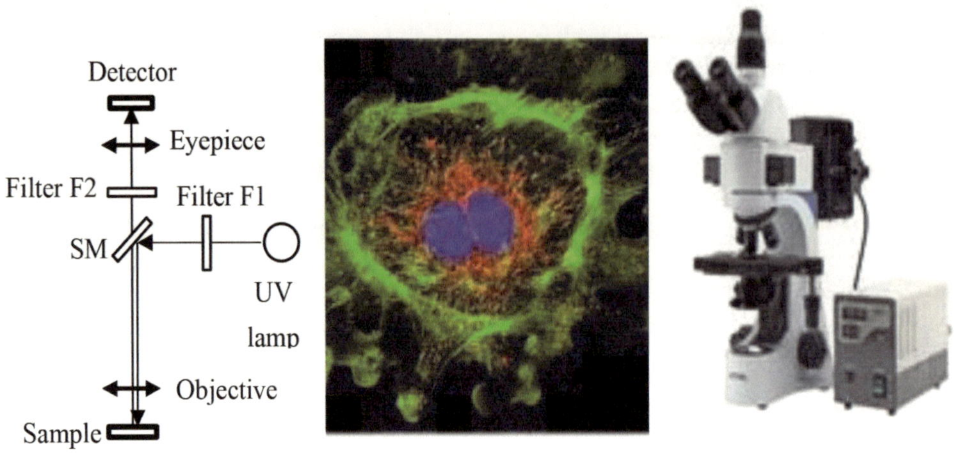

Figure 27.
Fluorescence microscope.

light with the selected wavelength proceeds to the semipermeable mirror SM and is reflected towards the sample. It induces fluorescence in the sample. The emitted visible light enters the microscope objective and passes through the SM to the optical filter F2, the eyepiece, and the detector. Filter F2 suppresses reflected UV radiation. The image is observed directly with eyes or captured with a digital camera. The parts of the sample containing a fluorescent substance are displayed markedly in the resulting image. Since different molecules or cellular components have different excitation energy, it is possible to change the display of the individual fluorescent components by retuning the F1 filter.

In **Figure 27** right is an apparatus for direct observation or with digital output and display of the observed sample on the LCD. The figure also shows an image of a cell with structures that emit light of different wavelengths (colours). In some cases, the primary fluorescence of certain molecules (e.g., some proteins—amino acids) is used. More often objects are "coloured" with fluorescent dyes, which penetrate biological structures and make them visible. In this way, the processes taking place in them can also be observed (for example, nucleic acids—DNA, RNA—are visualised). Fluorescence microscopes are mainly used in biological research laboratories.

6.3 Resolution of the wave imaging

If we use waves to image a certain structure, we are interested in what details can be observed, that is, resolution. Suppose we observe a small circular detail with radius r on the surface of the sample. The light reflected from the circle produces a characteristic diffraction pattern consisting of a zero maximum and higher-order diffraction maxima, see Section 5.1.2. For the reconstruction corresponding at least approximately to the observed formation, we must capture at least the main lobe of the spectrum, which contains the most significant spectral components, **Figure 13**. Therefore, if we want to distinguish the detail, we must capture a beam of the rays of the main lobe up to the first minimum, so-called *Airi disk*, which falls on the lens of the detection device (eye, microscope, camera lens), **Figure 28**.

For the first minimum, the relation (30) applies. If the lens is at a focal length f from the detail and R is the radius of the lens, the cut-off angle is $\varphi = \arctan (R/f)$. The requirement for the circle resolution (display resolution) is $\varphi \approx \varphi_{1\ min}$. If we consider the maximum value $\varphi \approx 45°$, that is, $R = f$, we get the resolution limit of a circular detail with diameter d the condition $d = 2R \approx 1.22\lambda$.

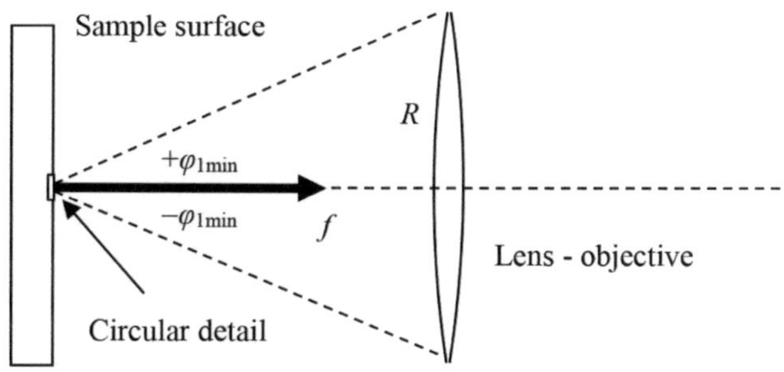

Figure 28.
Reconstruction of the diffraction pattern.

The main information of the zero-order lobe is in its width at the level of −3 dB (50%). The contours of the image of the circular detail will no longer be sharp but can still be distinguished. For $I/I_m = 0.5$, relation (29) and **Figure 13**, we get the value of the parameter $\gamma \approx 1.16$. Using (29) and estimating $\varphi = 45°$ we get the resolution limit of the circular detail $d_{min} \approx 0.37\lambda$.

It follows this analysis that wave imaging allows observing objects with minimum dimensions of about one-half of the wavelength of the used wave. With an optical microscope, details with dimensions of up to about 200 nm can be observed in blue light.

If we observe a sample with naked eyes, the radius of the pupil is approximately $R = 2$ mm and the distance of comfortable observation $f = 25$ cm, which corresponds to an angle $\varphi \approx 8 \times 10^{-3}$ rad. At the wavelength $\lambda = 500$ nm, the resolution is $d \approx 46\ \lambda \approx 0.02$ mm. A mesh having a fineness of about 0.05 mm can be seen with the naked eye. If we observe a finer structure, we cannot capture the diffraction maxima of small details with the eye lens, and thus we see only a homogeneous surface without any structure.

The resolution increases if the object can be observed from a closer distance so that the if angle φ is as large as possible. A magnifying glass or a microscope is used to increase the viewing angle of the observed object. Microscope objectives are therefore designed to meet the condition of maximum aperture, that is, $R \approx f$.

In edge cases, blue light is preferable to red one. X-rays provide greater resolution than light, but the device is technically more complicated. A significant rise in resolution provides electron beam imaging (electron microscopy), in which the electron wavelength λ can be set by the accelerating voltage U

$$\lambda = \frac{h}{\sqrt{2meU}}, \tag{77}$$

where h is the Planck constant, m and e are the mass and charge of the electron. For the voltage $U = 100$ kV we get the wavelength $\lambda \approx 4 \times 10^{-12}$ m, which is two orders of magnitude less than the size of individual atoms or interatomic distances in substances.

Bacteria, cells, larger viruses, etc., can be observed with an optical microscope. The electron microscope can image such small objects as macromolecules (e.g., DNA), proteins, small viruses, etc. The mentioned resolution rule also applies to ultrasound. USG imaging uses ultrasound with frequencies of 2–10 MHz. For fine structures, for example, eyes or nerves, higher frequencies > 10 MHz are used.

6.4 Focusing a wave beam

If the source is a strip, the wavefield described by the relation (26) arises. For a circular source (e.g., a circular hole or a laser output hole), the relevant relation (29) for the spatial distribution of the wavefield is similar, with Bessel functions instead of harmonic ones. We can see from the shape of the resulting relation for the strip source that the relation (25) for the angular dependence of the radiation characteristic corresponds to a Fourier image of a rectangular pulse with length a. If we do a reverse Fourier transform of this image, we get a reconstructed image that has the same structure as the source, that is, the strip with the width a. When reconstructing an impulse from its Fourier image, it is necessary to use at least the main part of the zero-lobe from the diffraction image according to the Eq. (27). The reverse transformation can be realised by a lens, cylindrical in the case of a strip, and spherical in the case of a circular source (**Figure 29**).

A lens with a circumference diameter D and a focal length f has a beam convergence angle $\Delta\varphi$ given by the relation when focusing a plane-wave beam

$$\tan\frac{\Delta\varphi}{2} = \frac{D}{2f}. \tag{78}$$

Using Eq. (27) we get a condition

$$\frac{\Delta\varphi}{2} = \arctan\frac{D}{2f} = \arcsin\left(0.44\frac{\lambda}{a}\right) \tag{79}$$

and after adjustment

$$a = 0.44\lambda\sqrt{1+\left(\frac{2f}{D}\right)^2}. \tag{80}$$

The $2f/D$ ratio acquires a real minimum value of about one, then the minimum width of the focused track is the $a_{min} \approx 0.6\lambda$. As the $2f/D$ ratio increases (i.e., the angle $\Delta\varphi$ decreases), the width of the focus track increases. In the case of a circular lens, the results are similar. In the optimal case, the wave beam can be focused on a track with a dimension equal to approximately half the wavelength. This phenomenon occurs regardless of the wavelength of the wave or its nature (mechanical or electromagnetic).

This fact must be respected, for example, in gentle operations with a laser scalpel in neurology, eye surgery, etc. We get a smaller focused track using blue light, in confront with a red light or IR radiation. The condition of the best focus applies to coherent waves, for example, laser. When using incoherent radiation, the possibility of focusing the beam is always worse (e.g., sunlight or LED).

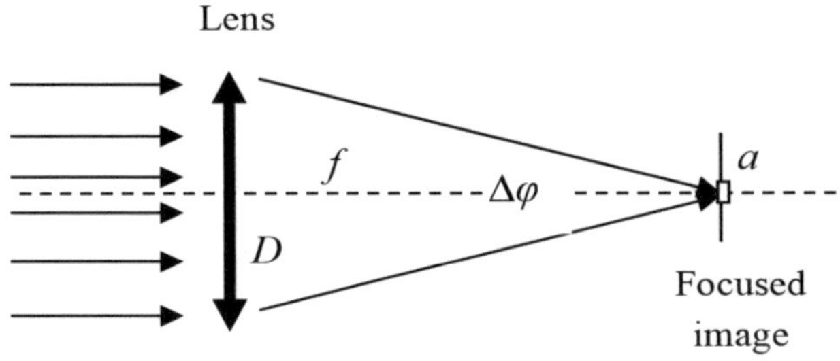

Figure 29.
Focusing a wave beam.

7. Non-linear phenomena

7.1 Non-linear wave interactions

In a linear medium, wave interference occurs, which means the waves add at the place of their common occurrence, but the waves themselves do not affect each other. However, if the medium is non-linear, the wave is deformed. It leads to arising higher harmonic components, and due to a non-linear interaction to different combination frequencies. These combination components may propagate in different directions relating to the direction of the original waves. These interactions are most often described by the quantum model. For example, the acoustic wave modulates the optical refractive index of the medium, and the electromagnetic wave thus passes through the medium with a periodic change of the propagation parameter, like through an optical grating. It causes a diffraction pattern, that is, the main lobe and lateral ones. Due to the movement of the grating at the speed of the acoustic wave, there arises also a shift of the EM wave frequency by the frequency of the acoustic wave.

Example 17 Acoustic modulator of the laser beam

In some information transmission by light, for example, optical fibre, it is necessary to modulate the light beam frequency. One way is an acoustic-optical modulator, which uses the nonlinearity of the modulation crystal, **Figure 30**. The carrier of the signal is a frequency-modulated acoustic wave, which causes a temporal change of the refractive index of the crystal corresponding to a transient change of the signal. A laser beam enters this crystal perpendicularly to the direction of propagation of the acoustic wave and is diffracted. The modulated first-order diffraction beam is used, which is angularly separated from the 0-order beam.

The principle of the deflector (modulator) is easily explained using the quantum concept of waves. EM waves represent photons with energy $E = \hbar\omega$ and momentum $\boldsymbol{p} = \hbar\boldsymbol{k}$, and acoustic waves phonons with energy $E_{ph} = \hbar\Omega$ and momentum $\boldsymbol{p}_{ph} = \hbar\boldsymbol{K}$.

In the interaction, where the photon captures the phonon, the law of conservation of energy and momentum is fulfilled.

$$\begin{aligned} \hbar\omega_0 + \hbar\Omega &= \hbar\omega \\ \hbar\mathbf{k}_0 + \hbar\mathbf{K} &= \hbar\mathbf{k} \end{aligned} \tag{81}$$

If we consider only a very small change in frequency $\Omega \ll \omega_0$ is $p \approx p_0$ and according to **Figure 30** is

$$\omega = \omega_0 + \Omega \tag{82}$$

and $2k \sin \frac{\varphi}{2} = K$, or $\varphi = 2 \arcsin\left(\frac{\lambda}{2\Lambda}\right)$, for $\lambda \ll \Lambda$ we have $\varphi \approx \frac{\lambda}{\Lambda}$.

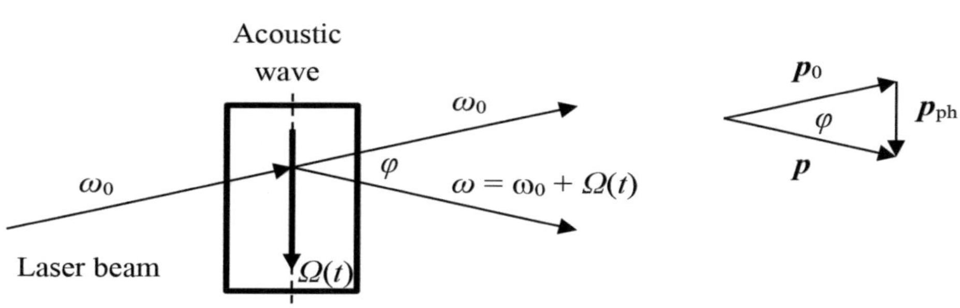

Figure 30.
Modulator of the laser beam.

The deflected beam is frequency modulated by an acoustic signal and angularly separated from the unmodulated 0-th order beam.

Example 18 Two-photon excitation microscopy

Another example of the nonlinear interaction of a laser beam with a substance is fluorescence microscopy used in biochemistry, which uses the principle of two-photon excitation of atoms. Conventional fluorescence microscopy—see Section 6.2.8, utilises excitation by high energy photons of UV radiation, which have a shorter depth of penetration into the sample due to the higher frequency and which produce a relatively strong white background of the image.

Two-photon excitation uses the excitation of molecules by a pair of low-energy photons. If we observe the fluorescence of the most common fluorophores (molecules exhibiting fluorescence) in the optical range of 400–500 nm, IR laser radiation of 800–1000 nm is used for excitation. If an electron captures a photon in the ground state, it is excited to a higher energy level. The electrons from this excitation level relax back to the ground state, emitting photons in the IR band, that is, optically invisible.

However, if it is excited again to the next higher energy level before relaxation, due to the relaxation from this second level photons of the visible light are re-emitted—fluorescence occurs. Each fluorescent molecule has its characteristic excitation energy, so that specific fluorophore can be discovered. The probability of double capture of excitation photons is very small and increases with an increasing energy density of radiation. The conditions for double excitation are only in the focus of the focused laser beam. In such a way, the location of the fluorophore can be precisely addressed. The method of scanning individual layers of the sample is used for the display. It permits creating a 3D image of the structure.

7.2 Photo-acoustic imaging

Other modern diagnostic tools use a nonlinear photoacoustic (PA) effect, for example, Xu [3], Beard [4]. As mentioned in Chapter 3, the ultrasound can be excited thermally (by thermal pulse) using a powerful pulse laser. The laser focuses at a location on or near the surface of the object and emits a very short (nanosecond) pulse of radiation. The absorbed energy causes a local increase in temperature, and thus a mechanical expansion of the material. This thermal deformation causes a mechanical shock wave to propagate from this point to all sides. If a series of pulses is applied, a series of shock waves is generated which has a harmonic ultrasonic component with a frequency equal to the repetition rate of the pulses. Since the pulse length is significantly shorter than the repetition period, it is sufficient to return the temperature to the original site temperature before the next pulse arrives. The amplitude of the generated mechanical wave depends on the amount of energy absorbed, and this is directly proportional to the absorption coefficient (absorbance) of the substance at a given location. The generated mechanical (ultrasonic) waves are detected by ultrasonic sensors. In this way, the absorbance distribution of the sample, which is related to the tissue structure, can be mapped using a photoacoustic phenomenon. For example, the blood has a large absorbance for a red light, and therefore the bloodstream and small blood capillaries are displayed very well. The method has a very good resolution due to the possibility of focusing the light beam on an area with dimensions of units of μm. Another advantage is that, unlike light, the attenuation of mechanical waves is relatively small and the generated wave shocks propagate well through an investigated sample. Some specific imaging devices work on the principle of the photoacoustic phenomenon. Some of them are listed below.

DOI: http://dx.doi.org/10.5772/intechopen.101653

7.2.1 Photoacoustic microscopy

The first method that uses the principle of the photoacoustic phenomenon is photoacoustic microscopy (PAM), for example, Wang [5]. The laser beam and the detection acoustic transducer are focused on the examined point of the sample. The energy of the laser beam is thus concentrated to one point and a shock wave with a repetition frequency of 500 MHz, is detected by an acoustic transducer focused at the same point. PAM is a scanning method. The sample is shifted in the transverse directions x, y, and the acoustic transducer signal is recorded. It is also possible to adjust the optical and acoustic lens holder perpendicularly to the sample surface and to image the sample structure at different depths below the surface.

PAM allows displaying a depth up 3–4 mm. By composing images from different depths, a 3D image can be created. **Figure 31** is the basic principle of PAM. The box with an optical lens and a focused acoustic transducer contains water as a transmission medium for the acoustic wave. The box is acoustically bound to the displayed object using a binding gel. Point A is the common focus and displayed point. The picture shows four scans from different depths and a 3D reconstruction.

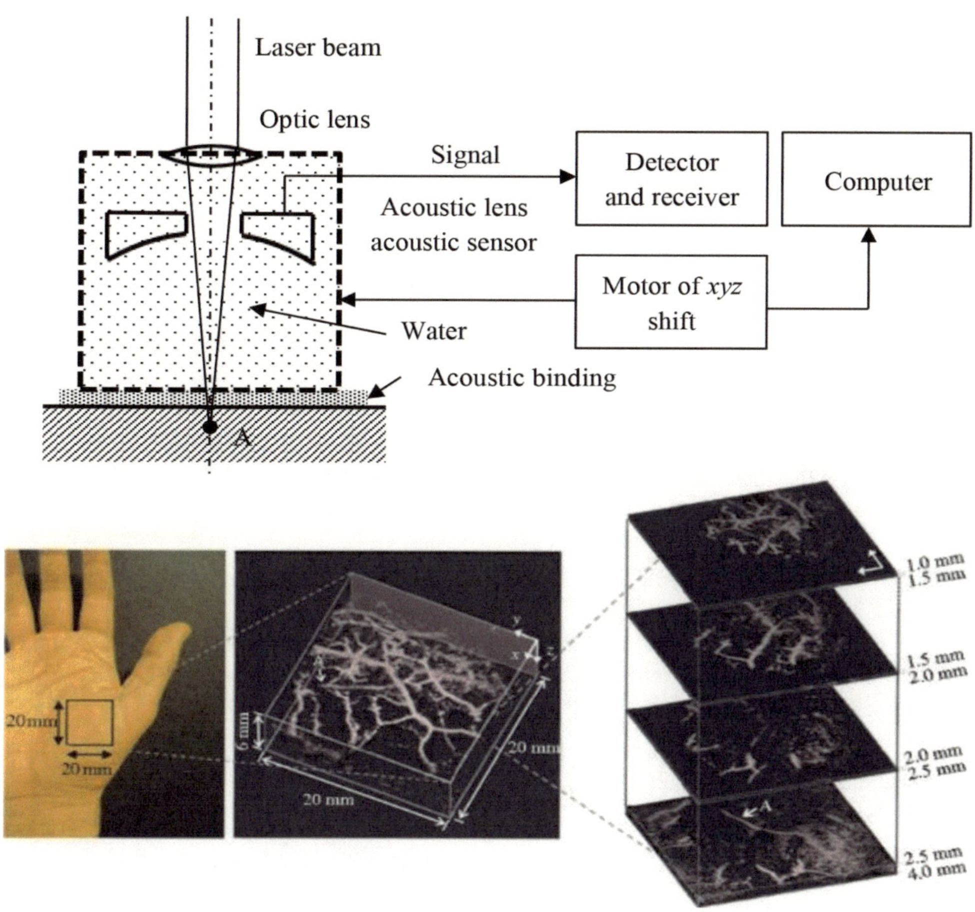

Figure 31.
Principal of photoacoustic imaging—PAM.

7.2.2 Photoacoustic computing tomography

The second principle of information processing of a photo-excited sample is photoacoustic computed tomography (PACT). Unlike PAM, the light pulse of the power laser illuminates the entire examined surface of the sample. As a result, all points with higher absorbance in the sample become a source of acoustic waves. The sample is surrounded by a system, for example, 512 small acoustic detectors, arranged on a hemisphere to obtain a 3D image, or on a circular ring around the sample to create a 2D image. The signals of all detectors are scanned and fed to a computer. They are converted by a complex integral transformation into a spatial or planar image of the distribution of points with different absorbances. In this way, different tissues in the surface layer of the sample are displayed. PACT can display the structure up to a depth of 50 mm, in the case of using a set of detectors arranged on a hemispherical surface, with a resolution of 0.5 mm at a pulse repetition frequency of 5 MHz.

In **Figure 32** on the left is a 3D image of the tissue perfusion of the top layer of the skin. Different levels of the signal are distinguished in colour, which corresponds to different absorbances of the cells. Such an image allows, for example, detection of skin tumour (melanoma)—the picture on the right.

PAM and PACT provide similar resolution as ultrasonography (USG). Against USG, they have a much smaller depth of view, which is limited by the attenuation of light in the tissue but allows seeing the information that USG does not provide. This is due to another mechanism of ultrasound generation. While different acoustic impedances of tissues are applied in USG, different absorbance of tissues is decisive for PA methods. Photoacoustic imaging methods are not yet widely used but are the subject of intensive research.

7.2.3 Photoacoustic spectroscopy

Another method that uses the photoacoustic phenomenon is photoacoustic spectroscopy (PAS), for example, West [6]. It uses different spectral compositions of absorbance of different substances in the tissue.

Figure 33 is the spectrum of various substances in the blood: melanin, Hb-haemoglobin, Mb-myoglobin, and others. The difference in the absorbance of HbO_2 and HbR (oxidised and reduced haemoglobin) at a light wavelength of about 680 nm can be used to distinguish oxygenated blood from deoxygenated blood. In this way, it is possible to determine the degree of oxygenation of the blood—*oximetry*.

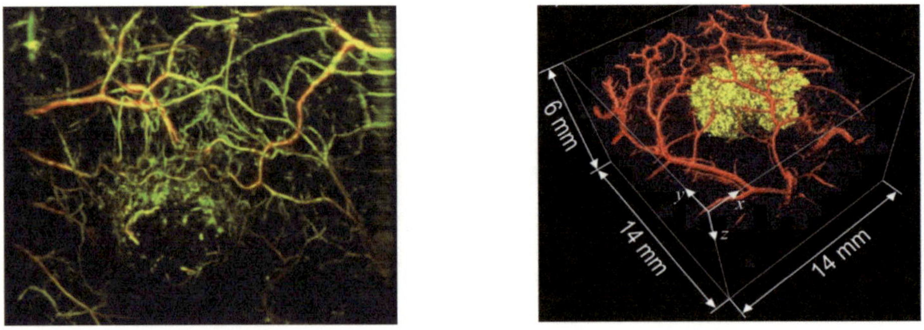

Figure 32.
PACT—on the left image of the surface layer of the skin, right view of melanoma cells (source: https://www.charite.de/en/service/press_reports/artikel/detail/photoakustische_bildgebung_ermoeglicht_tiefen_blick_ins_gewebe/).

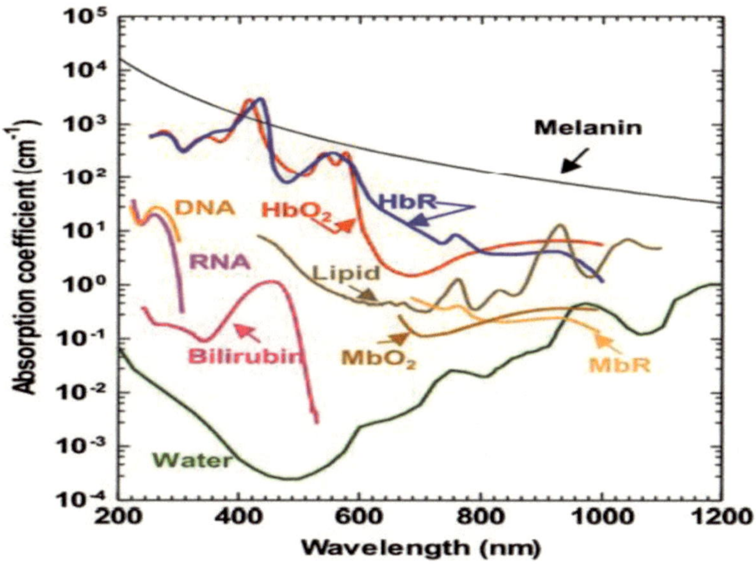

Figure 33.
The spectrum of absorbance of different substances in the blood.

Author details

Ivo Čáp*, Klára Čápová, Milan Smetana and Štefan Borik
Faculty of Electrical Engineering and Information Technology, University of Žilina, Slovakia

*Address all correspondence to: ivo.cap@fel.uniza.sk

References

[1] Wyatt CL. Electro-Optical System Design—For Information Processing. New York: McGraw-Hill; 1991. ISBN 978-0-0707-2184-5

[2] Splinter R, Hooper BA. An Introduction to Biomedical Optics. Boca Raton: CRC Press; 2007. ISBN 978-0-7503-0938-7

[3] Xu M, Wang LV. Photoacoustic imaging in biomedicine. Review of Scientific Instruments. 2006;**77**(4): 041101

[4] Beard P. Biomedical photoacoustic imaging. Interface Focus. 2011;**1**(4): 602-631

[5] Wang LV. Multiscale photoacoustic microscopy and computed tomography. Nature Photonics. 2009;**3**(9):503-509

[6] West GA et al. Photoacoustic spectroscopy. Review of Scientific Instruments. 1983;**54**:797-817

Chapter 7

Conclusion

Ivo Čáp, Klára Čápová, Milan Smetana and Štefan Borik

1. To conclude

This textbook aims to acquaint students and those interested in the field of use of technology in medicine with the elementary principles of operation of devices and tools based on the use of various wave phenomena.

In addition to the basic principles, this publication lists and explains some simple applications encountered in the field of biomedicine. However, modern science and technology provide many new sophisticated technical tools that go beyond the scope of this textbook. These are mainly devices of radiology and nuclear medicine. These are also applications of wave processes but in conjunction with sophisticated computational methods that require a more detailed explanation. These are mainly acoustic and optical imaging methods, USG, thermography, tomographic imaging methods, such as CT, MRI, PET, SPECT, and other methodologies, which use radioactive radiation in therapy and diagnostics. The description of these advanced methods will be the content of the prepared book - Technical means of biomedical engineering.

The present textbook uses basic knowledge of mathematics and physics. Special medical applications are going out of the personal experience of authors and current books and journals. Part of the information and most of the documentary images are from publicly available and freely usable Internet sources.

List of used symbols

A	voltage transmission (–)
$\mathbf{A}$	complex voltage transmission (–)
b	oscillation damping coefficient (s^{-1})
B	magnetic induction (T)
c	phase velocity ($m{\bullet}s^{-1}$), speed of light ($m{\bullet}s^{-1}$)
$c0$	speed of light in free space ($c0$ = 299,792,458 $m{\bullet}s^{-1}$ exactly)
C	capacitance (F)
D	electric displacement ($C{\bullet}m^{-2}$)
e	elementary charge (e = 1,602,177 × 10^{-19} C)
eV	electron-volt unit (1 eV = 1,602,177 × 10^{-19} J)
e_{EM}	electromagnetic field energy density ($J{\bullet}m^{-3}$)
E	energy (J, eV), e.g., Ep potential, Ek kinetic
E	illuminance (lx)
E	electric field strength ($V{\bullet}m^{-1}$)
f	frequency (Hz), focal length (m)
fL	Larmor frequency (Hz)
F	force vector (N)
g	gravity acceleration ($m{\bullet}s^{-2}$)
h	Planck's constant (h = 6,626,070 × 10–34 J•s)
H	loudness level (Ph – phon, dB)

H	magnetic field strength ($A \cdot m^{-1}$)
i	electric current (A)
$\mathbf{I}$	phasor of electric current (A)
I	rms value of electric current (A), luminous intensity (cd)
I	power density of wave (radiation) ($W \cdot m^{-2}$), *I*dB intensity level (dB)
j	imaginary unit ($j = \sqrt{-1}$)
J	current density ($A \cdot m^{-2}$)
$\mathbf{k}$	complex wave number (m^{-1})
l	length (m)
L	inductance (H), luminance ($cd \cdot m^{-2}$)
L	angular momentum (N•m•s)
m	mass (kg)
m	magnetic dipole moment ($N \cdot m \cdot T^{-1}$)
M	torque (N•m)
n	refractive index (–)
p	pressure (Pa), power density ($W \cdot m^{-3}$)
p_a	acoustic pressure (Pa)
p	linear momentum ($kg \cdot m \cdot s^{-1}$)
P	power (W), active power (W)
Q	electric charge (C), quality factor (–), reactive power (Var)
r	radius (m), distance (m)
r	wave reflection factor (–)
r	position vector (m)
R	electrical resistance (Ω)
S	apparent power (VA), area (m^2)
$\mathbf{S}$	complex power of the alternating current (VA)
t	time (s)
t	wave transition factor (–)
T	period (s), thermodynamic temperature (K)
u	voltage (V), acoustic displacement (m)
U	rms value of electric voltage (V)
$\mathbf{U}$	voltage phasor (V)
v	velocity vector ($m \cdot s^{-1}$)
V	volume (m^3)
W	work (J)
x_m	amplitude of oscillations (m)
x	coordinate (m), axis designation, displacement in the *x*- axis direction
y	coordinate (m), axis designation
z	coordinate (m), axis designation
Z	impedance, wave impedance (Ω)
$\mathbf{Z}$	complex impedance (Ω)
α	wavenumber (m^{-1}), angle (rad),
β	wave attenuation coefficient (m^{-1}), angle (rad)
δ	effective wave propagation length (m), wave penetration depth (m)
γ	conductivity ($S \cdot m^{-1}$), gyromagnetic ratio ($s^{-1} \cdot T^{-1}$)
ε	electric permittivity ($F \cdot m^{-1}$), strain (–)
ε_0	electric permittivity of free space (ε_0 = 8,854,187 × 10^{-12} $F \cdot m^{-1}$)
ε_r	relative permittivity (–)
λ	wavelength (m)
φ	plane angle (rad), phase shift (rad)

ρ	bulk density (kg•m^{-3}), electric charge density (C•m^{-3})
μ	magnetic permeability (H•m^{-1})
μ_0	permeability of free space (μ_0 = 4π × 10^{-7} H•m^{-1})
μ_r	relative permeability (–)
Π	Poynting vector (W•m^{-2})
τ	time constant (s)
τ	mechanical stress in shear (Pa)
σ	mechanical tensile stress (Pa)
Φ	magnetic flux (Wb), luminous flux (lm)
Φ_e	radiation flux density (W•m^{-2})
ω	angular frequency (s^{-1}), angular velocity (rad•s^{-1})
ω_L	Larmor angular frequency (s^{-1})
Ω	angular frequency of forced oscillations (s^{-1}), solid angle (sr)
$\dot{x} = \frac{dx}{dt}$	designation of the first derivative by time
$\ddot{x} = \frac{d^2x}{dt^2}$	designation of the second derivative by time
a, A	designation of a scalar quantity
a, A	designation of a vector quantity
a, A	designation of a complex quantity

Abbreviations

CCD	detection chip (Charge-Coupled Device)
CMOS	detection chip (Complementary Metal Oxide Semiconductor)
CMYK	subtractive colour composition (Cyan-Magenta-Yellow-Black)
CNT	Carbon Nano Tubes
CT	Computed Tomography
EM	electromagnetic
FID	magnetic resonance signal (Free Induction Decay)
IR	Infra-Red
LASER	Light Amplification by Stimulated Emission of Radiation
LCD	Liquid Crystals Display
LED	Light Emitting Diode
MR	Magnetic Resonance
MRI	Magnetic Resonance Imaging
MRS	Magnetic Resonance Spectroscopy
MW	Micro-Waves
PAM	Photo-Acoustic Microscopy
PET	Positron Emission Tomography
RGB	additive colour composition (Red-Green-Blue)
RF, RW	Radiofrequency, Radio-Waves
SPECT	Single Photon Emission Tomography
USG	Ultrasonography
UV	Ultra-Violet
UHF	Ultra-High Frequency
VSW	Very Short Waves
WIFI	wireless connection (Wireless Fidelity)
VL	Visible Light
X	X-rays (Roentgen radiation)
γ	gamma radiation
2D, 3D	two-, three-dimensional

Author details

Ivo Čáp*, Klára Čápová, Milan Smetana and Štefan Borik
Faculty of Electrical Engineering and Information Technology, University of Žilina, Slovakia

*Address all correspondence to: ivo.cap@fel.uniza.sk